Contemporary Abnormal Psychology

Selected Readings

Edited by Brendan Maher

Penguin Books

Penguin Books Ltd, Harmondsworth,
Middlesex, England
Penguin Books Inc, 7110 Ambassador Road,
Baltimore, Md 21207, USA
Penguin Books Australia Ltd,
Ringwood, Victoria, Australia

First published 1973
This selection copyright © Brendan Maher, 1973
Introduction and note copyright © Brendan Maher, 1973
Copyright acknowledgements for items in this volume
will be found on page 421

Made and printed in Great Britain by
Cox & Wyman Ltd,
London, Reading and Fakenham
Set in Monotype Times

Contents

Introduction

This is a book of readings about disordered human behaviour. Pathologies of human psychology are to be found in a wide range of systems and processes – cognitive, emotional, motivational and behavioural. Much human misery and social disruption has followed from these pathologies. Centuries of trial and error have gone into our attempts to understand and alleviate them. Abnormal psychology has been defined in many different ways, as a religious problem, as a legal and criminal problem, and as a problem of distorted instincts. None of these has been successful, although each has provided partial insights for later psychopathologists.

Abnormal psychology is now going through a period of rapid change. New theories, new techniques and new methods have arisen drawing not only upon the behavioural sciences but also upon the biological sciences. Perhaps the most important aspect of these developments is the rising emphasis upon controlled experimentation as a primary source of valid knowledge about psychopathology. Although there is a history of experimentation in research in abnormal psychology, it has been, until recently, a rather minor influence when viewed against the dominance of the classical methods of clinical observation and authoritarian teaching.

A full appreciation of changes that have occurred in abnormal psychology can best be provided by taking a brief look at the background from which it has emerged – and to which it presents a contrast.

To a large extent the recent history of psychopathology is the history of the rise, and current decline, of psychoanalytic influence in western psychiatry. From a research point of view, this influence operated in certain ways. First and foremost was the emphasis upon the observation of the single clinical case, coupled with the use of 'interpretation' of the objective data along lines predetermined by the hypotheses at test. The inevitable consequence of this was that, to a large extent, much of the research literature consisted of demonstrations of principles the validity of which was presupposed rather than the examination of them with the combination of enthusiasm and scepticism that science demands.

In a larger framework psychoanalytic influence led to a temporary repudiation of genetics and biopsychology generally. Although psychodynamic theory formally acknowledged the role of constitutional factors in contributing to a psychopathological outcome, this acknowledgement rarely produced any serious attempt to identify them. Indeed, as the American psychologist Meehl pointed out in 1962, it became commonplace to accept without serious question minimally significant data supporting a psychodynamic view of schizophrenia but to insist upon much higher standards of evidence when examining genetic data.

There were, of course, exceptions to all of this. Some psychodynamically-inclined research workers sought to put Freudian hypothesis to controlled test, but even as recently as 1970 it was possible for a leading psychoanalytic scholar to write:

But the question remains as to when ultimate experimental validation of psychoanalytic formulations should occur. The author of this book agrees that psychoanalytic formulations should be subjected to experimental or other empirical validation but favors a different timing than that demanded by a strict operational of positivistic approach. To guard against nipping preliminary exploration in the bud, there must be a period in which curiosity and inquiry into the unique and novel is fostered while the results of natural observations are awaited and then formalized.[1]

As over three-quarters of a century have passed since the first publications of psychoanalytic inquiry appeared one is tempted to wonder how long this 'preliminary' exploration might last!

Contemporary abnormal psychology has arisen in its present form as the result of several different influences. Some of these have been scientific and some have been social. At the scientific level the major impetus has come from certain developments of both biological and behavioural kinds. One of the most influential basic discoveries was heralded by the work of Moruzzi and Magoun in the early 1950s in their studies of the biology of con-

[1] See Holzman, 1970.

sciousness. As long as the study of consciousness had been limited to the recording of introspective personal reports it remained difficult to incorporate abnormal phenomena of consciousness to any general theory relating biology and behaviour. Inevitably this left the explanation of conscious states to concepts of 'unconscious' psychological forces or other motivational assumptions. Further evidence of the role of biology in the production of abnormal conscious states was provided shortly afterwards by the data from the effects of psychotomimetic drugs upon conscious states of awareness. The resemblance of these changes to certain clinical phenomena seen in the psychoses gave additional weight to the probability that both biological and environmental factors are involved in the etiology.

A second major determinant of the current state of research in psychopathology has been the kind of education that has been provided for the clinical psychologist. The power of the experimental method in the investigation of learning, perception, motivation and other psychological functions in normal people is clear to the student of psychology in his study of the fundamentals of his field. Thus the new complexion of abnormal psychology is, to a significant extent, a consequence of the rise of experimental psychology within the universities, and its influence upon the thinking of behavioural scientists generally.

The growth of research has not been uniform across the range of clinical problems that comprise the material of abnormal psychology. Some disorders have attracted more attention than others, either on the basis of their severity and frequency, or because of the fascination of the scientific problems that they present. Schizophrenia (or the schizophrenias) is a case in point. The sheer volume of research literature that has been published on this group of disorders makes it impossible to do other than select certain papers for inclusion in this present book. Those that have been included have been chosen because of the light that they shed upon the reawakened question of genetic versus environmental explanations or because they illustrate the most recent developments in research strategies in this field. Of particular significance is the increasing concern with the study of populations of children who are at risk for schizophrenia.

Garmezy summarizes succinctly the weaknesses inherent in data gathered retrospectively through the case-study of adult patients who are already schizophrenic. In the study of 'vulnerable' children there appears to be a viable and reliable alternative to this – and one that we might expect to bring very different perspectives of the parent-child interaction in the schizophrenogenic family than those reconstructed from parental memories.

Much the same is the case in the study of psychopathy (or *sociopathy*, to use an alternative term). Here, however, the general outlines of the etiological hypotheses to be tested are clearer than for the schizophrenias. So many of the clinical phenomena are susceptible to explanation in terms of diminished emotional responsiveness that the investigation of autonomic nervous system reactivity has become a natural strategy for research workers.

The shift of interest from psychodynamic formulations to experimental investigation is nowhere more clear than in the area of psychosomatic disorders. At the present time there is a more or less tacit acceptance of the view that psychosomatic disorders arise from a combination of biological predisposition and environmental stress, the so-called *diathesis-stress* model. From this model there arises several general lines of inquiry. One has to do with the nature of the biological factors in various disorders. Another is concerned with the question of the specificity of the stress involved. Is the predisposed patient likely to succumb only to certain rather circumscribed classes of stress, or will any stress suffice? If biological factors produce a predisposition to a biological breakdown, are there likewise childhood experiences that predispose to vulnerability to specific pathogenic stresses?

Amongst the many changes that have taken place recently in the applied aspects of psychopathology, none has been more striking than the rise of new approaches to treatment. The single greatest change is to be seen in the development of psychopharmacology. Here also the literature is enormous. We have decided, however, not to include readings from it in this book. Much of the literature is of great clinical interest from an empirical point of view, but of little significance yet for our understanding of abnormal psychology. A proper understanding of the technical reports of psychopharmacological research requires a familiarity with concepts and terms that lie outside the interest and training of many students of psychopathology. Given these considerations, and the inexorable pressures of limited space, the best that can be done is to refer the interested reader elsewhere through the list of further reading at the end of this volume.

Second only to the expansion of drug treatment is the shift in hospital practices. The pioneer in this is, without doubt, the British psychiatrist Maxwell Jones and we have included his early report on this as both a landmark itself and as an expression of the changing ideas of the time. Parallel, but separate, the work of the Skinnerian operant conditioners has produced innovative approaches to the therapeutic use of the hospital environment via the use of the 'token economy' plan.

Inevitably, several lively issues have had to be omitted for lack of space. Clinical research in the area of individual psychotherapy or individual behaviour therapy has been left out. The current controversy about the usefulness of the disease model as a basis for thinking about disordered behaviour has also been omitted. There is no doubt that this question is of great social importance, but there is little evidence as yet that any of the discussion has produced new scientific insights for psychopathologists. No space could be spared for inclusion of any of the many ingenious experimental analogues of psychopathology that have been reported in the past two or three decades.

The introduction of the experimental method into psychopathology has had an effect upon the style and format of the literature of the discipline. Empirical findings have a way of chastening the finder. Grand systems conceived in supportive surroundings of the study tend to have a rough time of it in the laboratory and the field. Hence the mood of the modern psychopathologist tends away from the comprehensive synthesis and towards the discovery of modest but reliable empirical relationships. The very heterogeneity of the variables that affect and impair behaviour presses us away from the goal of complete explanation through simple principles. It is now apparent that the theorizing of half a century ago was premature and that what is needed is more trustworthy data. In this spirit we find that the contemporary literature contains fewer theoretical papers and these are generally directed at limited topics. To know modern psychopathology is to know results of research and to understand the design and execution of empirical investigations. The several research reports that are included in this book have been chosen because they illustrate the application of objective techniques to the investigation of abnormal psychology and do so in ways that do not achieve precision at the expense of psychological significance.

It would be misleading to leave the reader with the impression that the main questions of psychopathology are being solved simply through the continued use of the experimental method in research. There are many important problems facing the psychopathologist some of which cannot readily be handled experimentally and others of which arise from the very changes that we have described.

Some kinds of critical clinical phenomena are seen only periodically and cannot be elicited 'on demand' for research purpose. Disordered speech, catatonic posture, anti-social activity, etc. are not present in the patient's behaviour at all times, nor can they be realistically generated in the laboratory. Much ingenuity is needed to devise objective methods of measurement for events such as these that occur only in the natural habitat of the patient. One consequence of the success of pharmacological methods of treatment is that it is becoming rare to find patients who are not on some form of medication. We are largely ignorant of the detailed mechanisms by which these drugs achieve their effects but it is reasonable to assume that they may alter psychological processes of all kinds. The behaviour of the medicated schizophrenic is almost certainly different from that of the unmedicated, a fact which makes the use of non-medicated subjects crucial in research, but hard to manage in practice.

Finally, it must be emphasized that clinical observation of the single case is the procedure from which most useful hypotheses about psychopathology have come. The fact that it is unsuited to establishing their validity must not obscure the central role of imaginative scrutiny in the forward progress of abnormal psychology.

This is a book of *contemporary* readings. We have been at pains to point out that we are in a period of change, with the excitement and challenge that change brings. We see many varied movements and developments, eclectic rather than monolithic. The shape of the future can be glimpsed in outline only: the safest prediction is that the changes we see now will continue to evolve for many years to come. Whatever the future may bring, however, it seems certain that psychopathology is becoming firmly rooted in general behavioural science. It is from this turn of events that we can derive the best hope of the alleviation of the human suffering that psychological abnormality inflicts.

Part One
Classification and Diagnosis

It is in the nature of the scientific enterprise that we must
define our problems clearly before we can hope to solve them.
In principle, it is necessary to have an unambiguous
classification scheme for the varieties of disordered behaviour
if we are to commence work on the task of discovering
etiology and treatment of any of them. Abnormal psychology
has been plagued by difficulties in establishing reliable
diagnostic categories. Kraepelin, the founder of the system of
categories currently employed (albeit with many series of
revisions), envisaged a two-stage process in the development
of classification. The first step would be descriptive – the
provision of a detailed and thorough description of all of the
features of each syndrome. Once these had been defined and
separated from each other the task of discovering the
aetiology of each syndrome could begin. With aetiologies
discovered, the categorization scheme could be transformed
into one based upon causative factors. Zigler and Phillips
review the history of this enterprise, noting the many
problems and criticisms that have been levelled against the
Kraepelinian plan but concluding that, none the less, it has
not yet been replaced any more viable programme.

Classificatory systems vary from one country to another,
even where the diagnostic labels employed appear to be the
same. The years since the Second World War have seen the
growth of organized international efforts, under the aegis of
the World Health Organization, to achieve the uniformity of
diagnosis that exists to a large degree in physical medicine.
This requires empirical examination of differences in
diagnostic usage, Sandifer and his colleagues report a study

examining the practices of British and American clinicians, one of the first organized attempts to do so.

While comparative studies are aimed at improving the current system, there are psychopathologists who have concluded that the basic error is in categorical classification of any kind. In the United States, such writers as Szasz and Sarbin[2] have rejected the notion of disease entities entirely, and in Britain, Laing has taken a similar tack although from different premises. Bindra's paper presents a behaviourist's view of the insufficiency of aetiological classification and a plea for explanation in terms of the general laws of learning.

1 E. Zigler and L. Phillips

Psychiatric Diagnosis: a Critique[1]

E. Zigler and L. Phillips, 'Psychiatric Diagnosis: a Critique', *Journal of Abnormal and Social Psychology*, vol. 63, 1961, pp. 607–8.

The inadequacies of conventional psychiatric diagnosis have frequently been noted (Ash, 1949; Cattell, 1957; Eysenck, 1952; Foulds, 1955; Harrower, 1950; Hoch and Zubin, 1953; Jellinek, 1939; King, 1954; Leary and Coffey, 1955; Mehlman, 1952; Menninger, 1955; Noyes, 1953; Phillips and Rabinovitch, 1958; Roe, 1949; Rogers, 1951; Rotter, 1954; Scott, 1958; Thorne, 1953; Wittenborn and Weiss, 1952; Wittman and Sheldon, 1948). The responses to this rather imposing body of criticism have ranged from the position that the present class-ificatory system is in need of further refinement (Caveny, Wittson, Hunt, and Herman, 1955; Foulds, 1955), through steps towards major revisions (Cattell, 1957; Eysenck, 1952; Leary and Coffey, 1955; Phillips and Rabinovitch, 1958; Thorne, 1953; Wittman and Sheldon, 1948), to a plea for the abolishment of all 'labeling' (Menninger, 1955; Noyes, 1953; Rogers, 1951). As other investigators have noted (Caveny *et al.*, 1955; Jellinek, 1939), this last position suggests that the classifi-catory enterprise is valueless. This reaction against classification has gained considerable popularity in clinical circles. The alacrity with which many clinicians have accepted this view seems to represent more than a disillusionment with the specific current form of psychiatric diagnosis. These negative attitudes appear to reflect a belief that diagnostic classification is inherently antithetical to such clinically favored concepts as 'dynamic', 'idiographic', etc. Thus, a question is raised as to

[1] This investigation was supported by the Dementia Praecox Research Project, Worcester State Hospital, and a research grant (M-896) from the National Institute of Mental Health, United States Public Health Service.

whether any diagnostic schema can be of value. Let us initially direct our attention to this question.

On classification

The growth among clinicians of sentiment against categorization has coincided with a period of critical reappraisal within the behavioral sciences generally (Beach, 1950; Brower, 1949; Cronbach, 1957; Guthrie, 1950; Harlow, 1953; Koch, 1951; MacKinnon, 1953; Marquis, 1948; Rapaport, 1947; Roby, 1959; Scott, 1955; Tolman, 1953; Tyler, 1959). This parallel development is more than coincidental. The reaction against 'labeling' can be viewed as an extreme outgrowth of this critical self-evaluation, i.e., that psychology's conceptual schemata are artificial in their construction, sterile in terms of their practical predictions, and lead only to greater and greater precision about matters which are more and more irrelevant. It is little wonder that, in this atmosphere, conceptualization has itself become suspect nor that Maslow's (1948) exposition of the possible dangers of labeling or naming has been extended (Rotter, 1954) as a blanket indictment of the categorizing process.

The error in this extension is the failure to realize that what has been criticized is not the conceptual process but only certain of its products. The criticisms mentioned above have not been in favor of the abolishment of conceptualization, but have rather been directed at the prematurity and rarifications of many of our conceptual schemata and our slavish adherence to them. Indeed, many of these criticisms have been accompanied by pleas for lower-order conceptualization based more firmly on observational data (Koch, 1951; MacKinnon, 1953; Tolman, 1953).

In the clinical area, the sentiment against classification has become sufficiently serious that several investigators (Cattell, 1957; Caveny et al., 1955; Eysenck, 1952; Jellinek, 1939) have felt the need to champion the merits of psychiatric categorization. They have pointed out that diagnosis is a basic scientific classificatory enterprise to be viewed as essentially the practice of taxonomy, which is characteristic of all science. Eysenck (1952) puts the matter quite succinctly in his statement,

'Measurement is essential to science, but before we can measure, we must know what it is we want to measure. Qualitative or taxonomic discovery must precede quantitative measurement' (p. 34).

Reduced to its essentials, diagnostic classification involves the establishment of categories to which phenomena can be ordered. The number of class systems that potentially may be constructed is limited only by man's ability to abstract from his experience. The principles employed to construct such classes may be inductive, deductive, or a combination of both, and may vary on a continuum from the closely descriptive to the highly abstract.

Related to the nature of the classificatory principle are the implications to be derived from class membership. Class membership may involve nothing more than descriptive compartmentalization, its only utility being greater ease in the handling of data. Obversely, the attributes or correlates of class membership may be widespread and far-reaching in their consequences. The originators of a classificatory schema may assert that specified behavioral correlates accompany class membership. This assertion is open to test. If the hypothesized correlates represent the full heuristic value of the diagnostic schema and class membership is found not to be related to these correlates, then revision or discard is in order. A somewhat different type of problem may also arise. With the passage of time, correlates not originally related to the schema may erroneously be attributed to class membership. Nevertheless, the original taxonomy may still possess a degree of relevance to current objectives in a discipline. In these circumstances, its maintenance may be the rational choice, although a clarification and purification of categories is called for. The relationship of the two problems outlined here to the criticism of contemporary psychiatric diagnosis will be discussed later. What should be noted at this point is that the solution to neither problem implies the abolishment of the attempt at classification.

Another aspect of taxonomy is in need of clarification. When a phenomenon is assigned to a class, certain individual characteristics of that phenomenon are forever lost. No two class members are completely identical. Indeed, a single class member may be viewed as continuously differing from itself over time. It is this loss of uniqueness and an implied unconcern with process that have led many clinicians to reject classification in principle. While classificatory schemata inevitably involve losses of this type, it must be noted that they potentially offer a more than compensatory gain. This gain is represented in the significance of the class attributes and correlates. Class membership conveys information ranging from the descriptive similarity of two phenomena to a knowledge of the common operative processes underlying the phenomena.

A conceptual system minimizes the aforementioned loss to the extent that only irrelevant aspects of a phenomenon are deleted in the classificatory process. The implicit assumption is made that what is not class relevant is inconsequential. The dilemma, of course, lies in our lacking divine revelation as to what constitutes inconsequentiality. It is this issue which lies at the heart of the idiographic versus nomothetic controversy (Allport, 1937, 1946; Beck, 1953; Eysenck, 1954; Falk, 1956; Hunt, 1951a, 1951b; Skaggs, 1945, 1947). The supporters of the idiographic position (Allport, 1937; Beck, 1953) have criticized certain conceptual schemata for treating idiosyncratic aspects of behavior as inconsequential when they are in fact pertinent data which must be utilized if a comprehensive and adequate view of human behavior is to emerge. However, the idiographic position is not a movement toward the abolishment of classification, a fact emphasized by Allport (1937) and Falk (1956). Rather, it represents a plea for broader and more meaningful classificatory schemata.

A conceptually different type of argument against the use of any diagnostic classification has been made by the adherents of nondirective psychotherapy (Patterson, 1948; Rogers, 1946, 1951). This position has advanced the specific contention that differential diagnosis is unnecessary for, and perhaps detrimental to, successful psychotherapy. This attitude of the non-directivists has been interpreted (Thorne, 1953) as an attack on the entire classificatory enterprise. To argue against diagnosis on the grounds that it affects therapeutic outcome is to confuse diagnosis as an act of scientific classification with the present clinical practice of diagnosis with its use of interviewing, psychological testing, etc. The error here lies in turning one's attention away from diagnosis as an act of classification, a basic scientific enterprise, and attending instead to the immediate and prognostic consequences of some specific diagnostic technique in a specific therapeutic situation, i.e., an applied aspect. To reject the former on the basis of the latter would appear to be an unsound decision.

Although the nondirectivists' opposition to diagnosis seems to be based on a confusion between the basic and applied aspects of classification, implicitly contained within their position is a more fundamental argument against the classificatory effort. Undoubtedly, diagnosis both articulates and restricts the range of assumptions which may be entertained about a client. However, the philosophy of the nondirectivist forces him to reject any theoretical position which violates a belief in the unlimited psychological growth of the client. It would appear that this position represents the rejection, in principle, of the view that any individual can be like another in his essential characteristics, or that any predictable relationship can be established between a client's current level of functioning and the ends which may be achieved. In the setting of this assumption, a transindividual classificatory schema is inappropriate. There is no appeal from such a judgement, but one should be cognizant that it rejects the essence of a scientific discipline. If one insists on operating within the context of a predictive psychology, one argues for the necessity of a classificatory system, even though particular diagnostic schemata may be rejected as irrelevant, futile, or obscure.

Let us now direct our discussion toward some of the specific criticisms of conventional psychiatric diagnosis – that the categories employed lack homogeneity, reliability, and validity.

Homogeneity

A criticism often leveled against the contemporary diagnostic system is that its categories encompass heterogeneous groups of individuals, i.e., individuals varying in respect to symptomatology, test scores, prognosis, etc. (King, 1954; Rotter, 1954; Wittenborn, 1952; Wittenborn and Bailey, 1952; Wittenborn and Weiss, 1952). Contrary to the view of one investigator

(Rotter, 1954), a lack of homogeneity does not necessarily imply a lack of reliability. King (1954) has clearly noted the distinction between these two concepts. Reliability refers to the agreement in assigning individuals to different diagnostic categories, whereas homogeneity refers to the diversity of behavior subsumed within categories. While the two concepts may be related, it is not difficult to conceptualize categories which, though quite reliable, subsume diverse phenomena.

King (1954) has argued in favor of constructing a new diagnostic classification having more restrictive and homogeneous categories. He supports his argument by noting his own findings and those of Kantor, Wallner, and Winder (1953), which have indicated that within the schizophrenic group subcategories may be formed which differ in test performance. King found further support for the construction of new and more homogeneous diagnostic categories in a study by Windle and Hamwi (1953). This study indicated that two subgroups could be constructed within a psychotic population which was composed of patients with diverse psychiatric diagnoses. Though matched on the distribution of these diagnostic types, the subgroups differed in the relationship obtained between test performance and prognosis. On the basis of these studies, King suggests that the type of homogeneous categories he would favor involves such classificatory dichotomies as reactive versus process schizophrenics and chronic versus nonchronic psychotics.

An analysis of King's (1954) criticism of the present diagnostic system discloses certain difficulties. The first is that King's heterogeneity criticism does not fully take into consideration certain basic aspects of classification. A common feature of classificatory systems is that they utilize classes which contain subclasses. An example drawn from biology would be a genus embracing a number of species. If schizophrenia is conceptualized as a genus, it cannot be criticized on the grounds that all its members do not share a particular attribute. Such a criticism would involve a confusion between the more specific attributes of the species and the more general attributes of the genus. This is not to assert that schizophrenia does in fact possess the characteristics of a genus. It is, of course, possible that a careful analysis will reveal that it does not, and the class schizophrenia will have to be replaced by an aggregate of entities which does constitute a legitimate genus. However, when a genus is formulated, it cannot be attacked because of its heterogeneous nature since genera are characterized by such heterogeneity.

A more serious difficulty with King's (1954) heterogeneity criticism lies in the inherent ambiguity of a homogeneity-heterogeneity parameter. To criticize a classificatory system because its categories subsume heterogeneous phenomena is to make the error of assuming that homogeneity is a quality which inheres in phenomena when in actuality it is a construction of the observer or classifier. In order to make this point clear, let us return to King's argument. What does it mean to assert that chronic psychosis is an example of an homogeneous class, while schizophrenia is an example of an heterogeneous one? In terms of the descriptively diverse phenomena encompassed, the latter would appear to have the greater homogeneity. The statement only has meaning insofar as a particular correlate – for instance, the relationship of test score to prognosis – is shared by all members of one class but not so shared by the members of the other class. Thus, the meaningfulness of the homogeneity concept is ultimately dependent on the correlates or attributes of class membership or to the classificatory principle related to these correlates or attributes. The intimacy of the relationship between the attributes of classes and the classificatory principle can best be exemplified by the extreme case in which a class has but a single attribute, and that attribute is defined by the classificatory principle, e.g., the classification of plants on the basis of the number of stamens they possess. Therefore, the heterogeneity criticism of a classificatory system is nothing more than a plea for the utilization of a new classificatory principle so that attention may be focused on particular class correlates or attributes not considered in the original schema. While this plea may be a justifiable one, depending on the significance of the new attributes, it has little to do with the homogeneity, in an absolute sense, of phenomena. Indeed, following the formulation of a new classificatory schema, the heterogeneity criticism could well be leveled against it by the adherents of the old system, since the phenomena encompassed by the new categories would probably not be considered homogeneous when evaluated by the older classificatory principle.

Although differing in its formulation, the heterogeneity criticism of present psychiatric classification made by Wittenborn and his colleagues (Wittenborn, 1952; Wittenborn and Bailey, 1952; Wittenborn and Weiss, 1952) suffers from the same difficulties as does King's (1954) criticism. Wittenborn's findings indicated that individuals given a common diagnosis showed differences in their symptom cluster score profiles based on nine symptom clusters isolated earlier by means of factor analytic techniques (Wittenborn, 1951; Wittenborn and Holzberg, 1951). It is upon the existence of these different profiles within a diagnostic category that Wittenborn bases his heterogeneity criticism. Here again the homogeneity-heterogeneity distinction is only meaningful in terms of an independent criterion, a particular symptom cluster score profile. Had it been discovered that all individuals placed into a particular diagnostic category shared a common symptom cluster score profile, then this category would be described as subsuming homogeneous phenomena. But the phenomena – the symptoms mirrored by the symptom profile – are not homogeneous in any absolute sense because the pattern of symptoms may involve the symptoms in descriptively diverse symptom clusters. Thus, the homogeneity ascribed to the category would refer only to the fact that individuals within the category homogeneously exhibited a particular pattern of descriptively diverse behaviors. However, the organization of symptoms mirrored by the symptom cluster profiles is not in any fundamental sense different from that observed in conventional diagnostic syndromes. Both methods of categorization systematize diverse behaviors because of an observed regularity in their concurrent appearance.

The difference between these two approaches, then, lies only in the pattern of deviant behaviors that define the categories. Indeed, Eysenck (1953) has noted that both the clinician and the factor analyst derive syndromes in essentially the same manner, i.e., in terms of the observed intercorrelations of various symptoms. It is the difference in method, purely observational versus statistical, that explains why the final symptom structure may differ. The assumption must not be made that the advantage lies entirely with the factor analytic method. The merit accruing through the greater rigor of factor analysis may be outweighed by the limitations imposed in employing a restricted group of symptoms and a particular sample of patients. Thus, the factor analyst cannot claim that the class-defining symptom pattern he has derived is a standard of homogeneity against which classes within another schema can be evaluated. The plea that symptom cluster scores, derived from factor analytic techniques, substitute for the present method of psychiatric classification has little relevance to the heterogeneity issue.

In the light of this discussion we may conclude that the concept of homogeneity has little utility in evaluating classificatory schemata. Since the heterogeneity criticism invariably involves an implicit preference for one classificatory principle over another, it would perhaps be more fruitful to dispense entirely with the homogeneity-heterogeneity distinction, thus, allowing us to direct our attention to the underlying problem of the relative merits of different classificatory principles.

Reliability and validity

A matter of continuing concern has been the degree of reliability of the present diagnostic system. Considerable energy has been expended by both those who criticize the present system for its lack of reliability (Ash, 1949; Boisen, 1938; Eysenck, 1952; Mehlman, 1952; Roe, 1949; Rotter, 1954; Scott, 1958) and those who defend it against this criticism (Foulds, 1955; Hunt, Wittson, and Hunt, 1953; Schmidt and Fonda, 1956; Seeman, 1953). Certain investigators (Foulds, 1955; Schmidt and Fonda, 1956) who have offered evidence that the present system is reliable have also pointed out that the earlier studies emphasizing the unreliability of psychiatric diagnosis have suffered from serious conceptual and methodological difficulties.

In evaluating the body of studies concerned with the reliability of psychiatric diagnosis, one must conclude that so long as diagnosis is confined to broad diagnostic categories, it is reasonably reliable, but the reliability diminishes as one proceeds from broad, inclusive class categories to narrower, more specific ones. As finer discriminations are called for, accuracy in diagnosis becomes increasingly difficult. Since this latter characteristic appears to be common to the classificatory efforts in many areas of knowledge, it would appear to be inappropriate to criticize psychiatric diagnosis on the grounds that it is less than perfectly reliable. This should not lead to an underestimation of the importance of reliability. While certain extra-classificatory factors, e.g., proficiency of the clinicians, biases of the particular clinical settings, etc., may influence it, reliability is primarily related to the precision with which classes of a schema are defined. Since the defining characteristic of most classes in psychiatric diagnosis is the occurrence of symptoms in particular combinations, the reliability of the system mirrors the specificity with which the various combinations of symptoms (syndromes) have been spelled out. It is mandatory for a classificatory schema to be reliable since reliability refers to the definiteness with which phenomena can be ordered to classes. If a system does not allow for such a division of phenomena, it can make no pretense of being a classificatory schema.

While reliability is a prerequisite if the diagnostic system is to have any value, it must not be assumed that if human effort were to make the present system perfectly reliable, it could escape all the difficulties attributed to it. This perfect reliability would only mean that individuals within each class shared a particular commonality in relation to the classificatory principle of symptom manifestation. If one were interested in attributes unrelated or minimally related to the classificatory principle employed, the perfect reliability of the system would offer little cause for rejoicing. Perfect reliability of the present system can only be the goal of those who are interested in nothing more than the present classificatory principle and the particular attributes of the classes constructed on the basis of this principle.

When attention is shifted from characteristics which define a class to the correlates of class membership, this implies a shift in concern from the reliability of a system to its validity. The distinction between the reliability and validity of a classificatory system would appear to involve certain conceptual difficulties. It is perhaps this conceptual difficulty which explains why the rather imposing body of literature concerned with diagnosis has been virtually silent on the question of the validity of the present system of psychiatric diagnosis. Only one group of investigators (Hunt, 1951a; Hunt, Wittson, and Barton, 1950a, 1950b; Hunt, Wittson, and Hunt, 1953; Wittson and Hunt, 1951) has specifically been concerned with the predictive efficacy of diagnoses and, thus, to the validity of psychiatric classifications; and even in this work, the distinction between validity and reliability is not clearly drawn.

In order to grasp the distinction between the reliability and the validity of a classificatory schema, one must differentiate the defining characteristics of the classes from the correlates of the classes. In the former case, we are interested in the principles upon which classes are formed; in the latter, in the predictions or valid statements that can be made about phenomena once they are classified. The difficulty lies in the overlap between the classifying principles and the class correlates. If a classificatory system is reliable, it is also valid to the extent that we can predict that the individuals within a class will exhibit certain characteristics, namely, those behaviors or attributes which serve to define the class.

It is the rare class, however, that does not connote correlates beyond its defining characteristics. The predictions associated with class membership may vary from simple extensions of the classificatory principles to correlates which would appear to have little connection with these principles. Let us examine a simple illustration and see what follows from categorizing an individual. Once an individual has been classified as manifesting a manic-depressive reaction, depressed type on the basis of the symptoms of depression of mood, motor retardation, and stupor (American Psychiatric Association, 1952), the prediction may be made that the individual will spend a great deal of time in bed, which represents an obvious extension of the symptom pattern. One may also hypothesize that the patient will show improvement if electro-shock therapy is employed. This is a correlate which has little direct connection with the symptoms themselves. These predictions are open to test, and evidence may or may not be found to support them. Thus, measures of validity may be obtained which are independent of the reliability of the system of classification.

The problem of validity lies at the heart of the confusion which surrounds psychiatric diagnosis. When the present diagnostic schema is assailed, the common complaint is that class membership conveys little information beyond the gross symptomatology of the patient and contributes little to the solution of the pressing problems of etiology, treatment procedures, prognosis, etc. The criticism that class membership does not predict these important aspects of a disorder appears to be a legitimate one. This does not mean the present system has no validity. It simply indicates that the system may be valid in respect to certain correlates but invalid in respect to others. Much confusion would be dispelled if as much care were taken in noting the existing correlates of classes as is taken in noting the classificatory principles. A great deal of effort has gone into the formalization of the defining characteristics of classes (American Psychiatric Association, 1952), but one looks in vain for a formal delineation of the extraclassificatory attributes and correlates of class membership. As a result, the various diagnostic categories have been burdened with correlates not systematically derived from a classificatory principle but which were attributed to the classes because they were the focal points of clinical interest. A major question is just what correlates can justifiably be attributed to the class categories. To answer this question we must turn our attention to the purposes and philosophy underlying contemporary psychiatric diagnosis.

Philosophy and purpose of conventional diagnosis

The validity of the conventional diagnostic system is least ambiguous and most free from potential criticism as a descriptive schema, a taxonomy of mental disorders analogous to the work of Ray and Linnaeus in biology. In this sense, class membership confirms that the inclusion of an individual within a class guarantees only that he exhibit the defining characteristics of that class. Only a modest extension of this system, in terms of a very limited number of well-established correlates, makes for a system of impressive heuristic value, even though it falls considerably short of what would now be considered an optimal classificatory schema. As has been noted (Caveny et al., 1955; Hunt et al., 1953), the present diagnostic system is quite useful when evaluated in terms of its administrative and, to a lesser extent, its preventive implications, Caveny *et al.* (1955) and Wittenborn, Holzberg, and Simon (1953) should be consulted for a comprehensive list of such uses, but examples would include legal determination of insanity, declaration of incompetence, type of ward required for custodial care, census figures and statistical data upon which considerable planning is based, screening devices for the military services or other agencies, etc. In view of the extensive criticism of contemporary diagnosis, the surprising fact is not that so few valid predictions can be derived from class membership, but that so many can.

The value of the present psychiatric classification system would be further enhanced by its explicit divorcement from its Kraepelinian heritage by an emphasis on its descriptive aspect and, through careful empirical investigation, the cataloguing of the reliable correlates of its categories. That this catalogue of correlates would be an impressive one is expressed in Hoch's (1953) view that the present system is superior to any system which has been evolved to replace it. It is an open question whether the system merits this amount of praise. In general, however, the defense of the present system – or, for that matter, diagnosis in general (Caveny *et al.*, 1955; Eysenck, 1952; Hunt *et al.*, 1953; Jellinek, 1939) – tends to rest on the merits of its descriptive, empirical, and nondynamic aspects.

The present classificatory system, even as a purely descriptive device, is still open to a certain degree of criticism. Its classificatory principle is organized primarily about symptom manifestation. This would be adequate for a descriptive system if this principle were consistently applied to all classes of the schema and if the symptoms associated with each diagnostic category were clearly specified. There is some question, however, whether the system meets these requirements (Phillips and Rabinovitch, 1958; Rotter, 1954). The criticism has been advanced that the present system is based on a number of diverse principles of classification. Most classes are indeed defined by symptom manifestation, but the organic disorders, for example, tend to be identified by aetiology, while such other factors as prognosis, social conformity, etc. are also employed as classificatory principles. This does not appear, however, to be an insurmountable problem, for the system could be made a completely consistent one by explicitly defining each category by the symptoms encompassed. The system would appear to be eminently amenable to the unitary application of this descriptive classificatory principle, for there are actually few cases where classes are not so defined. Where reliable relations between the present categories and aetiology and prognosis have been established, these also could be incorporated explicitly within the system. Aetiology and prognosis would be treated not as inherent attributes of the various classifications, but rather as correlates of the particular classes to which their relationship is known. They would, thus, not be confounded with the classificatory principle of the system.

This course of action would satisfy the requirement of consistency in the application of the classificatory principle. A remaining area of ambiguity would be the lack of agreement in what constitutes a symptom. In physical medicine, a clear distinction has been made between a symptom, which is defined as a subjectively experienced abnormality, and a sign, which is considered an objective indication of abnormality (Holmes, 1946). This differentiation has not, however, been extended to the sphere of mental disorders. A source of difficulty may lie in the definition of what is psychologically abnormal. In psychiatric terminology, symptoms include a wide range of phenomena from the grossest type of behavior deviation, through the complaints of the patient, to events almost completely inferential in nature. One suggestion (Yates, 1958) has been to eliminate the term 'symptom' and direct attention to the manifest responses of the individual. This suggestion appears to be embodied in the work of Wittenborn and his colleagues (Wittenborn, 1951, 1952; Wittenborn and Bailey, 1952; Wittenborn and Holzberg, 1951; Wittenborn et al., 1953; Wittenborn and Weiss, 1952). Wittenborn's diagnostic system, in which symptoms are defined as currently discernible behaviors, represents a standard of clarity for purely descriptive systems of psychiatric classification. This clarity was achieved by clearly noting and limiting the group of behaviors which would be employed in the system. But even here a certain amount of ambiguity remains. The number of responses or discernible behaviors which may be considered for inclusion within a diagnostic schema borders on the infinite. The question arises, then, as to how one goes about the selection of those behaviors to be incorporated in the classificatory system. Parsimony demands that only 'meaningful' items of behavior be chosen for inclusion, and this selective principle has certainly been at work in the construction of all systems of diagnosis. In this sense, the present method of psychiatric classification is not a purely descriptive one, nor can any classification schema truly meet this criterion of purity. Meaning and utility inevitably appear among the determinants of classificatory systems.

Several investigators (Cameron, 1953; Jellinek, 1939; Magaret, 1952) have stressed the inappropriateness of discussing diagnosis in the abstract, pointing out that such a discussion should center around the question of 'diagnosis for what?' Indeed, a diagnostic system cannot be described as 'true' or 'false,' but only as being useful or not useful in attaining prescribed goals. Therefore, when a system is devised, its purposes should be explicitly stated so that the system can be evaluated in terms of its success or failure in attaining these objectives. Furthermore, these goals should be kept explicit throughout the period during which the system is being employed. The present diagnostic schema has not met this requirement. Instead, its goals have been carried along in an implicit manner and have been allowed to become vague. The result has been that some see the purpose of the schema as being an adequate description of mental disorders (Hunt *et al.*, 1953), others view it as being concerned with prognosis (Hoch, 1953), and still others view the schemata goal as the discovery of aetiology (Cameron, 1953).

Typically, the present schema has been conceptualized as descriptive in nature, but a brief glance at its history indicates that the original purposes and goals in the construction of this schema went far beyond the desire for a descriptive taxonomy. As Zilboorg and Henry (1941) clearly note, Kraepelin not only studied the individual while hospitalized, but also the patient's premorbid history and post-hospital course. His hope was to make our understanding of all mental disorders as precise as our knowledge of the course of general paresis. He insisted on the classification of mental disorders according to regularities in symptoms and course of illness, believing this would lead to a clearer discrimination among the different disease entities. He hoped for the subsequent discovery of a specific somatic malfunction responsible for each disease. For Kraepelin, then, classification was related to etiology, treatment, and prognosis. Had the system worked as envisaged, these variables would have become the extra-classificatory attributes of the schema. When matched against this aspiration, the present system must be considered a failure since the common complaint against it is that a diagnostic label tells us very little about etiology, treatment, or prognosis (Miles, 1953). However, it would be erroneous to conclude that the present system is valueless because its classes are only minimally related to etiology and prognosis.

What should be noted is that etiology and prognosis, though important, are but two of a multitude of variables of interest. The importance of these variables should not obscure the fact that their relationship to a classificatory system is exactly the same as that of any other variables. This relationship may take one of two forms. Etiology and prognosis may be the correlates of the classes of a diagnostic system which employs an independent classificatory principle like symptom manifestation. Optimally, we should prefer a classificatory schema in which the indices of etiology and preferred modes of treatment would be incorporated (Hunt *et al.*, 1953; Pepinsky, 1948). In essence, this was Kraepelin's approach, and it continues to underlie some promising work in the area of psychopathology. Although Kraepelin's disease concept is in disrepute (Hoch and Zubin, 1953; Marzoff, 1947; Rotter, 1954), it is the opinion of several investigators (Eysenck, 1953; Phillips and Rabinovitch, 1958; Wittenborn *et al.*, 1953) that further work employing the descriptive symptomatic approach could well lead to a greater understanding of the etiology underlying abnormal 'processes'.

Another manner in which etiology, treatment, or prognosis could be related to a classificatory schema is by utilizing each of these variables as the classificatory principle for a new diagnostic system. For instance, we might organize patients into groups which respond differentially to particular forms of treatment like electroshock, drugs, psychotherapy, etc. The new schemata which might be proposed could be of considerable value in respect to certain goals but useless in regard to others. Since we do not possess a diagnostic system based on all the variables of clinical interest, we might have to be satisfied with the construction of a variety of diagnostic systems, each based on a different principle of classification. These classificatory techniques would exist side by side, their use being determined by the specific objectives of the diagnostician.

Etiology versus description in diagnosis

The classical Kraepelinian classification schema shows two major characteristics: a commitment to a detailed description of the individual and an underlying assumption that such a descriptive classification would be transitory, eventually leading to and being replaced by a system whose classificatory principle was the etiology of the various mental disorders. Major criticism of this classificatory effort has been directed at the first of these. The reservations are that, in practice, such a descriptive effort allows no place for a process interpretation of psychopathology and that it has not encouraged the development of prevention and treatment programs in the mental disorders.

The authors do not feel that the failure of the Kraepelinian system has demonstrated the futility of employing symptoms as the basis for classification. It does suggest that if one approaches the problem of description with an assumption as to the necessary correlates of such descriptions, then the diagnostic system may well be in error. Kraepelin's empiricism is contaminated in just this way. For example, he refused to accept as cases of dementia praecox those individuals who recovered from the disorder, since he assumed irreversibility as a necessary concomitant of its hypothesized neurophysiological base. Bleuler, on the other hand, who was much less committed to any particular form of causality in this illness, readily recognized the possibility of its favorable outcome. It is not, then, the descriptive approach itself which is open to criticism, but description contaminated by preconception. An unfettered description of those schizophrenics with good prognosis in contrast to those with poor prognosis reveals clear differences in the symptom configuration between these kinds of patients (Farina and Webb, 1956; Phillips, 1953).

Kraepelin's basic concern with the problem of etiology has remained a focus of efforts in the clinical area. Although his postulate of central nervous system disease as the basis of mental disorder is in disrepute, and his systematic classificatory efforts are assailed, one nevertheless finds a striking congruence between Kraepelin's preconceptions and certain current attempts at the solution of the problem of psychopathology. There is an unwavering belief that some simple categorical system will quickly solve the mysteries of etiology. The exponents of these newer classificatory schemata have merely replaced symptoms by other phenomena like test scores (King, 1954), particular patterns of interpersonal relations (Leary and Coffey, 1955), etc. It is the authors' conviction that these new efforts to find short-cut solutions to the question of etiology will similarly remain unsuccessful. The amount of descriptive effort required before etiological factors are likely to be discovered has been underestimated (Kety, 1959a, 1959b), and the pursuit of aetiology should represent an end point rather than a beginning for classificatory systems. The process of moving from an empirical orientation to an etiological one is, of necessity, inferential and therefore susceptible to the myriad dangers of premature inference. We propose that the greatest safeguard against such prematurity is not to be found in the scrapping of an empirical descriptive approach, but in an accelerated program of empirical research. What is needed at this time is a systematic, empirical attack on the problem of mental disorders. Inherent in this program is the employment of symptoms, broadly defined as meaningful and discernible behaviors, as the basis of a classificatory system. Rather than an abstract search for etiologies, it would appear more currently fruitful to investigate such empirical correlates of symptomatology as reactions to specific forms of treatment, outcome in the disorders, case history phenomena, etc.

The pervasive concern with etiology may derive from a belief that if this were known, prevention would shortly be forthcoming, thus, making the present complex problems of treatment and prognosis inconsequential. Unfortunately, efforts to short-circuit the drudgery involved in establishing an empirically founded psychiatry has not resulted in any major breakthroughs. Etiology is typically the last characteristic of a disorder to be discovered. Consequently, we would suggest the search for etiology be put aside and attempted only when a greater number of the correlates of symptomatic behaviors have been established.

The authors are impressed by the amount of energy that has been expended in both attacking and defending various contemporary systems of classification. We believe that a classificatory system should include any behavior or phenomenon that appears promising in terms of its significant correlates. At this stage of our investigations, the system employed should be an open and expanding one, not one which is closed and defended on conceptual grounds. Systems of classification must be treated as tools for further discovery, not as bases for polemic disputation.

As stated above, it is possible that a number of systems of classification may be needed to encompass the behaviors presently of clinical interest. It may appear that the espousal of this position, in conjunction with a plea for empirical exploration of the correlates of these behaviors, runs headlong into a desire for conceptual neatness and parsimony. It may be feared that the use of a number of classificatory systems concurrently, each with its own correlates, may lead to the creation of a gigantic actuarial table of unrelated elements. However, the authors do not feel that such a fear is well founded because it assumes that the correlates of these systems have no eventual relation one to the other.

We believe that this latter view is unnecessarily pessimistic. While in principle a multiplicity of classificatory systems might be called for, results from the authors' own research program suggests that a single, relatively restricted and coherent classification system can be derived from an empirical study of the correlates of symptomatic behaviors (Phillips and Rabinovitch, 1958; Zigler and Phillips, 1960), Such a system might serve a number of psychiatrically significant functions, including the optimum selection of patients for specific treatment programs and the prediction of treatment outcomes. In conclusion, a descriptive classificatory system appears far from dead, and if properly employed, it can lead to a fuller as well as a more conceptually based understanding of the psychopathologies.

References

ALLPORT, G. (1937), *Personality: A Psychological Interpretation*, Holt, Rinehart & Winston.

ALLPORT, G. (1946), 'Personalistic psychology as science: a reply', *Psychol. Rev.*, vol. 53, pp. 132–5.

AMERICAN PSYCHIATRIC ASSOCIATION (1952), Mental Hospital Service, Committee on Nomenclature and Statistics of the American Psychiatric Association. *Diagnostic and Statistical Manual: Mental Disorders*, A.P.A.

ASH, P. (1949), 'The reliability of psychiatric diagnosis', *J. abnorm. soc. Psychol.*, vol. 44, pp. 272–7.

BEACH, F. (1950), 'The snark was a boojum', *Amer. Psycholst*, vol. 5, pp. 115–24.

BECK, S. (1953), 'The science of personality: nomothetic or idiographic?' *Psychol. Rev.*, vol. 60, pp. 353–9.

BOISEN, A. (1938), 'Types of dementia praecox: a study in psychiatric classification', *Psychology*, vol. 1, pp. 232–6.

BROWER, D. (1949), 'The problem of quantification in psychological science', *Psychol. Rev.*, vol. 56, pp. 325–33.

CAMERON, D. (1953), 'A theory of diagnosis', in P. Hoch and J. Zubin (eds.), *Current Problems in Psychiatric Diagnosis*, Grune & Stratton, pp. 33–45.

CATTELL, R. (1957), *Personality and Motivation Structure and Measurement*, World Book.

CAVENY, E., WITTSON, C., HUNT, W., and HERMAN, R. (1955), 'Psychiatric diagnosis, its nature and function', *J. nerv. ment. Dis.*, vol. 121, pp. 367–80.

CRONBACH, L. (1957), 'The two disciplines of scientific psychology', *Amer. Psycholst*, vol. 12, pp. 671–84.

EYSENCK, H. (1952), *The Scientific Study of Personality*, Routledge & Kegan Paul.

EYSENCK, H. (1953), 'The logical basis of factor analysis', *Amer. Psycholst*, vol. 8, pp. 105–13.

EYSENCK, H. (1954), 'The science of personality: nomothetic', *Psychol. Rev.*, vol. 61, pp. 339–41.

FALK, J. (1956), 'Issues distinguishing idiographic from nomothetic approaches to personality theory', *Psychol. Rev.*, vol. 63, pp. 53–62.

FARINA, A. and WEBB, W. (1956), 'Premorbid adjustment and subsequent discharge', *J. nerv. ment. Dis.*, vol. 124, pp. 612–13.

FOULDS, G. (1955), 'The reliability of psychiatric and the validity of psychological diagnosis', *J. ment. Sci.*, vol. 101, pp. 851–2.

GUTHRIE, E. (1950), 'The status of systematic psychology', *Amer. Psycholst*, vol. 5, pp. 97–101.

HARLOW, H. (1953), 'Mice, monkeys, men, and motives,' *Psychol. Rev.* vol. 60, pp. 23–32.

HARROWER, MOLLY (ed.) (1950), *Diagnostic Psychological Testing*, Charles C. Thomas.

HOCH, P. (1953), 'Discussion', in P. Hoch and J. Zubin (eds.), *Current Problems in Psychiatric Diagnosis*, Grune & Stratton, pp. 46–50.

HOCH, P. and ZUBIN, E. (eds.) (1953), *Current Problems in Psychiatric Diagnosis*, Grune & Stratton.

HOLMES, G. (1946), *Introduction to Clinical Neurology*, Livingstone.

HOLZMAN, P. S. (1970), *Psychoanalysis and Psychopathology*, McGraw-Hill.

HUNT, W. (1951a), 'Clinical psychology – science or superstition', *Amer. Psycholst*, vol. 6, pp. 683–7.

HUNT, W. (1951b), 'An investigation of naval neuropsychiatric screening procedures', in H. Gruetskaw (ed.), *Groups, Leadership and Men*, Carnegie Press, pp. 245–56.

HUNT, W., WITTSON, C. and BARTON, H. (1950a), 'A further validation of naval neuropsychiatric screening', *J. consult. Psychol.*, vol. 14, pp. 485–588.

HUNT, W., WITTSON, C. and BARTON, H. (1950a), 'A validation study of naval neuropsychiatric screening,' *J. consult. Psychol.*, vol. 14, pp. 35–9.

HUNT, W., WITTSON, C. and HUNT, E. (1953), 'A theoretical and practical analysis of the diagnostic process', in P. Hoch and J. Zubin (eds.), *Current Problems in Psychiatric Diagnosis*, Grune & Stratton, pp. 53–65.

JELLINEK, E. (1939), 'Some principles of psychiatric classification', *Psychiatry*, vol. 2, pp. 161–5.

KANTOR, R., WALLNER, J. and WINDER, C. (1953), 'Process and reactive schizophrenia', *J. consult. Psychol.*, vol. 17, pp. 157–62.

KETY, S. (1959a), 'Biochemical theories of schizophrenia', part I, *Science*, vol. 129, pp. 1528–32.

KETY, S. (1959a), 'Biochemical theories of schizophrenia', part II, *Science*, vol. 129, pp. 1590–1956.

KING, G. (1954), 'Research with neuropsychiatric samples', *J. Psychol.*, vol. 38, pp. 383–7.

KOCH, S. (1951), 'The current status of motivational psychology', *Psychol. Rev.*, vol. 58, pp. 147–54.

LEARY, T. and COFFEY, H. (1955), 'Interpersonal diagnosis: Some problems of methodology and validation', *J. abnorm. soc. Psychol.*, vol. 50, pp. 110–26.

MACKINNON, D. (1953), 'Fact and fancy in personality research', *Amer. Psycholst*, vol. 8, pp. 138–46.

MARGARET, ANN (1952), 'Clinical methods: psychodiagnostics', *Ann. Rev. Psychol.*, vol. 3, pp. 283–320.

MARQUIS, D. (1948), 'Research planning at the frontiers of science', *Amer. Psycholst*, vol. 3, pp. 430–38.

MARZOFF, S. S. (1947), 'The disease concept in psychology,' *Psychol. Rev.*, vol. 54, pp. 211–21.

MASLOW, A. (1948), 'Cognition of the particular and of the generic,' *Psychol. Rev.*, vol. 55, pp. 22–40.

MEHLMAN, B. (1952), 'The reliability of psychiatric diagnosis', *J. abnorm. soc. Psychol.*, vol. 47, pp. 577–8.

MENNINGER, K. (1955), 'The practice of psychiatry', *Dig. Neurol. Psychiat.*, vol. 23, p. 101.

MILES, H. (1953), 'Discussion', in P. Hoch and J. Zubin (eds.), *Current Problems in Psychiatric Diagnosis*, Grune & Stratton, pp. 107–111.

NOYES, A. (1953), *Modern Clinical Psychiatry*, Saunders, 1953.

PATTERSON, C. (1948), 'Is psychotherapy dependent on diagnosis?' *Amer. Psycholst*, vol. 3, pp. 155–9.

PEPINSKY, H. B. (1948), 'Diagnostic categories in clinical counseling', *Appl. Psychol. Monogr.*, No. 15.

PHILLIPS, L. (1953), 'Case history data and prognosis in schizophrenia', *J. nerv. ment. Dis.*, vol. 117, pp. 515–25.

PHILLIPS, L. and RABINOVITCH, M. (1958), 'Social role and patterns of symptomatic behaviors', *J. abnorm. soc. Psychol.*, vol. 57, pp. 181–6.

RAPAPORT, D. (1947), 'The future of research in clinical psychology and psychiatry', *Amer. Psycholst*, vol. 2, pp. 167–72.

ROBY, T. (1959), 'An opinion on the construction of behavior theory', *Amer. Psychologist*, vol. 14, pp. 129–34.

ROE, ANNE (1949), 'Integration of personality theory and clinical practice', *J. abnorm. soc. Psychol.*, vol. 44, pp. 36–41.

ROGERS, C. (1946), 'Significant aspects of client-centered therapy', *Amer. Psycholst*, vol. 1, pp. 415–22.

ROGERS, C. (1951), *Client-centered Therapy*, Houghton Mifflin.

ROTTER, J. (1954), *Social Learning and Clinical Psychology*, Prentice-Hall.

SCHMIDT, H. and FONDA, C. (1956), 'The reliability of psychiatric diagnosis: a new look', *J. abnorm. soc. Psychol.*, vol. 52, pp. 262–7.

SCOTT, J. (1955), 'The place of observation in biological and psychological science', *Amer. Psycholst*, vol. 10, pp. 61–3.

SCOTT, W. (1958), 'Research definitions of mental health and mental illness', *Psychol. Bull.*, vol. 55, pp. 1–45.

SEEMAN, W. (1953), 'Psychiatric diagnosis: an investigation of interperson-reliability after didactic instruction', *J. nerv. ment. Dis.*, vol. 118, pp. 541–4.

SKAGGS, E. (1945), 'Personalistic psychology as science', *Psychol. Rev.*, vol. 52, pp. 234–8.

SKAGGS, E. (1947), 'Ten basic postulates of personalistic psychology', *Psychol. Rev.*, vol. 54, pp. 255–62.

THORNE, F. (1953), 'Back to fundamentals', *J. clin. Psychol.*, vol. 9, pp. 89–91.

TOLMAN, R. (1953), 'Virtue rewarded and vice punished', *Amer. Psycholst*, vol. 8, pp. 721–33.

TYLER, LEONA (1959), 'Toward a workable psychology of individuality', *Amer. Psycholst*, vol. 14, pp. 75–81.

WINDLE, C. and HAMWI, V. (1953), 'An explanatory study of the prognostic value of the complex reaction time tests in early and chronic psychotics', *J. clin. Psychol.*, vol. 9, pp. 156–61.

WITTENBORN, J. (1951), 'Symptom patterns in a group of mental hospital patients', *J. consult. Psychol.*, vol. 15, pp. 290–302.

WITTENBORN, J. (1952), 'The behavioral symptoms for certain organic psychoses', *J. consult. Psychol.*, vol. 16, pp. 104–6.

WITTENBORN, J. and BAILEY, C. (1952), 'The symptoms of involutional psychosis', *J. consult. Psychol.*, vol. 16, pp. 13–17.

WITTENBORN, J. and HOLZBERG, J. (1951), 'The generality of psychiatric syndromes', *J. consult. Psychol.*, vol. 15, pp. 372–80.

WITTENBORN, J., HOLZBERG, J. and SIMON, B. (1953), 'Symptom correlates for descriptive diagnosis', *Genet. Psychol. Monogr.*, vol. 47, pp. 237–301.

WITTENBORN, J. and WEISS, W. (1952), 'Patients diagnosed manic-depressive psychosismanic state', *J. consult. Psychol.*, vol. 16, pp. 193–8.

WITTMAN, P. and SHELDON, W. (1948), 'A proposed classification of psychotic behavior reactions', *Amer. J. Psychiat.*, vol. 105, pp. 124–8.

WITTSON, C. and HUNT, W. (1951), 'The predictive value of the brief psychiatric interview', *Amer. J. Psychiat.*, vol. 107, pp. 582–5.

YATES, A. (1958), 'Symptoms and symptom substitution', *Psychol. Rev.*, vol. 65, pp. 371–4.

ZIEGLER, E. and PHILLIPS, L. (1960), 'Social effectiveness and symptomatic behaviours', *J. abnorm. soc. Psychol.*, vol. 61, pp. 231–8.

ZILBOORG, G. and HENRY, G. W. (1941), *History of Medical Psychology*, Norton.

2 M. G. Sandifer, A. Hordern, G. C. Timbury and L. M. Green

Psychiatric Diagnosis: A Comparative Study in North Carolina, London and Glasgow[1]

M. G. Sandifer, A. Hordern, G. C. Timbury and L. M. Green, 'Psychiatric diagnosis: a comparative study in North Carolina, London and Glasgow', *British Journal of Psychology*, 1968, vol. 114, pp. 1–9.

'What's the use of their having names,' the Gnat said, 'if they won't answer to them?' 'No use to *them*', said Alice, 'but it's useful to the people that name them, I suppose. If not, why do things have names at all?'

Lewis Carroll, *Through the Looking Glass*

Better communication and the demonstration of cross-national differences in admissions by diagnosis to public mental hospitals (Brooke, 1959; Kramer, 1961, 1965) have recently stimulated

1. This study was supported in part by U.S. Public Health Service Research Grants 08800 and Fr 00021. The authors gratefully acknowledge the support of Dr Walter Sikes, Superintendent of Dorothea Dix Hospital, Dr D. W. Liddell, Head of the Department of Psychological Medicine at King's College Hospital, London and Dr T. Ferguson Rodger, Professor of Psychiatry at the University of Glasgow. In addition to the authors, the following diagnosticians, whose help was invaluable, participated: in North Carolina, Drs Thad J. Barringer, Wilmer C. Betts, Lloyd C. Brannon, Thomas Curtis, Edward F. Doehne, C. W. Erwin, John A. Ewing, George C. Ham, George W. Hamby, Robert N. Harper, Peter L. Hein, William G. Hollister, Richard W. Hudgens, Francis J. Kane, Jr, Richard D. Knapp, Bruce Kyles, Albert A. Kurland, Morris Lipton, Demmie G. Mayfield, Milton L. Miller, John T. Monroe, Jr, Charles W. Neville, Jr, Kurt Nussbaum, Nicholas Pediaditakis, Alex D. Pokorny, Arthur Prange, Clifford B. Reifler, Mario Perez-Reyes, Stanley J. Rogers, Julian W. Selig, Walter A. Sikes, James E. Somers, Roger F. Spencer, Nicholas E. Stratas, D. Frederic Thompson, A. Granville Tolley, John W. Varner, Fred A. Vinson, Thomas G. Webster, Ian C. Wilson, N. P. Zarzar, William Zung; in London, Drs P. K. Bridges, H. S. Greer, and I. S. Kreeger; and in Glasgow, I. M. Ingram, A. N. Munro and J. M. Carlisle.

Thanks are due to Mr J. L. Fleiss for his help with statistics; and to Mr Jerry Woodward, Mr Landis Bennett and Mr Kent Whitfield for their part in filming and projection, as well as to Mr C. T. Harlow in London and Mrs M. Murray in Glasgow. Dr Thomas Buie prepared the histories. Miss Eva Schloss and Mrs Mary Norton kindly prepared the manuscript.

an increased interest in international psychiatric nomenclature; indeed, standardizing such nomenclature and establishing appropriate international criteria for psychiatric diagnosis is now an activity of the World Health Organization. Whilst a definitive assessment of international diagnostic similarities and differences can hardly be obtained from a single investigation, this paper presents a contribution to what may become a growing field. It examines the diagnoses made by groups of psychiatrists in North Carolina, London and Glasgow, who independently studied sound films of initial psychiatric interviews conducted on thirty patients admitted to a large public mental hospital in the United States.[1]

Methodology

This comprised: (1) selection of patients, (2) filming of diagnostic interviews, (3) choice of diagnostician, and (4) provision of clinical data. The setting of the presentations and the method used for recording diagnostic opinions also deserve mention.

Selection of patients

Any patient admitted to the hospital who gave consent was regarded as eligible for the study. Only two patients refused to participate. Convenience in filming the diagnostic interview was the primary factor used in selection. Usually one or two films were made each week and the first patients admitted the day before filming were asked to participate. Films were made of thirty patients, by chance evenly divided between males and females. Their age range was fifteen to seventy-six, with a mean age of thirty-nine.

Individual characteristics of the patients, diagnostic or otherwise, played no part in case selection. Subsequent comparison showed that the sample was diagnostically representative (by U.S. diagnostic opinion) of admissions to Dorothea Dix Hospital.

Filming of diagnostic interviews

Except for two interviews conducted by one of the authors (A.H.), all the diagnostic interviews were conducted by psy-

1. The Dorothea Dix Hospital, Raleigh, North Carolina.

chiatrists living in North Carolina. Six interviewers participated in the study. The only instructions they were given were to conduct diagnostic interviews in their customary manner. 16 mm. black-and-white film was used, and most of the films ran for about twenty-five minutes.

Choice of diagnostician

In North Carolina, between six and ten psychiatrists from a pool of forty-three observers were chosen to report on each film. Every diagnostician had had three years of formal psychiatric training and two further years of additional experience. Although the majority of the forty-three psychiatrists came from within fifty miles of Dorothea Dix Hospital, they included ten engaged in private practice, thirteen working in three public mental hospitals, sixteen from universities (principally Duke and North Carolina), and four from Veterans Administration Hospitals. The mean age of the North Carolina psychiatrists was forty; and they had a mean of eleven years of combined training and experience.

In London four psychiatrists were selected to report on each film. All had had at least five years of training and experience in psychiatry, and all belonged to the staff of the Department of Psychological Medicine of a London Undergraduate Teaching Hospital. Of these four observers, three had eclectic orientations with a bias towards an organic-descriptive approach: one had worked in the United States and Australia as well as England, whilst the second had worked in Australia and London; the third had worked in Army psychiatry in Malaysia as well as in London. The fourth observer was an experienced psychoanalyst with a dynamic orientation who had spent his professional life in London. The mean age of the London psychiatrists was thirty-seven; and they had a mean of eleven years of training and experience.

In Glasgow, four psychiatrists reported on each film. All had at least four years of training and experience in psychiatry and all were working in the University Department of Psychological Medicine and the University of Glasgow. All four observers had been trained exclusively in Scotland, but one had worked in Dumfries with the late Dr W. Mayer-Gross and another in

Dundee with Professor I. R. C. Batchelor – i.e. two distinguished psychiatrists associated with the authorship of two standard British textbooks of psychiatry. All four had an eclectic orientation and none was strongly psychoanalytically orientated. The mean age of the group was thirty-three years and they had a mean of seven years of experience and training. All were in whole time hospital practice.

Provision of clinical data

The study of psychiatric diagnosis described in the present paper represented one aspect of a larger project in which the diagnostic process itself was investigated. To this end it was considered important that the individual diagnosticians viewed and commented on each filmed interview with open minds, i.e., with no preliminary information other than the age, sex, marital and admission status (first admission or readmission) of the patient. In other words the situation filmed resembled, as closely as possible, the psychiatrist's initial contact with a patient – the time during which he ascertains the mental state and takes the detailed history. After observing the film the diagnosticians received, in written form, a résumé of the present and past history of the patient, the relevant family history, the physical examination and laboratory findings, the Wechsler Adult Intelligence Scale score, the (uninterpreted) Minnesota Multiphasic Personality Inventory Profile, a description of the treatment given during the first two weeks in hospital, and extracts from the case notes on the patient's course during this period. Each observer made his final diagnosis on the basis of the film and the additional written information. It has been noted that the filmed interview was shown first, to give the observing psychiatrist an opportunity to view this initial contact with the patient without the possible bias of another observer's résumé of the history and mental status. However, on the conviction that an adequate clinical diagnosis frequently cannot be made on the basis of a single interview alone, the additional data were considered essential. The inclusion of an observation period of two weeks was chosen, in one sense arbitrarily, but in another sense as a reasonable period of observation which did not postpone diagnostic decision immediately.

Setting of the presentations

In North Carolina all film presentations were made to individual diagnosticians, and an observer had no knowledge of his co-observers on a particular film. In both London and Glasgow, the films were shown to groups of two to four observers. There was, however, no communication during the process of observation, and only minimal conversation concerning diagnosis on completion. By design, there was no attempt to resolve individual differences of diagnostic viewpoint.

The diagnoses made were recorded according to the nomenclature of the American Psychiatric Association.

Results: general observations

To the UK observers, the American patients appeared to be representative of the diagnostic types seen in the United Kingdom. There was some initial difficulty in applying the American Psychiatric Association nomenclature, but this was resolved by use of the handbook (Diagnostic Manual, 1952). There was frequent difficulty in understanding the patient's speech (but not the interviewer's). The same problem occurred to some extent amongst the US observers, and was, in part, related to low audio fidelity of optical sound on the film. But, even more, difficulties in understanding were due to phrases and accents which were strange to the UK observers. (More recently, the converse problem has been noted by US observers listening to audio tapes of British patients.) Interestingly, a process of adaptation appeared to occur wherein observers understood better after two or three minutes of listening.

Most observers appeared satisfied with the style of the interviews themselves, generally preferring those which were moderately structured. The UK observers apparently did not find the psychological tests (WAIS and MMPI) of particular value in diagnosis. All groups of observers would have preferred more detailed histories.

Specific findings

Diagnostic agreement within observer groups

Table 1 is a cumulative tabulation of agreement within local diagnostic groups. The Glasgow diagnosticians achieved a higher consensus than the London group, which in turn had more cases with high consensus than the North Carolina group. The Glasgow group, in fact, had complete concordance on almost half the sample.

Table 1 **Levels of agreement among diagnosticians** (cumulative cases and percentages) total N = 30 cases

	North Carolina	London	Glasgow
Complete agreement	3	6	14
	(10%)	(20%)	(47%)
At least three out of four	14	20	22
	(47%)	(67%)	(74%)
At least half	27	30	29
	(90%)	(100%)	(97%)
Remainder	30	—	30
	(100%)		(100%)

In terms of attaining a majority diagnosis, the results from the thirty cases were: Glasgow twenty-two patients, London twenty patients, and North Carolina twenty-two patients.[1] This finding – a majority opinion on two out of three cases – is in agreement with the results of an earlier study by the senior author (Sandifer, Pettus and Quade, 1964).

A comparison of within- and across-observer group agreement

Table 2 gives the percentage agreement on the twelve major diagnostic categories within and across all three groups of diagnosticians. In each instance the within-group agreement is better than the cross-group agreement, and there is a descending order of within-group agreement from Glasgow (73 per cent) to London (64 per cent) to North Carolina (58 per cent). Cross-group agreement was rather similar (44 per cent, 48 per cent and 49 per cent) in the three comparisons.[2]

1. On eight cases, the North Carolina group had levels of agreement better than half but less than three out of four.
2. The computation for within-group agreements was made by dividing the sum of the squares of all concurring opinions on a case by the square of total opinions and averaging over all cases; the cross-group agreements were computed by dividing the sum of all concurring cross-matchings on a case

Table 2 **Within- and cross-group diagnostic agreement**
(Figures in parentheses are the number of agreeing pairs
divided by total pairs)

	North Carolina	London	Glasgow
North Carolina	58% (922/1702)	49% (434/884)	44% (398/896)
London		64% (300/466)	48% (227/472)
Glasgow			73% (352/480)

Diagnostic trends within specific diagnostic categories

Table 3 shows the proportion of patients assigned to the twelve
diagnostic categories by the three groups of diagnosticians.
There is little difference across the groups on the first two
categories ('Organic' diagnoses). On the third category, Schizophrenia, the North Carolina and London groups are in close
agreement, whilst the Glasgow group diagnosed a lower percentage of patients as having this disorder. On Manic Depres-
sives the London and Glasgow groups agreed on proportions,
and used this category twice as frequently as did the group from
North Carolina. The three groups differed on the Involutional
category, but they were in agreement on the next four – Psychotic Depressive, Paranoia, Psychotic 'Other', and Psycho-
physiologic. There was a pronounced tendency for the group
from North Carolina to employ the category Neurotic, which
the Glasgow group was much less prone to use. On the other
hand, the Glasgow diagnosticians used the category Personality
Disorder approximately twice as frequently as either of the
other two groups of diagnosticians. There was little disagreement on the last category – Mental Deficiency.

---

by the total number of all cross-matchings, and averaging over all cases.
Thus, if eight US psychiatrists rendered six Diagnoses A and two Diagnoses B, the within-group agreement would be $(6^2+2^2)/8^2$, or 62·5 per cent.
By the same token, three As and one B by the London psychiatrists would
yield $(3^2+1^2)/4^2$, or again 62·5 per cent. The cross-group agreement on this
case for these two groups would then be $(6 \times 3 + 2 \times 1)/32$ or yet again 62·5
per cent.

There were seven cases which showed a high concordance on diagnoses for all observers. The diagnoses of these seven patients were: Chronic Brain Syndrome (two cases), Schizophrenia (two cases), Manic Depressive, Manic (one case), Manic Depressive, Depressed (one case), and Alcoholism (one case).

Table 3 **Proportions of diagnoses by specific categories**

	North Carolina		London		Glasgow	
	%	actual number	%	actual number	%	actual number
1. Acute Brain Syndrome	2	(5)	0	(0)	1	(1)
2. Chronic Brain Syndrome	8	(18)	10	(12)	12	(14)
3. Schizophrenia	18	(40)	20	(24)	13	(15)
4. Manic Depressive (all types)	9	(20)	18	(21)	18	(22)
5. Involutional	4	(9)	8	(9)	0	(0)
6. Psychotic Depressive	5	(11)	4	(5)	4	(5)
7. Paranoia	1	(3)	0	(0)	0	(0)
8. Psychotic 'Other'	0	(0)	0	(0)	0	(0)
9. Psychophysiological	2	(4)	2	(2)	2	(2)
10. Neurotic	29	(64)	15	(18)	10	(12)
11. Personality Disorder	18	(41)	22	(26)	37	(45)
12. Mental Deficiency	4	(8)	1	(1)	3	(4)
Total	100	(223)	100	(118)	100	(120)

Table 4 **Depressive disorders**
Diagnostic categories allocated in twelve cases

	North Carolina		London		Glasgow	
	%	No.	%	No.	%	No.
Neurotic Depressed	46	(40)	17	(8)	15	(7)
Combined ('Endogenous' Psychotic Involutional and Manic Depressed)	26	(23)	48	(22)	25	(12)
Total 'Depressives'	72	(63)	65	(30)	40	(19)
Personality Disorder	8	(7)	11	(5)	40	(19)
Other (nine categories)	20	(17)	24	(11)	20	(10)
	100	(87)	100	(46)	100	(48)

Depressive cases

Among the thirty cases there were twelve in which the majority diagnosis, by at least one of the observer groups, was a depressive diagnosis (Neurotic, Psychotic, Involutional or Manic Depressive). Table 4 shows the distribution of diagnoses by observer groups on these twelve cases. North Carolina and London were not far apart on the proportion of depressive diagnoses on these cases, but the proportions between neurotic-endogenous were reversed. London and Glasgow were more similar on their neurotic-endogenous ratio, but the Glasgow psychiatrists used a very much smaller proportion of depressive diagnoses on these cases. As can be seen from the table, most of the Glasgow non-depressive diagnoses were Personality Disorders.

The 'Schizophrenia versus Manic Depressive' conflict

One interesting area of alleged international diagnostic disagreement is the diagnosis of Schizophrenia *vis-à-vis* Manic Depressive. The earlier study (Sandifer, Pettus and Quade, 1964) had demonstrated that this particular conflict did not occur frequently amongst observers in North Carolina; thus, if Schizophrenia was taken as a first opinion, the likelihood of the second opinion being Manic Depressive was less than 5 per cent; and similarly if Manic Depressive was taken as the first diagnosis, the likelihood of Schizophrenia as a second diagnosis was only 7 per cent.[5]

Using the same method, a series of questions concerning the 'Schizophrenia versus Manic Depressive' conflict was posed on the results yielded by the present investigation. These questions

5. The calculation is as follows: Given a diagnosis on a case (e.g., Schizophrenia), the number of Schizophrenia–Schizophrenia pairings, Schizophrenia–Manic Depressive pairings, and Schizophrenia–Other Diagnoses pairings on that case is computed. For example, on a case in which the opinions are Schizophrenia seven, Manic Depressive two and Other Diagnoses one, there are forty-two Schizophrenia–Schizophrenia pairings, fourteen Schizophrenia–Manic Depressive pairings and seven Schizophrenia–Other Diagnoses pairings. In this example, Schizophrenia is designated the 'first diagnosis', but the same procedure can be used for any category. The frequency of such pairings is summed over all cases, and the proportions of each type are expressed in percentages.

are explored in Tables 5 and 6, in which the London and Glasgow diagnosticians are combined to form a single UK group.

Table 5 **Concurrence on Schizophrenia *v*. Schizophrenia-Manic Depressive**

| | Matched opinions | | | | | |
| | Schizophrenia | | Manic Depressive | | All others | |
	US	UK	US	UK	US	UK
Schizophrenia – US	62%	56%	3%	20%	35%	24%
Schizophrenia – UK	60%	57%	4%	16%	35%	28%

If a diagnosis of Schizophrenia was made, by either a US psychiatrist or a UK pyschiatrist, this opinion was matched (Table 5) against every psychiatrist's opinion on the same case. Data from individual cases were then combined to obtain overall proportions for various types of matching. The proportion of agreeing matched opinions – i.e., Schizophrenia–Schizophrenia – are shown in the first two columns. Proportions of Schizophrenia–Manic Depressive matchings are shown in the middle two columns. The remaining, heterogeneous matchings (Schizophrenia – all others) are shown in the fifth and sixth columns. For example, individual diagnoses of Schizophrenia by US psychiatrists were found to be concordantly matched 62 per cent of the time amongst their US colleagues and 56 per cent of the time amongst UK colleagues. Starting with a UK diagnosis of Schizophrenia, the concordant matches are 60 per cent amongst US psychiatrists and 57 per cent amongst UK psychiatrists. Examination of these four figures (columns one and two) reveals that a diagnosis of Schizophrenia, irrespective of where it originates, is slightly more apt to receive support amongst US psychiatrists than among UK psychiatrists. However, the differences are rather small, It is also to be noted that the cross-group matches (56 per cent and 60 per cent) are quite similar to the within-group matches (57 per cent, and 62 per cent).

In contrast, however, in the third and fourth columns the

Schizophrenia–Manic Depressive matches show a very different pattern. There is roughly a five-fold (16 per cent and 20 per cent versus 3 per cent and 4 per cent) greater likelihood among United Kingdom psychiatrists that if the second diagnosis is not Schizophrenia, it will be Manic Depressive disorder. Further, it does not appear to matter greatly from which team of observers the diagnosis of Schizophrenia originates; in each instance the UK psychiatrists use Manic Depressive disorder more frequently as an alternative diagnosis. The fifth and sixth columns simply make up the heterogeneous remainder (Schizophrenia–all other diagnoses), no one category predominating.

Table 6 Concurrence on Manic Depressive v. Manic Depressive, Other Depressive and Schizophrenia

| | Matched opinions | | | | | |
| | Manic Depressive | | Other Depressive | | Schizophrenia | |
	US	UK	US	UK	US	UK
Manic Depressive – US	63%	78%	16%	3%	7%	8%
Manic Depressive – UK	38%	58%	27%	15%	20%	15%

In Table 6, the matching process is again examined, starting now with an individual diagnosis of Manic Depressive disorder. In this table an additional match, 'Manic Depressive–Other Depressive', has been added and the heterogeneous remainder has been omitted. Comparing across the figures in the first and second columns (63 per cent versus 78 per cent and 38 per cent versus 58 per cent) it is immediately apparent that a Manic Depressive–Manic Depressive match is much more likely to be obtained if the *matching opinion* comes from the UK. It may seem paradoxical that the highest proportion of concordance (78 per cent) occurs when the initial diagnosis of Manic Depressive disorder comes from the US. However, this only confirms the general trend. The US psychiatrists used this category much more sparingly, thus presumably only on more obvious cases. It is therefore not surprising that their UK colleagues concurred when the diagnosis did appear amongst US diagnosticians. Of considerable importance is that a UK Manic Depressive diagnosis found only 38 per cent concordance among US psychiatrists. As an alternative diagnosis, the US opinion was quite likely to be another depressive disorder (27 per cent) or Schizophrenia (20 per cent). Thus, a UK diagnosis of Manic Depressive disorder finds a substantial likelihood of being called Manic Depressive, Other Depressive or Schizophrenia by American colleagues. Amongst his own colleagues, a United Kingdom psychiatrist has a much better chance (58 per cent) of concurrence on Manic Depressive, as compared to Other Depressive (15 per cent) or Schizophrenia (15 per cent).

From Tables 5 and 6 two general conclusions emerge, namely:

1. That a diagnosis of Schizophrenia from either group is more likely to have Manic Depressive as an alternative diagnosis amongst UK psychiatrists than among US psychiatrists.

2. That a UK diagnosis of Manic Depressive is more likely to have an alternative diagnosis of Schizophrenia from either group than a US diagnosis of Manic Depressive. American psychiatrists also show a greater tendency to use another depressive category as an alternative diagnosis. Thus the earlier findings that Manic Depressive disorder and Schizophrenia were infrequent alternative diagnoses (among a group of American psychiatrists) were *not* replicated in this study. In this cross-national study, the Manic Depressive versus Schizophrenia conflict was found to be much more substantial, and was found to occur in directions that might have been presumed from knowledge of national vital statistics.

Discussion

As was shown in Tables 1 and 2 there were differences in proportions in diagnostic agreement both within and across groups. Whilst on *a priori* grounds the two groups from the United Kingdom might be expected to agree with each other better than would either with the United States group, this was found only on particular categories rather than generally. The numbers of diagnosticians in the groups and their background and experience may have played a part in the differential group agreement values. The higher level of consensus found in the Glasgow group could have been due to its consisting of four relatively homogeneous observers who had had similar Scottish backgrounds of psychiatric training and experience. In contrast, in the London group three of the four diagnosticians had spent appreciable periods working abroad. Finally, the lower level of consensus attained by the North Carolina group may have been related to its having been made up of a larger number of observers whose backgrounds and experience were quite dissimilar (private practice, mental hospital, Veterans Hospitals and work in university departments). To the extent that these explanations are accurate they would confirm the commonsense observation that consensus on diagnosis is positively related to similarity of background and training.

The findings on specific diagnostic categories are, we feel, of greater interest.

Whilst the US and UK groups did differ, as noted, on alternative diagnoses to Schizophrenia, the proportionate use of the category Schizophrenia in the US compared to the UK was rather similar (US 18 per cent, UK 16 per cent). This finding is in opposition to the widely held belief that Schizophrenia is more readily diagnosed in the United States than in the United Kingdom. It may be, of course, that in some of the major North American psychiatric training centres – those that are most frequently visited by British observers – the category Schizophrenia is more readily employed than amongst the North Carolina diagnosticians. The figure rendered by the North Carolina observers – 18 per cent – is consistent with the annual percentage of admissions diagnosed as Schizophrenic at Dorothea Dix Hospital.

On Manic Depressive the findings are more in line with expectation, the two UK groups agreeing on the proportions and using the category twice as frequently as their US counterparts. The 'Manic Depressive Trend' is apparent across all subtypes (Manic, Depressive, and Mixed) but the figures are too small to make specific generalizations possible. Whilst the US–UK difference is perhaps somewhat less than might have been expected from reported figures for public mental hospitals in the two countries (Kramer, 1961), it is true that, observing the same patients, the London and Glasgow psychiatrists used the

Manic Depressive category more frequently than their American colleagues.

On the cases of depression we can only point to the complexity of findings in that each group of observers resembled another group in some respects but was very different in others. The similarity of the North Carolina and London groups on total proportion of depressive diagnoses, however, emphasizes the importance of considering Neurotic Depressive Reaction in cross-national comparisons of admissions for affective disorders.

Summary and conclusions

It is worth reiterating that the formidable problem of cross-national differences in diagnostic styles cannot be resolved by a single study. Such an investigation would require not only an enormous, really representative sample of patients, but also a huge sample of diagnosticians. In order to obtain meaningful conclusions, the present report has focused on group performance on diagnosis, but a review of the tables demonstrates that there are substantial variations within groups of observers. Within these limitations, the study shows:

1. Cross-national exceed within-national differences in diagnosis. Since diagnosis is a function of training and experience any other finding would have been surprising indeed.

2. The major differences in the utilization of diagnostic categories were a greater use of Neurotic (especially Neurotic Depressive) by North Carolina psychiatrists, a greater use of Personality Disorder by the Glasgow psychiatrists, and greater use of Manic Depressive by both UK groups of diagnosticians.

3. Whilst the differences in the proportionate use of the diagnosis Schizophrenia were unimpressive, the London and Glasgow groups tended to use Manic Depressive more frequently as an alternative or second opinion.

The trends in diagnosis that have been reported are consistent with comparative statistics for mental hospital admissions. The national statistical differences, however, are greater than those found in the present study, which was carried out by a group of investigators with a better-than-average knowledge of each other's countries, and a shared interest in the problems of psychiatric diagnosis. The role of other factors, such as the methods employed to code the admission diagnosis, differential selectivity of admissions or 'true' differences in incidence, await further exploration.

References

BROOKE, E. M. (1959), 'National (British) statistics in the epidemiology of mental illness', *J. ment. Sci.*, vol. 105, pp. 893–908.

Diagnostic and Statistical Manual, Mental Disorders, (1952), American Psychiatric Association.

KRAMER, M. (1961), 'Some problems for international research suggested by observations on differences in first admission rates to the mental hospitals of England and Wales and of the United States', *Proc. Third World Congress Psychiat.*, vol. 3, pp. 153–60.

KRAMER, M. (1965), 'Classification of mental disorders', Paper presented at American Psychiatric Association Conference on Nosology, Washington, D.C.

SANDIFER, M. G., PETTUS, C. and QUADE, D. (1964), 'A study of psychiatric diagnosis', *J. nerv. ment. Dis.*, vol. 139, pp. 350–6.

3 D. Bindra

Experimental Psychology and the Problem of Behaviour Disorders

D. Bindra, 'Experimental psychology and the problem of behaviour disorders', *Canadian Journal of Psychology*, vol. 13, 1959, pp. 135–50.

The purpose of this paper is to suggest a set of principles that might serve as useful guidelines for further research in the area of behaviour disorders or mental illness. These principles are derived mainly from experimental psychology and are opposed to the currently popular 'psychodynamic approach'. The thesis of this paper is that they provide the only sure way of accumulating reliable knowledge that could serve as a basis for the diagnosis and treatment of behaviour disorders.

The accumulation of reliable and accurate information is, of course, a slow process. However, for better or worse, society's demand for the diagnosis and treatment of man's ills has seldom waited upon the accumulation of scientifically impeccable knowledge. Typically, the professions have developed before the sciences with which they have come to be associated: engineering is older than physics, medicine than physiology and bacteriology, and surgery than anatomy. Thus, it should surprise no one that, although the science of psychology is still in its infancy, there exist two socially recognized professions concerned with the diagnosis and treatment of behaviour disorders. One is psychiatry; the other, clinical psychology. Though the stated aims of and training in the fields of psychiatry, clinical psychology, and experimental psychology are different from each other, many psychiatrists and clinical psychologists are engaged in experimental research. Thus, when I label psychiatrists and clinical psychologists as clinical workers, I shall be referring only to the clinical part of their work; at other times the same persons may function as experimental researchers.

Evaluation of current status

I shall begin by posing the problem presented by behaviour disorders and evaluating the contribution of the 'psychodynamic approach' to the study of their nature, diagnosis, and treatment.

The problem

A person with a behaviour disorder is one whose behaviour is persistently and markedly different from that of the majority of his cultural group, in a way that is considered undesirable by the group or its appointed experts. Whether it arises from a series of anxiety-linked experiences, or from brain impairment, or from abnormalities of body chemistry, the basic identifying feature of any behaviour disorder lies in the frequencies of occurrence of various individual and social activities relative to the frequencies of occurrence of the same activities in a defined relevant group. Clearly, then, the central problem in understanding the causes or psychopathology of a disorder is one of delineating the relevant categories of activities and experimentally analysing the factors that control them.

At the more practical level of dealing with patients, one faces two separate problems. The first of these is that of finding reliable measures obtainable from a small sample of behaviour which, together with other information about the age, sex, past history, employment, present complaint, and so on, would enable one to make with some assurance certain predictive statements about classification, aetiology, therapeutic action, or prognosis, or any combination of these. For convenience, the development of reliable methods for making such predictive statements about a patient may be referred to as the problem of diagnosis. The second practical problem is that of finding, for each type of patient, a course of therapeutic action that will change the patient's frequencies of occurrence of the various classes of activities in the direction of the pattern of activities of the group norm. This is the problem of treatment.

Now, what has the currently popular research approach yielded by way of reliable knowledge about the problems of causation or psychopathology, diagnosis, and treatment of behaviour disorders?

For the past two or three decades discussions of the problems of causation, diagnosis, and treatment of behaviour disorders have been dominated by what may be called the 'psycho-dynamic approach'. It is difficult to give a precise and generally acceptable definition of the psychodynamic approach, but perhaps everyone would agree that it refers to a view of behaviour which stresses 'motivation'. A large number of conscious and unconscious motivational entities, wishes, desires, tendencies, complexes, frustrations, anxieties, and so on, are considered as the crucial variables determining both normal and abnormal behaviour. These motivational entities are said to develop through the interaction of constitution and experience; however, in practice, experience or learning is looked upon as the more variable and, therefore, as the more important factor in determining individual differences in the quality, aim, and intensity of the motivational entities. In the area of behaviour disorders, the answer to the problem of psychopathology is said to lie in the 'psychodynamics' of the case, and diagnosis is looked upon as the process of discovering the 'psychodynamics', that is, of determining the dominant motivations of the patient and the circumstances in which they were acquired. The problem of treatment is then considered as one of altering the patient's behaviour through changing the aims or directions of his motivations.

Anyone who has carefully looked through the last three decades of psychodynamically oriented research knows that it does not provide an occasion for rejoicing and self-congratulation. In fact it seems to have produced findings that, for the most part, either are unreliable (that is, cannot be reproduced) or are of little positive significance. Consider, for example, the mass of research with the Rorschach and other similar personality tests designed to yield meaningful predictive statements about a person on the basis of an assessment of 'his psychodynamics'. The negative verdict on the claims of psychodynamically oriented tests arrived at in the reviews of Windle (1952), and Zubin and Windle (1954), and in reviews of the literature on personality assessment techniques published in the recent volumes of the *Annual Review of Psychology*, is well known by now. There are also a number of negative findings obtained in carefully controlled recent studies of investigators such as Holtzman and Sells (1954), Kelly and Fiske (1951), Kostlan (1954) and Sines (1957). In general, these studies show that the increment in predictive accuracy made when the results of the psychodynamic type of psychological tests are added to certain data of an actuarial type – age, education, referral source, etc. – is close to nil; indeed, sometimes the predictions become less accurate when psychodynamical interpretations are added to the actuarial data. Rapid accumulation of negative results of this type has led Meehl to challenge anyone to cite a consistent body of published evidence showing that predictions based on 'psychodynamics' or 'the structure and dynamics of an individual's motivations' are superior to the predictions based on information of an actuarial type. In spite of the great confidence that many clinical workers place in the value of psychodynamics to them, no one to my knowledge has accepted Meehl's challenge.

Turn now to psychotherapy, which is the main procedure of treatment typically followed by clinical workers who subscribe to the psychodynamic approach. The label 'psychotherapy' includes a variety of methods involving social interaction and systematic use by the therapist of any one or more of the techniques labelled catharsis, suggestion, interpretation, and insight. Though strong opinions are held by many concerning the effectiveness of psychotherapy, at present there appears to be no unequivocal evidence that psychotherapy, as defined above, contributes to recovery from behaviour disorders (Bindra 1956). Meehl, who is both a critical scientist and a practising psychotherapist, has summed up the current evidence of psychotherapy in one schizophrenic statement: 'Like all therapists, I personally experience an utter inability not to believe I effect results in individual cases; but as a psychologist I know it is foolish to take this conviction at face value' (Meehl 1955, p. 373). Meehl goes on to say, 'Our daily therapeutic experiences . . . can be explained within a crude statistical model of the patient-therapist population that assigns very little specific "power" to therapeutic intervention' (Meehl, 1955, pp. 373–4).

By way of conclusion, it may be said that it is not possible to *prove* that the psychodynamic approach will never produce any reliable information or useful techniques; it is conceivable that in the next ten, twenty, or fifty years it may yield something worthwhile. However, in view of the available published research it appears that the confidence which many workers place in the value of the psychodynamic approach in their research and practice is misplaced; the ritual of going through the psychodynamic test and therapeutic procedures may impress the patient, may give the clinical worker a *feeling* of 'understanding', and may increase the confidence he places in his own predictions and treatments, but it has no demonstrable clinical or research value. The available research also suggests that the psychodynamic approach, like so many other ideas in the history of science, has turned out to be a wrong 'lead'. Thus it seems to me that any further work along this approach would not constitute the most efficient strategy of research.

Some guidelines for future research

In the remainder of this paper I shall attempt to indicate a strategy of research which might prove more fruitful than the psychodynamic approach. I shall do no more than attempt to make explicit and bring together those principles in psychological and medical research that are particularly relevant to the study of behaviour disorders.

Principle 1

Research on the problems of causation, diagnosis, and treatment of behaviour disorders should concentrate, not on 'psychodynamics' or other hypothetical processes, but on observed behaviour.

Typically, a clinical report consists of two parts. In the first part the clinical worker describes the behaviour of the patient as he has observed it or as it has been described to him. He follows this with certain facts about the present circumstances of the patient and information about the family and personal histories. These data consist of such items as age, socio-economic level, performance at school, the symptoms as observed, and circumstances of onset of the disorder. All these items of information can be, and usually are, determined in a fairly objective and reliable way. In the second part of the clinical report the worker reports the results of some personality tests of questionable reliability and validity, and then adds his over-all impression of the 'psychodynamics' of the case. Statements in this part of the report may read as 'Marked anxiety reaction in an immature individual with passive dependent needs' (Garfield, 1957, p. 225), or 'strong pent-up aggressions are indicated and, although the aggressions appear to be absorbed to a large extent in fantasy, the poor controls implied in his impulsiveness probably permit aggressive, anti-social out-bursts' (Schafer, 1948, p. 232). Such statements obviously lack any precise, operational meaning. Thus, the clinical worker often moves from reliable data in the first part of his report to vague, interpretative statements about hypothetical processes in the second part.

No matter how vague and untidy these interpretative statements may be, they do serve an important function for the clinical worker. They provide him with some sort of a rationale for deciding upon a course of therapeutic action, and, in the absence of exact knowledge of the aetiology of most behaviour disorders, there is no other basis for making the administrative decisions as to which one of several treatments to give a patient. Thus, so far as the objectives of clinical work are concerned, it may be desirable to postulate hypothetical psychodynamic processes as temporary and tentative substitutes for exact know-ledge of aetiology. However, whatever the requirements of practical, administrative decisions, there can be no doubt that for purposes of research on psychopathology, and for develop-ing improved methods of diagnosis and treatment, one must concentrate on behaviour as observed. For, in moving from observed behaviour to the type of hypothetical processes usually postulated, one abandons the more reliable in favour of the less reliable; error and vagueness are introduced. And this is no way to develop reliable knowledge. Therefore, as far as possible we should minimize the use of hypothetical entities, and link behavioural data directly to other empirical variables, such as the course of a disorder, environmental and physiological factors that produce fluctuations in symptoms, and effects of particular treatments. The practical implication of this principle is that those clinicians who also function as research workers must work with different sets of concepts and must step outside the framework of psychodynamic theory and practice for improving their diagnostic and therapeutic techniques for the future.

Principle 2

Descriptions of subjective states, not being subject to publicly observable or objective reliability checks, should not be considered as statements about crucial psychopathological events; however, verbal statements about such states may, under certain conditions, serve as reliable data.

Subjective states such as those of pain, anxiety, depression, elation, triumph, jealousy, helplessness, and dejection are reported by almost all human beings, and, in a common sense sort of way, it appears reasonable that personal descriptions of such states be considered as evidence in discussions of psychopathology. One often hears that the diagnostician or the therapist should aim at determining not what the patient does but what he 'feels', not how the investigator manipulates the patient's environment but what the change 'means' to the patient, not what the patient is but what he 'perceives' himself to be. Now, as everyone knows, scientific evidence must be open to objective reliability checks. Therefore, no personal descriptions of subjective states can be employed as evidence in discussions of hypotheses concerning psychopathology, no matter how 'real' such states may be to the patients describing them.

It is hardly necessary to review at length the utter confusion that resulted from the introspectionist schools of Titchener and Külpe in their attempts to answer psychological questions by regarding descriptions of subjective states as crucial evidence. Two sentences from Boring's paper (1953) on the history of introspection tell the story:

Classical introspection, it seems to me, went out of style after Titchener's death [1927] because it had demonstrated no functional use and therefore seemed dull, and also because it was unreliable. Laboratory atmosphere crept into the descriptions, and it was not possible to verify, from one laboratory to another, the introspective accounts of the consciousnesses of action, feeling, choice and judgment (Boring, 1953, p. 174).

In view of this historical lesson it is regrettable that many workers in the field of psychopathology continue to consider descriptions of subjective states as evidence, and often formulate diagnostic and therapeutic questions in terms of such states.

It should be noted that the above statement does not deny the possibility of the use of verbal statements about subjective states as data in their own right. Indeed, it is quite legitimate to consider statements such as 'I am depressed' and 'I feel anxious' as dependent variables and to investigate the frequency of occurrence of these responses under different experimental conditions. An analysis of the conditions which determine the occurrence of such verbal responses would be a contribution to the study of linguistic behaviour, and might also provide the knowledge necessary to link meaningfully verbal data with causal, diagnostic, and therapeutic considerations in the area of behaviour disorders. However, these types of correlations can be established only by treating verbal statements as data rather than as crucial evidence, and completely ignoring the subjective connotations of the statements.

Principle 3

The aim of diagnostic and research testing procedures should be the measurement of significant aspects of behaviour: that is, tests should measure variables whose relations with other dependent and independent variables in general psychology have been well established experimentally rather than *ad hoc* variables which appear temporarily to be of some practical significance.

By a significant psychological variable I mean nothing more than a variable which has been studied extensively and has been shown to be related to a variety of other behavioural, social, or biological variables. Any variable that is meaningfully related to a large number of other empirical variables may be considered as a more significant variable than one that is not so related. This criterion for determining whether a variable can be considered 'fundamental' is closer to Margenau's (1950) concept of basic validity than to Cronbach and Meehl's (1955) and Loevinger's (1957) concept of construct validity.

Recent experimental work in both animal and human laboratories has delineated many significant variables that are of direct relevance to the problems of behaviour disorders, that is, they appear to be meaningfully related to the variable of presence versus absence of particular symptoms. For instance, Malmo and Shagass (1949) have shown that normals, neurotics, and psychotics differ from each other in the increase in muscle tension brought about by noxious stimulation; furthermore, they have shown a clear relation between a patient's symptoms and the pattern of increases in muscle tension in different parts of the body. Other recently delineated significant variables, which can be objectively and reliably measured and which are relevant to behaviour disorders, include relative response specificity (Lacey et al., 1953), sedation threshold (Shagass, 1956), susceptibility to arousal and avoidance tendency (Kamin et al., 1955), rate of operant responding (Skinner et al., 1954) and (Lindsley, 1956), time estimation (Stern, 1959), suggestibility and persistence (Eysenck, 1952), and rate of conditioning (Taylor, 1951). Fundamental variables of this type are already providing a basis for conducting reliable and significant investigations and for developing diagnostic procedures for use in clinical work. It should be noted that research of this type is initially aimed not at developing tests for practical purposes but at delineating fundamental aspects of behaviour through detailed experimental analysis of relevant phenomena. The laboratory is the best place for this type of analysis.

The fact that the currently popular personality tests fail significantly to increase the validity of diagnostic decisions is partly attributable to their failure to sample fundamental aspects of behaviour: they bear no established relation to the main body of psychological knowledge. Thus, it is hard to see why, for example, a small 'd' response on the Rorschach, or agreement with the statement 'I find it hard to keep my mind on a task or job' on the Taylor Scale of anxiety, should have any general diagnostic capacity. The fact that these responses are given more frequently by neurotics than by normals may be practically useful information, but it is not clear how these responses are related to other variables of greater empirical and theoretical significance. Since the relation of such responses to a criterion variable remains an isolated fact, it is likely that even the practical utility of this relation lacks cross-situational power, being dependent upon the operation of some adventitious factors peculiar to a particular time and place. Thus, if in 1954 disagreement with the item 'I prefer a bath to a shower' was a characteristic response of successful graduate students of the University of California at Berkeley, it is unlikely that the same item would differentiate between successful and unsuccessful graduate students at the University of Edinburgh, or that it would differentiate between these groups today, five years later, even at Berkeley. What is worse is that such test items may cease to correlate with the validating criterion with variations of time and place without the investigator being any the wiser.

In view of these considerations, it is important to concentrate on developing reliable, objective measures of fundamental aspects of behaviour rather than on developing tests which may, for some unknown reason, temporarily appear to be useful. Once some reliable measures of significant variables have been found, the measures are bound to be of significance for both research and clinical purposes. This suggestion is supported by a study of the diagnostic and research tests employed in the field of general medicine. Such widely used medical tests as body temperature, pulse rate, blood pressure, and blood count are all tests that measure fundamental physiological aspects of the body, aspects that are equally relevant to the description of the physiology of normal and sick persons. Take body temperature, for instance. Though there had been some interest in the use of the thermometer in medical diagnosis, it was not until the middle of the last century that variations in body temperature came to be regarded as an index of a fundamental physiological property of the organism (Mettler, 1947, p. 312). Thus, it was only after an instrument for reliably measuring body temperature was available, and only after the mean body temperature of the normal man was established, that it was possible to do the kind of validation study that laid the foundation of modern clinical thermometry. The pioneering validation study was carried out by Wunderlich (*see* Mettler, 1926) who, after studying hundreds of typhoid patients during an epidemic was able to give an affirmative answer to the question of the existence of a significant relation between the course of the disease and variations in body temperature. I think it is high time that in the field of behaviour disorders it was also recognized that only the fundamental behavioural properties of the organism constitute a reasonable basis for developing tests for clinical and other applied psychological purposes.

Principle 4

The crucial psychological problem in understanding behaviour disorders is that of determining the laws which govern the interaction between habit strength and other factors that control the occurrence of responses.

It must be recognized once and for all that the behaviour on the basis of which we classify a person as, for example, a neurotic or an organic psychotic is not determined solely by a particular set of anxiety-related experiences or by a particular type of brain damage. As has been pointed out by so many, the functional-organic dichotomy of behaviour disorders does not correspond to facts of psychopathology. Not all those who have undergone anxiety-producing experiences become neurotics, nor do all with a certain type of brain damage show identical behavioural deviations. In the case of a compulsive neurotic, for example, though the specific compulsions could undoubtedly be shown to be related to the life experiences of the patient, a psychologist must still face the problem that not all persons with similar experiences develop the same compulsions, and, indeed, many do not develop any compulsions at all. Similarly, the various activities that characterize the general paretic do not result from brain damage alone; there is no specific type of brain damage that will cause a person to propose marriage to the ward nurse three times a day, or to walk the hospital wards wearing nothing except a hat and a cigar. Of course, since the existence of tertiary syphilitic infection in general paretics has been established, general paresis has come to be defined in terms of the syphilitic damage to brain cells. However, this happy finding, no matter how useful it may be practically, leaves unanswered the psychological question of why the general paretic behaves as he does. What I am saying is that explaining neurotic or psychotic behaviour involves more than linking it to some aetiological factor, such as particular antecedent experiences or the abnormality of brain function. The medical concept of aetiology is too narrow to cover all aspects of scientific inquiry. In analysing and explaining behaviour disorders, the psychologist faces many subtle problems which go beyond the interests of the practising clinicians.

The essential problem in developing explanations of behaviour disorders seems to reside in the interaction between habit strength, on the one hand, and, on the other, the so-called aetiological factors, be they chemical, organic, or experiential in origin. I employ the term 'habit strength' to refer to nothing more than the degree of prepotence acquired by a particular activity. The variable of habit strength occupies a special place among the factors that control behaviour, for, as the habit strength of an activity increases, it seems to become functionally autonomous, or relatively independent of the chemical, situational, and other factors that initially controlled it (Bindra, 1959). Thus, what I consider to be the crucial interaction is the one between the habit strengths of the various activities that exist in an individual's repertoire and the operation of the so-called aetiological factors such as anxiety-producing experiences, brain damage, and changes in body chemistry. This type of interaction may be illustrated with reference to the recent studies with the psychotomimetic drug, adrenochrome (Hoffer *et al.*, 1954).

Suppose that the presence of a certain amount of adrenochrome, or some related substance, is a necessary factor in making a person behave in a way that would lead to his classification as a schizophrenic. Now, as has been pointed out by Hoffer *et al.* (1954), the exact effects on behaviour of any experimentally administered adrenochrome are typically not uniform from individual to individual. This variability seems to persist even when an equivalent amount is injected into every subject, and when the behaviour is observed after approximately the same post-injection interval. Some of the reported variability is undoubtedly due to individual differences in the reactivity of the relevant tissues to the drug, but another equally important source of variability seems to lie in the initial differences between subjects in the habit strength of the relevant responses. Thus, assuming adrenochrome to be the necessary factor in schizophrenia, one must ask how the specific activities shown by different schizophrenics are related to the relative strengths of the activities existing in their repertoires at the time of the disease onset (i.e. operation of the 'etiological factor'), as well as to the new responses acquired after the onset. Specifically, the psychologist must learn (a) the exact way in which adrenochrome affects the occurrence of activities of varying habit strength that already exist in a person's repertoire, (b) how adrenochrome affects the acquisition of new activities, and (c) what the behavioural characteristics of high adrenochrome individuals reared in different environmental ('cultural') settings are. Knowledge of such interaction between habit strength and adrenochrome will tell us not only what the exact effects of a given dosage of adrenochrome will be, but also how, through appropriate combinations of drugs and psychological training, one could minimize the occurrence of given (undesirable) types of activities.

I believe that some fundamental experimental research designed to determine the general laws which govern the interaction between habit strength on the one hand and factors such as body chemistry, arousal, and sensory cues on the other is the most important single problem facing psychologists who are interested in understanding the phenomena of behaviour disorders. Any systematic therapeutic use of drugs or psychological retraining, or a combination of the two, presupposes a knowledge of the laws that govern these interactions.

Principle 5

Research on treatment of behaviour disorders should concentrate on developing techniques of manipulating the conditions that currently control the patient's undesirable responses rather than on unearthing the conditions which initially produced his disorder.

This principle represents a finding that has been repeatedly corroborated in a variety of areas of research. It is what Allport

(1937) referred to as 'functional autonomy of motives', and what, in my recent book (1959), I have rechristened as 'partial autonomy of activities'. In that book I have collated considerable evidence supporting the generalization that with increasing practice an activity becomes relatively independent of the conditions under which that activity was initially acquired or practised. For example, the alteration of certain sensory cues will disrupt the normal sexual responses of a sexually inexperienced male rat, but will not affect the sexual performance of a sexually sophisticated (i.e., high habit-strength) rat. Similarly, the greater the habit strength of a dominance or aggressive activity the more likely is it to withstand variations in gonadal hormones and in other blood factors. The same relation also holds between habit strength and the level of arousal of the organism: the greater the habit strength of an activity the greater appears to be the range of variation of the organism's level of arousal within which that activity will occur without disruption. Clearly, through repeated performance, activities tend to become relatively independent of the conditions which were initially necessary for their performance. This means that the chemical, situational, and reinforcement factors that maintain an activity after it has been well practised may be different from those that were crucial in its acquisition and early performance.

The phenomenon of partial autonomy of activities implies that in order to eliminate or to decrease the frequency of occurrence of an undesirable activity, it is more important to know and to manipulate the conditions that currently control that activity than to unearth the factors under which it was first acquired. The success of some recent attempts at purely symptomatic treatment, for example Jones (1956), Malmo *et al.* (1952), Wolpe (1958) and Yates (1958) indicate that Freud was too hasty, and wrong, in concluding that unearthing the developmental conditions of a neurotic disorder (hysteria) was necessary for its successful treatment (1953, pp. 253–4). Of course, knowledge of the historical factors which led to the development of an undesirable activity may be sought for its own sake, and such knowledge will undoubtedly increase our understanding of behaviour disorders; however, so far as the practical aim of modifying behaviour is concerned, the factors that currently control it are the more, if not the only, important ones.

These considerations point to one of the reasons for the doubtful efficacy of psychotherapy. Typically, one of the major undertakings in the psychotherapeutic situation is what is called 'interpretation'. To a large extent interpretation involves linking the patient's symptoms to the factors which did operate or may have operated at the onset of his behaviour disorder. Now, it is certainly doubtful whether it is possible to unearth the factors which actually determined the onset of the symptoms through the social interaction of a psychotherapeutic situation. But even if it is possible, this knowledge on the part of either the therapist or the patient would have little bearing on any attempt to discover and manipulate the variables that currently control the disordered aspects of the patient's behaviour. Perhaps the best course of action would be, first, to subject the patient to some semi-experimental situations to determine the factors that currently control the undesirable activities, and then to consider which factors, situational, chemical, or experiential, or which combination of these, are likely to constitute the most effective treatment. 'Interpretation' and 'insight', in the sense in which these terms are employed in psychotherapy, have little bearing on this procedure.

A recent study by Coons (1957) is relevant to this point. Coons compared the effects on hospital patients of two types of group psychotherapy. In one type the technique stressed interaction among members of the group without reference to personal difficulties of individual patients. In the other condition the technique stressed 'cognitive understanding of personal difficulties (insight)'. Coons found that the interaction group showed significantly greater improvement in adjustment than did the insight group; the insight group did not differ from a control group which had received no treatment at all. Thus, Coons concludes that interaction rather than insight seems to be the essential condition for therapeutic change. The failure of insight by itself to produce any favourable change is consistent with the proposition that getting to know the factors that initially produced a disorder may have little bearing upon treatment of that disorder. The efficacy of the interaction procedure may be attributed to the fact that the patients were made to engage in the very types of activities which are considered as representing improved adjustment.

The work of Wolpe (1958) and Ferster (1958) also bears on this issue. Both have shown how experimental findings in the field of learning may be used as a basis for modifying the behaviour of patients without getting involved in interpretation, insight, or other similar procedures employed in traditional psychotherapy. Some would claim that traditional psychotherapy also seeks to employ the principles of learning but does so at a verbal, symbolic level. But the fact that psychotherapy has not been shown to constitute an effective treatment of behaviour disorders means that the current psychodynamically oriented techniques of re-education (catharsis, interpretation, insight, etc.) apparently fail to make use of those principles of learning which might constitute a sound basis for effecting change in behaviour. Indeed, the procedures suggested by Wolpe and Ferster are so different from those currently subsumed under the rubric of 'psychotherapy' that they should probably be given a separate name – perhaps 'retraining' or 'response re-education'.

To recapitulate, treatment of behaviour disorders must necessarily involve replacing undesirable activities with desirable ones. This can be done by subjecting the patient to the type of procedures – and these include situational, chemical, surgical and all other types of factors that control response – that would increase the probability of occurrence of the desired activities. Such procedures must involve the active manipulation of real, palpable conditions that currently control his behaviour, rather than merely the indirect, symbolic re-education that may take place in the conventional psychotherapist's office.

Summary and conclusion

Three decades of psychodynamically oriented research, which stresses conscious and unconscious wishes, desires, frustrations, anxieties, and other motivational entities as the determiners of normal and abnormal behaviour, have failed to contribute significantly to the problems of causation or psychopathology, diagnosis, and treatment of behaviour disorders or mental illness. This paper suggests a set of principles that are likely to serve as useful alternative guidelines for further research in the area of behaviour disorders. The principles are derived mainly from the research experience of experimental psychologists. The proposed principles are:

1. Research on the problems of causation, diagnosis, and treatment of behaviour disorders should concentrate, not on 'psychodynamics' or other hypothetical processes, but on observed behaviour.

2. Descriptions of subjective states, not being subject to publicly observable or objective reliability checks, should not be considered as statements about crucial psychopathological events; however, verbal statements about such states may, under certain conditions, serve as reliable data.

3. The aim of diagnostic and research testing procedures should be the measurement of significant aspects of behaviour: that is, tests should measure variables whose relations with other dependent and independent variables in general psychology have been well established experimentally rather than *ad hoc* variables which appear temporarily to be of some practical significance.

4. The crucial psychological problem in understanding behaviour disorders is that of determining the laws which govern the interaction between habit strength and other factors that control the occurrence of responses.

5. Research on treatment of behaviour disorders should concentrate on developing techniques of manipulating the conditions that currently control the patient's undesirable responses rather than on unearthing the conditions which initially produced his disorder.

Only if these principles are followed in research is there any hope of accumulating a systematic body of reliable knowledge about behaviour disorders, knowledge which would be not only scientifically sound but also practically useful. It is to be hoped that more and more mental hospitals will start laboratories for experimental research and that more and more experimental psychologists will interest themselves in the field of behaviour disorders. If this happens, there can be no doubt that psychology will, in the near future, provide the practice of psychiatry and clinical psychology with the same type of reliable scientific foundation as physiology has provided for the practice of general medicine.

D. Bindra 73

References

ALLPORT, G. W. (1937), *Personality*, Holt Rinehart & Winston.

BINDRA, D. (1956), 'Psychotherapy and the recovery from neurosis', *J. abnorm. soc. Psychol.*, vol. 53, pp. 251–4.

BINDRA, D. (1959), *Motivation: A Systematic Reinterpretation*, Ronald Press.

BORING, E. G. (1953), 'A history of introspection', *Psychol. Bull.*, vol. 50, pp. 168–89.

COONS, W. H. (1957), 'Interaction and insight in group psychotherapy', *Canad. J. Psychol.*, vol. 11, pp. 1–8.

CRONBACH, L. J. and MEEHL, P. L. (1955), 'Construct validity in psychological tests', *Psychol. Bull.*, vol. 52, pp. 281–302.

EYSENCK, H. L. (1952), *The Scientific Study of Personality*, Routledge & Kegan Paul.

FERSTER, C. B. (1958), 'Reinforcement and punishment in the control of human behavior by social agencies', *Psychiatric Research Reports*, vol. 10, pp. 101–18.

FREUD, S. (1953), *Collected Papers*, vol. I., Hogarth Press and Institute of Psychoanalysis.

GARFIELD, S. L. (1957), *Introductory Clinical Psychology*, Macmillan.

HOFFER, A., OSMOND, H. and SMYTHIES, J. (1954), 'Schizophrenia: a new approach. II. Result of a year's research', *J. ment. Sci.*, vol. 100, pp. 29–45.

HOLTZMAN, W. H. and SELLS, S. B. (1954), 'Prediction of flying success by clinical analysis of test protocols', *J. abnorm. soc. Psychol.*, vol. 49, pp. 485–90.

JONES, H. W. (1956), 'The application of conditioning and learning techniques to the treatment of a psychiatric patient', *J. abnorm. soc. Psychol.*, vol. 52, pp. 414–19.

KAMIN, L. J., BINDRA, D., CLARK, J. W. and WAKSBERG, H. (1955) 'The inter-relations among some behavioural measures of anxiety', *Canad. J. Psychol.*, vol. 9, pp. 79–83.

KELLY, E. L. and FISKE, D. W. (1951), *The Prediction of Performance in Clinical Psychology*, University of Michigan Press.

KOSTLAN, A. (1954), 'A method for the empirical study of psychodiagnosis', *J. consult. Psychol.*, vol. 18, pp. 83–88.

LACEY, J. I., BATEMAN, D. E. and VAN LEHN, R. (1953), 'Autonomic response specificity: an experimental study', *Psychosom. Med.*, vol. 15, pp. 8–21.

LINDSLEY, O. R. (1956), 'Operant conditioning methods applied to research in chronic schizophrenia', *Psychiatric Research Reports*, vol. 5, pp. 118–39.

LOEVINGER, J. (1957), 'Objective tests as instruments of psychological theory', *Psychol. Reports. Monogr. Supplement 9*, vol. 3, pp. 635–94.

MALMO, R. B., DAVIS, J. F. and BARZA, S. (1952), 'Total hysterical deafness: an experimental case study', *J. Person.*, vol. 21, pp. 188–20.

MALMO, R. B. and SHAGASS, C. (1949a), 'Physiologic studies of reaction to stress in anxiety and early schizophrenia', *Psychosom. Med.*, vol. 11, pp. 9–24.

MALMO, R. B. and SHAGASS, C. (1949b), 'Physiologic study of symptom mechanisms in psychiatric patients under stress', *Psychosom. Med.*, vol. 11, pp. 25–9.

MARGENAU, H. (1950), *The Nature of Physical Reality*, McGraw-Hill.

MEEHL, P. E. (1955), 'Psychotherapy', *Ann. Rev. Psychol.*, vol. 6, pp. 357–78.

MEEHL, P. E. (1959), 'Some ruminations on the validation of clinical procedures', *Canad. J. Psychol.*, vol. 13, pp. 102–126.

METTLER, C. C. (1947), *History of Medicine*, Blakiston.

SCHAFER, R. (1948), *The Clinical Application of Psychological Tests*, International Universities Press.

SHAGASS, C. (1956), 'Sedation threshold: a neurophysiological tool for psychosomatic research', *Psychosom. Med.*, vol. 18, pp. 410–19.

SINES, L. K. (1957), 'An experimental investigation of the relative contribution to clinical diagnosis and personality description of various kinds of pertinent data', unpublished Ph.D. thesis, University of Minnesota.

SKINNER, B. F., SOLOMON, H. C. and LINDSLEY, O. R. (1954), 'A new method for the experimental analysis of the behavior of psychotic patients', *J. nerv. ment. Dis.*, vol. 120, pp. 403–6.

STERN, M. H. (1959), 'Thyroid function and activity, speed and timing aspects of behaviour', *Canad. J. Psychol.*, vol. 13, pp. 43–8.

TAYLOR, J. A. (1951), 'The relationship of anxiety to the conditioned eyelid response', *J. exp. Psychol.*, vol. 41, pp. 81–90.

WINDLE, C. (1952), 'Psychological tests in psychopathological prognosis', *Psychol. Bull.*, vol. 49, pp. 451–82.

WOLPE, J. (1958), *Psychotherapy By Reciprocal Inhibition*, Stanford University Press.

YATES, A. J. (1958), 'The application of learning theory to the treatment of tics', *J. abnorm. soc. Psychol.*, vol. 56, pp. 175–82.

ZUBIN, J. and WINDLE, C. (1954), 'Psychological prognosis of outcome in the mental disorders', *J. abnorm. soc. Psychol.*, vol. 49, pp. 272–81.

Part Two
Schizophrenia

Current research into schizophrenia has focused on two or three major issues. The first, and classic, question has been that of genetic or environmental explanations of the origin of the disorder. The pioneer in the use of twin comparisons in psychogenetic studies was Franz Kallman but his work has been both improved upon, and more widely accepted, than was the case when it first appeared. It is, however, improper to put this question as one of heredity *versus* environment. Most sophisticated psychopathologists accept the notion of a genetic predisposition coupled with environmental precipitants of the overt pathology. Acceptance of this model is one thing; implementation of it into detailed theory is another. Meehl's paper represents one of the first systematic attempts to do so. His interest in the concept of defective inhibition as one of the primary sources of the disorder is paralleled by the paper by the British psychiatrist, Fish. Both of them can be seen as the direct consequence of the work on the neurophysiology of consciousness and attention. Neither could have been written without this knowledge.

A similar picture, in many essentials, emerges from the work of McGhie, even though the method used is that of obtaining phenomenological descriptions from patients.

All of these papers are directed towards a general theory of schizophrenic aetiology. Their approach consists of identifying a central psychological process that leads to schizophrenic deficit and hypothesizing a biopsychological mechanism that might account for this process. However, many psychopathologists continue to direct their attention to the social environment in which the future schizophrenic grows up.

Environmental explanations of schizophrenia have centred upon the role of parent–child relations as the pathogenic agent. Examination of this general proposition is fraught with methodological dangers, and it seems likely that the longitudinal study of children at risk for schizophrenia will hold the only completely satisfactory possibility of a resolution of the question. The papers by Drs Heston, Fontana and Garmezy examine these considerations from different viewpoints.

4 P. E. Meehl

Schizotaxia, Schizotypy, Schizophrenia[1]

P. E. Meehl, 'Schizotaxia, schizotypy, schizophrenia', *American Psychologist*, vol. 17, 1962, pp. 827–831.

In the course of the last decade, while spending several thousand hours in the practice of intensive psychotherapy, I have treated – sometimes unknowingly except in retrospect – a considerable number of schizoid and schizophrenic patients. Like all clinicians, I have formed some theoretical opinions as a result of these experiences. While I have not until recently begun any systematic research efforts on this baffling disorder, I felt that to share with you some of my thoughts, based though they are upon clinical impressions in the context of selected research by others, might be an acceptable use of this occasion.

Let me begin by putting a question which I find is almost never answered correctly by our clinical students on doctoral oral examinations, and the answer to which they seem to dislike when it is offered. Suppose that you were required to write down a procedure for selecting an individual from the population who would be diagnosed as schizophrenic by a psychiatric staff; you have to wager $1,000 on being right; you may not include in your selection procedure any behavioral fact, such as a symptom or trait, manifested by the individual. What would you write down? So far as I have been able to ascertain, there is only one thing you could write down that would give you a better than even chance of winning such a bet – namely, 'Find an individual X who has a schizophrenic identical twin.' Admittedly, there are many other facts which would raise your odds somewhat above the low base rate of schizophrenia. You might, for example, identify X by first finding mothers who have certain unhealthy child-bearing attitudes; you might enter a

1. Address of the President to the seventh Annual Convention of the American Psychological Association, St Louis, September 2, 1962.

subpopulation defined jointly by such demographic variables as age, size of community, religion, ethnic background, or social class. But these would leave you with a pretty unfair wager, as would the rule, 'Find an X who has a fraternal twin, of the same sex, diagnosed as schizophrenic' (Fuller and Thompson, 1960, pp. 272–83; Stern, 1960, pp. 581–4).

Now the twin studies leave a good deal to be desired methodologically (Rosenthal, 1962); but there seems to be a kind of 'double standard of methodological morals' in our profession, in that we place a good deal of faith in our knowledge of schizophrenic dynamics, and we make theoretical inferences about social learning factors from the establishment of group trends which may be statistically significant and replicable although of small or moderate size; but when we come to the genetic studies, our standards of rigor suddenly increase. I would argue that the concordance rates in the twin studies need not be accepted uncritically as highly precise parameter estimates in order for us to say that their magnitudes represent the most important piece of etiological information we possess about schizophrenia.

It is worthwhile, I think, to pause here over a question in the sociology of knowledge, namely, why do psychologists exhibit an aversive response to the twin data? I have no wish to argue *ad hominem* here – I raise this question in a constructive and ironic spirit, because I think that a substantive confusion often lies at the bottom of this resistance, and one which can be easily dispelled. Everybody readily assents to such vague dicta as 'heredity and environment interact', 'there need be no conflict between organic and functional concepts', 'we always deal with the total organism', etc. But it almost seems that clinicians do not fully believe these principles in any concrete sense, because they show signs of thinking that *if* a genetic basis were found for schizophrenia, the psychodynamics of the disorder (especially in relation to intrafamilial social learnings) would be somehow negated or, at least, greatly demoted in importance. To what extent, if at all, is this true?

Here we run into some widespread misconceptions as to what is meant by *specific etiology* in nonpsychiatric medicine. By postulating a 'specific etiology' one does *not* imply any of the following:

1. The etiological factor always, or even usually, produces clinical illness.

2. If illness occurs, the particular form and content of symptoms is derivable by reference to the specific etiology alone.

3. The course of the illness can be materially influenced only by procedures directed against the specific etiology.

4. All persons who share the specific etiology will have closely similar histories, symptoms, and course.

5. The largest single contributor to symptom variance is the specific etiology.

In medicine, not one of these is part of the concept of specific aetiology, yet they are repeatedly invoked as arguments against a genetic interpretation of schizophrenia. I am not trying to impose the causal model of medicine by analogy; I merely wish to emphasize that *if* one postulates a genetic mutation as the specific aetiology of schizophrenia, he is not thereby committed to any of the above as implications. Consequently such familiar objections as, 'Schizophrenics differ widely from one another' or 'Many schizophrenics can be helped by purely psychological methods' should not disturb one who opts for a genetic hypothesis. In medicine, the concept of specific etiology means the *sine qua non* – the causal condition which is necessary, but not sufficient, for the disorder to occur. A genetic theory of schizophrenia would, in this sense, be stronger than that of 'one contributor to variance'; but weaker than that of 'largest contributor to variance.' In analysis of variance terms, it means an interaction effect such that no other variables can exert a main effect when the specific etiology is lacking.

Now it goes without saying that 'clinical schizophrenia' as such cannot be inherited, because it has behavioral and phenomenal contents which are learned. As Bleuler says, in order to have a delusion involving Jesuits one must first have learned about Jesuits. It seems inappropriate to apply the geneticist's concept of 'penetrance' to the crude statistics of formal diagnosis – if a specific genetic etiology exists, its phenotypic expression in *psychological* categories would be a quantitative aberration in some parameter of a behavioral acquisition function. What could possibly be a genetically determined functional parameter capable of generating such diverse behavioral outcomes, including the preservation of normal function in certain domains?

The theoretical puzzle is exaggerated when we fail to conceptualize at different levels of molarity. For instance, there is a tendency among organically minded theorists to analogize between catatonic phenomena and various neurological or chemically induced states in animals. But Bleuler's masterly *Theory of Schizophrenic Negativism* (1912) shows how the whole range of catatonic behavior, including diametrically opposite modes of relating to the interpersonal environment, can be satisfactorily explained as instrumental acts; thus even a convinced organicist, postulating a biochemical defect as specific etiology, should recognize that the causal linkage between this etiology and catatonia is indirect, requiring for the latter's derivation a lengthy chain of statements which are not even formulable except in molar psychological language.

What kind of behavioral fact about the patient leads us to diagnose schizophrenia? There are a number of traits and symptoms which get a high weight, and the weights differ among clinicians. But thought disorder continues to hold its own in spite of today's greater clinical interest in motivational (especially interpersonal) variables. If you are inclined to doubt this for yourself, consider the following indicators: Patient experiences intense ambivalence, readily reports conscious hatred of family figures, is pananxious, subjects therapist to a long series of testing operations, is withdrawn, and says 'Naturally, I am growing my father's hair.'

While all of these are schizophrenic indicators, the last one is the diagnostic bell ringer. In this respect we are still Bleulerians, although we know a lot more about the schizophrenic's psychodynamics than Bleuler did. The significance of thought disorder, associative dyscontrol (or, as I prefer to call it so as to include the very mildest forms it may take, 'cognitive slippage'), in schizophrenia has been somewhat de-emphasized in recent years. Partly this is due to the greater interest in interpersonal dynamics, but partly also to the realization that much of our earlier psychometric assessment of the thought disorder was mainly reflecting the schizophrenic's tendency to underperform because uninterested, preoccupied, resentful, or frightened. I suggest that this realization has been overgeneralized and led us to swing too far the other way, as if we had shown that there really *is* no cognitive slippage factor present. One rather common assumption seems to be that if one can demonstrate the potentiating effect of a motivational state upon cognitive slippage, light has thereby been shed upon the etiology of schizophrenia. Why are we entitled to think this? Clinically, we see a degree of cognitive slippage not found to a comparable degree among nonschizophrenic persons. Some patients (e.g., pseudoneurotics) are highly anxious and exhibit minimal slippage; others (e.g., burnt-out cases) are minimally anxious with marked slippage. The demonstration that we can intensify a particular patient's cognitive dysfunction by manipulating his affects is not really very illuminating. After all, even ordinary neurological diseases can often be tremendously influenced symptomatically via emotional stimuli; but if a psychologist demonstrates that the spasticity or tremor of a multiple sclerotic is affected by rage or fear, we would not thereby have learned anything about the etiology of multiple sclerosis.

Consequent upon our general assimilation of the insights given us by psychoanalysis, there is today a widespread and largely unquestioned assumption that when we can trace out the motivational forces linked to the content of aberrant behavior, then we understand why the person has fallen ill. There is no compelling reason to assume this, when the evidence is mainly our dynamic understanding of the patient, however valid that may be. The phrase 'why the person has fallen ill' may, of course, be legitimately taken to include these things; an account of how and when he falls ill will certainly include them. But they may be quite inadequate to answer the question, 'Why does X fall ill and not Y, granted that we can understand both of them?' I like the analogy of a color psychosis, which might be developed by certain individuals in a society entirely oriented around the making of fine color discriminations. Social, sexual, economic signals are color mediated; to misuse a color word is strictly taboo; compulsive mothers are horribly ashamed of a child who is retarded in color development, and so forth. Some color-blind individuals (not all, perhaps not most) develop a color psychosis in this culture; as adults, they are found on the couches of color therapists, where a great deal of *valid* understanding is achieved about color dynamics. Some of them make a social recovery. Nonetheless, if we ask, 'What was basically the matter with these patients?' meaning, 'What is the specific etiology of the color psychosis?' the answer is that mutated gene on the X chromosome. This is why my own therapeutic experience with schizophrenic patients has not yet convinced me of the schizophrenogenic mother as a specific etiology, even though the picture I get of my patients' mothers is pretty much in accord with the familiar one. There is no question here of accepting the patient's account; my point is that *given* the account, and taking it quite at face value, does not tell me why the patient is a patient and not just a fellow who had a bad mother.

Another theoretical lead is the one given greatest current emphasis, namely, *interpersonal aversiveness.* The schizophrene suffers a degree of social fear, distrust, expectation of rejection, and conviction of his own unlovability which cannot be matched in its depth, pervasity, and resistance to corrective experience by any other diagnostic group.

Then there is a quasi-pathognomonic sign, emphasized by Rado (1956; Rado and Daniels, 1956) but largely ignored in psychologists' diagnostic usage, namely, *anhedonia* – a marked, widespread, and refractory defect in pleasure capacity which, once you learn how to examine for it, is one of the most consistent and dramatic behavioral signs of the disease.

Finally, I include *ambivalence* from Bleuler's cardinal four (1950). His other two, 'autism' and 'dereism', I consider derivative from the combination of slippage, anhedonia, and aversiveness. Crudely put, if a person cannot think straight, gets little pleasure, and is afraid of everyone, he will of course learn to be autistic and dereistic.

If these clinical characterizations are correct, and we combine them with the hypothesis of a genetic specific etiology, do they give us any lead on theoretical possibilities?

Granting its initial vagueness as a construct, requiring to be filled in by neurophysiological research, I believe we should take seriously the old European notion of an 'integrative neural defect' as the only direct phenotypic consequence produced by the genic mutation. This is an aberration in some parameter of single cell function, which may or may not be manifested in the functioning of more molar CNS systems, depending upon the organization of the mutual feedback controls and upon the stochastic parameters of the reinforcement regime. This neural integrative defect, which I shall christen *schizotaxia*, is all that can properly be spoken of as inherited. The imposition of a social learning history upon schizotaxic individuals results in a personality organization which I shall call, following Rado, the *schizotype*. The four core behavior traits are obviously not innate; but I postulate that they are universally learned by schizotaxic individuals, given any of the actually existing social reinforcement regimes, from the best to the worst. If the inter-personal regime is favorable, and the schizotaxic person also has the good fortune to inherit a low anxiety readiness, physical vigor, general resistance to stress and the like, he will remain a well-compensated 'normal' schizotype, never manifesting symptoms of mental disease. He will be like the gout-prone male whose genes determine him to have an elevated blood uric acid titer, but who never develops clinical gout.

Only a subset of schizotypic personalities decompensate into clinical schizophrenia. It seems likely that the most important causal influence pushing the schizotype toward schizophrenic decompensation is the schizophrenogenic mother.

I hope it is clear that this view does not conflict with what has been established about the mother-child interaction. If this interaction were totally free of maternal ambivalence and aversive inputs to the schizotaxic child, even compensated schizotypy might be avoided; at most, we might expect to find only the faintest signs of cognitive slippage and other minimal neurological aberrations, possibly including body image and other proprioceptive deviations, but not the interpersonal aversiveness which is central to the clinical picture.

Nevertheless, while assuming the etiological importance of mother in determining the course of aversive social learnings, it is worthwhile to speculate about the modification our genetic equations might take on this hypothesis. Many schizophreno-genic mothers are themselves schizotypes in varying degrees of compensation. Their etiological contribution then consists jointly in their passing on the gene, *and* in the fact that being schizotypic, they provide the kind of ambivalent regime which potentiates the schizotypy of the child and raises the odds of his decompensating. Hence the incidence of the several parental genotypes among parent pairs of diagnosed proband cases is not calculable from the usual genetic formulas. For example, given a schizophrenic proband, the odds that mother is homozygous (or, if the gene were dominant, that it is mother who carries it) are different from those for father; since we have begun by selecting a decompensated case, and formal diagnosis as the phenotype involves a potentiating factor for mother which is psychodynamically greater than that for a schizotypic father. Another important influence would be the likelihood that the lower fertility of schizophrenics is also present, but to an unknown degree, among compensated schizotypes. Clinical experience suggests that in the semicompensated range, this lowering of fertility is greater among males, since many schizotypic women relate to men in an exploited or exploitive sexual way, whereas the male schizotype usually displays a marked deficit in heterosexual aggressiveness. Such a sex difference in fertility among decompensated cases has been reported by Meyers and Goldfarb (1962).

Since the extent of aversive learnings is a critical factor in decompensation, the inherited anxiety readiness is presumably greater among diagnosed cases. Since the more fertile mothers are likely to be compensated, hence themselves to be relatively low anxiety if schizotaxic, a frequent parent pattern should be a compensated schizotypic mother married to a neurotic father, the latter being the source of the proband's high-anxiety genes (plus providing a poor paternal model for identification in male patients, and a weak defender of the child against mother's schizotypic hostility).

These considerations make ordinary family concordance studies, based upon formal diagnoses, impossible to interpret. The most important research need here is development of high-validity indicators for compensated schizotypy. I see some evidence for these conceptions in the report of Lidz and co-workers, who in studying intensively the parents of fifteen schizophrenic patients were surprised to find that 'minimally, nine of the fifteen patients had at least one parent who could be called schizophrenic, or ambulatory schizophrenic, or clearly paranoid in behavior and attitudes' (Lidz, Cornelison, Terry, and Fleck, 1958, p. 308). As I read the brief personality sketches presented, I would judge that all but two of the probands had a clearly schizotypic parent. These authors, while favoring a 'learned irrationality' interpretation of their data, also recognize the alternative genetic interpretation. Such facts do not permit a decision, obviously; my main point is the striking difference between the high incidence of parental schizotypes, mostly quite decompensated (some to the point of diagnosable psychosis), and the zero incidence which a conventional family concordance study would have yielded for this group.

Another line of evidence, based upon a very small sample but exciting because of its uniformity, is McConaghy's report (1959) that among non-diagnosed parent pairs of ten schizophrenics, subclinical thought disorder was psychometrically detectable in at least one parent of every pair. Rosenthal (1962) reports that he can add five tallies to this parent-pair count, and suggests that such results might indicate that the specific heredity is dominant, and completely penetrant, rather than recessive. The attempt to replicate these findings, and other psychometric efforts to tap subclinical cognitive slippage in the 'normal' relatives of schizophrenics, should receive top priority in our research efforts.

Summarizing, I hypothesize that the statistical relation between schizotaxia, schizotypy, and schizophrenia is class inclusion: All schizotaxics become, *on all actually existing social learning regimes*, schizotypic in personality organization; but most of these remain compensated. A minority, disadvantaged by other (largely polygenically determined) constitutional weaknesses, and put on a bad regime by schizophrenogenic mothers (most of whom are themselves schizotypes) are thereby potentiated into clinical schizophrenia. What makes schizotaxia etiologically specific is its role as a *necessary* condition. I postulate that a non-schizotaxic individual, whatever his other genetic makeup and whatever his learning history, would at most develop a character disorder or a psychoneurosis; but he would not become a schizotype and therefore could never manifest its decompensated form, schizophrenia.

What sort of quantitative aberration in the structural or functional parameters of the nervous system can we conceive to be directly determined by a mutated gene, and to so alter initial dispositions that affected individuals will, in the course of their childhood learning history, develop the four schizotypal source traits: cognitive slippage, anhedonia, ambivalence, and interpersonal aversiveness? To me, the most baffling thing about the disorder is the phenotypic heterogeneity of this tetrad. If one sets himself to the task of doing a theoretical Vigotsky job on this list of psychological dispositions, he may manage part of it by invoking a sufficiently vague kind of descriptive unity between ambivalence and interpersonal aversiveness; and perhaps even anhedonia could be somehow subsumed. But the cognitive slippage presents a real roadblock. Since I consider cognitive slippage to be a core element in schizophrenia, any characterization of schizophrenic or schizotypic behavior which purports to abstract its essence but does not include the cognitive slippage must be deemed unsatisfactory. I believe that an adequate theoretical account will necessitate moving downward in the pyramid of the sciences to invoke explanatory constructs not found in social, psychodynamic, or even learning theory language, but instead at the neurophysiological level.

Perhaps we don't know enough about 'how the brain works' to theorize profitably at that level; and I daresay that the more a psychologist knows about the latest research on brain function, the more reluctant he would be to engage in aetiological speculation. Let me entreat my physiologically expert listeners to be charitable toward this clinician's premature speculations about how the schizotaxic brain might work. I feel partially justified in such speculating because there are some well-attested general truths about mammalian learned behavior which could almost have been set down from the armchair, in the way engineers draw block diagrams indicating what kinds of parts or subsystems a physical system *must* have, and what their interconnections *must* be, in order to function 'appropriately'. Brain research of the last decade provides a direct neurophysiological substrate for such cardinal behavior requirements as avoidance, escape, reward, drive differentiation, general and specific arousal or activation, and the like (see Delafresnaye, 1961; Ramey and O'Doherty, 1960). The discovery in the limbic system of specific positive reinforcement centers by Olds and Milner in 1954, and of aversive centers in the same year by Delgado, Roberts, and Miller (1954), seems to me to have an importance that can scarcely be exaggerated; and while the ensuing lines of research on the laws of intracranial stimulation as a mode of behavior control present some puzzles and paradoxes, what *has* been shown up to now may already suffice to provide a theoretical framework. As a general kind of brain model let us take a broadly Hebbian conception in combination with the findings on intracranial stimulation.

To avoid repetition I shall list some basic assumptions first but introduce others in context and only implicitly when the implication is obvious. I shall assume that:

When a presynaptic cell participates in firing a postsynaptic cell, the former gains an increment in firing control over the latter. Coactivation of anatomically connected cell assemblies or assembly systems therefore increases their stochastic control linkage, and the frequency of discharges by neurons of a system may be taken as an intensity variable influencing the growth rate of intersystem control linkage as well as the momentary activity level induced in the other systems. (I shall dichotomize acquired cortical systems into 'perceptual-cognitive', including central representations of goal objects; and 'instrumental', including overarching monitor systems which select and guide specific effector patterns.)

Most learning in mature organisms involves altering control linkages between systems which themselves have been consolidated by previous learnings, sometimes requiring thousands of activations and not necessarily related to the reinforcement operation to the extent that perceptual-to-instrumental linkage growth functions are.

Control linkage increments from coactivation depend heavily, if not entirely, upon a period of reverberatory activity facilitating consolidation.

Feedback from positive limbic centers is facilitative to concurrent perceptual-cognitive or instrumental sequences, whereas negative center feedback exerts an inhibitory influence. (These statements refer to initial features of the direct wiring diagram, not to all long-term results of learning.) Aversive input also has excitatory effects via the arousal system, which maintain activity permitting escape learning to occur because the organism is alerted and keeps doing things. But I postulate that this overall influence is working along with an opposite effect, quite clear from both molar and intracranial experiments, that a major biological function of aversive-center activation is to produce 'stoppage' of whatever the organism is currently doing.

Perceptual-cognitive systems and limbic motivational control centers develop two-way mutual controls (e.g., discriminative stimuli acquire the reinforcing property; 'thoughts' become pleasantly toned; drive-relevant perceptual components are 'souped-up').

What kind of heritable parametric aberration could underlie the schizotaxic's readiness to acquire the schizotypic tetrad? It would seem, first of all, that the defect is much more likely to reside in the neurone's synaptic control function than in its storage function. It is hard to conceive of a general defect in storage which would on the one hand permit so many perceptual-cognitive functions, such as tapped by intelligence tests, school learning, or the high order cognitive powers displayed by some schizotypes, and yet have the diffuse motivational and emotional effects found in these same individuals. I am not saying that a storage deficit is clearly excludable, but it hardly seems the best place to look. So we direct our attention to parameters of control.

One possibility is to take the anhedonia as fundamental. What is *phenomenologically* a radical pleasure deficiency may be roughly identified *behaviorally* with a quantitative deficit in the positive reinforcement growth constant, and each of these – the 'inner' and 'outer' aspects of the organism's appetite control system – reflect a quantitative deficit in the limbic 'positive' centers. The anhedonia would then be a direct consequence of the genetic defect in wiring. Ambivalence and interpersonal aversiveness would be quantitative deviations in the balance of appetitive-aversive controls. Most perceptual-cognitive and instrumental learnings occur under mixed positive and negative schedules, so the normal consequence is a collection of habits and expectancies varying widely in the intensity of their positive and negative components, but mostly 'mixed' in character. Crudely put, everybody has *some* ambivalence about almost everything, and everybody has *some* capacity for 'social fear.' Now if the brain centers which mediate phenomenal pleasure and behavioral reward are numerically sparse or functionally feeble, the aversive centers meanwhile functioning normally, the long-term result would be a general shift toward the aversive end, appearing clinically as ambivalence and exaggerated interpersonal fear. If, as Brady believes, there is a wired-in reciprocal inhibiting relation between positive and negative centers, the long-term aversive drift would be further potentiated (i.e., what we see at the molar level as a sort of 'softening' or 'soothing' effect of feeding or petting upon anxiety elicitors would be reduced).

Cognitive slippage is not as easy to fit in, but if we assume that normal ego function is acquired by a combination of social reinforcements and the self-reinforcements which become available to the child via identification; then we might say roughly that 'everybody has to learn *how* to think straight'. Rationality is socially acquired; the secondary process and the reality principle are slowly and imperfectly learned, by even the most clear headed. Insofar as slippage is manifested in the social sphere, such an explanation has some plausibility. An overall aversive drift would account for the paradoxical schizotypic combination of interpersonal distortions and acute perceptiveness of others' unconscious, since the latter is really a hypersensitivity to aversive signals rather than an overall superiority in realistically discriminating social cues. On the output side, we might view the cognitive slippage of mildly schizoid speech as originating from poorly consolidated second-order 'monitor' assembly systems which function in an editing role, their momentary regnancy constituting the 'set to communicate'. At this level, selection among competing verbal operants involves slight differences in appropriateness for which a washed-out social reinforcement history provides an insufficiently refined monitor system. However, if one is impressed with the presence of a pervasive and primary slippage, showing up in a diversity of tests (cf. Payne, 1961) and also on occasions when the patient is desperately trying to communicate, an explanation on the basis of deficient positive center activity is not too convincing.

This hypothesis has some other troubles which I shall merely indicate. Schizoid anhedonia is mainly interpersonal, i.e., schizotypes seem to derive adequate pleasure from aesthetic and cognitive rewards. Secondly, some successful psychotherapeutic results include what appears to be a genuine normality of hedonic capacity. Thirdly, regressive electroshock sometimes has the same effect, and the animal evidence suggests that shock works by knocking out the aversive control system rather than by souping up appetitive centers. Finally, if the anhedonia is really general in extent, it is hard to conceive of any simple genetic basis for weakening the different positive centers, whose reactivity has been shown by Olds and others to be chemically drive specific.

A second neurological hypothesis takes the slippage factor as primary. Suppose that the immediate consequence of whatever biochemical aberration the gene directly controls were a specific alteration in the neurone's membrane stability, such that the distribution of optional transmission probabilities is more widely dispersed over the synaptic signal space than in normals. That is, presynaptic input signals whose spatio-temporal configuration locates them peripherally in the neurone's signal space yield transmission probabilities which are relatively closer to those at the maximum point, thereby producing a kind of de-differentiation or flattening of the cell's selectivity. Under suitable parametric assumptions, this synaptic slippage would lead to a corresponding dedifferentiation of competing interassembly controls, because the elements in the less frequently or intensely coactivated control assembly would be accumulating control increments more rapidly than normal. Consider a perceptual-cognitive system whose regnancy is preponderantly associated with positive-center co-activation but sometimes with aversive. The cumulation of control increments will draw these apart; but if synaptic slippage exists, their difference, at least during intermediate stages of control development, will be attenuated. The intensity of aversive-center activation by a given level of perceptual-cognitive system activity will be exaggerated relative to that induced in the positive centers. For a preponderantly aversive control this will be reversed. But now the different algebraic sign of the feedbacks introduces an important asymmetry. Exaggerated negative feedback will tend to lower activity level in the predominantly appetitive case, retarding the growth of the control linkage; whereas exaggerated positive feedback in the predominantly aversive case will tend to heighten activity levels, accelerating the linkage growth. The long-term tendency will be that movement in the negative direction which I call *aversive drift*. In addition to the asymmetry generated by the difference in feedback signs, certain other features in the mixed-regime setup contribute to aversive drift. One factor is the characteristic difference between positive and negative reinforcers in their role as strengtheners. It seems a fairly safe generalization to say that positive centers function only weakly as strengtheners when 'on' continuously, and mainly when they are turned on as terminators of a cognitive or instrumental sequence; by contrast, negative centers work mainly as 'off' signals, tending to inhibit elements while steadily 'on'. We may suppose that the former strengthen mainly by facilitating post-activity reverberation (and hence consolidation) in successful systems, the latter mainly by holding down such reverberation in unsuccessful ones. Now a slippage-heightened aversive steady state during predominantly appetitive control sequences reduces their activity level, leaves fewer recently active elements available for a subsequent Olds-plus 'on' signal to consolidate. Whereas a slippage-heightened Olds-plus steady state during predominantly aversive control sequences (a) increases their negative control *during* the 'on' period and (b) leaves relatively more of their elements recently active and hence further consolidated by the negative 'off' signal when it occurs. Another factor is exaggerated competition by aversively controlled sequences, whereby the appetitive chains do not continue to the stage of receiving socially mediated positive reinforcement, because avoidant chains (e.g., phobic behavior, withdrawal, intellectualization) are getting in the way. It is worth mentioning that the schizophrenogenic mother's regime is presumably 'mixed' not only in the sense of the frequent and unpredictable aversive inputs she provides in response to the child's need signals, but also in her greater tendency to present such aversive inputs *concurrently* with drive reducers – thereby facilitating the 'scrambling' of appetitive-and-aversive controls so typical of schizophrenia.

The schizotype's dependency guilt and aversive overreaction to offers of help are here seen as residues of the early knitting together of his cortical representations of appetitive goals with punishment-expectancy assembly systems. Roughly speaking, he has learned that to want anything interpersonally provided is to be endangered.

The cognitive slippage is here conceived as a direct molar consequence of synaptic slippage, potentiated by the disruptive effects of aversive control and inadequate development of inter-personal communication sets. Cognitive and instrumental link-ages based upon sufficiently massive and consistent regimes, such as reaching for a seen pencil, will converge to asymptotes hardly distinguishable from the normal. But systems involving closely competing strengths and automatized selection among alternatives, especially when the main basis of acquisition and control is social reward, will exhibit evidences of malfunction.

My third speculative model revives a notion with a long history, namely, that the primary schizotaxic defect is a quanti-tative deficiency of inhibition. (In the light of Milner's revision of Hebb, in which the inhibitory action of Golgi Type II cells is crucial even for the formation of functionally differentiated cell assemblies, a defective inhibitory parameter could be an alter-native basis for a kind of slippage similar in its consequences to the one we have just finished discussing.) There are two things about this somewhat moth-eaten 'defective inhibition' idea which I find appealing. First, it is the most direct and uncompli-cated neurologizing of the schizoid cognitive slippage. Schizoid cognitive slippage is neither an incapacity to link, nor is it an unhealthy overcapacity to link; rather it seems to be a defective *control* over associations which are also accessible to the healthy (as in dreams, wit, psychoanalytic free association, and certain types of creative work) but are normally 'edited out' or 'auto-matically suppressed' by those superordinate monitoring

neurotic cases, where the diffuse withdrawal and deactivation factor would not provide the explanation it does in the chronic, burnt-out case (cf. Collins, Crampton and Posner, 1961). Another line of evidence is in the work of King (1954) on psychomotor deficit, noteworthy for its careful use of task simplicity, asymptote performance, concern for patient co-operation, and inclusion of an outpatient pseudoneurotic sample. King himself regards his data as indicative of a rather basic behavior defect, although he does not hold it to be schizophrenia-specific. Then we have such research as that of Barbara Fish (1961) indicating the occurrence of varying signs of perceptual-motor maldevelopment among infants and children who subsequently manifest clinical schizophrenia. The earlier work of Schilder and Bender along these lines is of course well known, and there has always been a strong minority report in clinical psychiatry that many schizophrenics provide subtle and fluctuating neurological signs of the 'soft' variety, if one keeps alert to notice or elicit them. I have myself been struck by the frequent occurrence, even among pseudoneurotic patients, of transitory neurologic-like complaints (e.g. diplopia, localized weakness, one-sided tremor, temperature dyscontrol, dizziness, disorientation) which seem to lack dynamic meaning or secondary gain and whose main effect upon the patient is to produce bafflement and anxiety. I have seen preliminary findings by J. McVicker Hunt and his students in which a rather dramatic quantitative deficiency in spatial cognizing is detectable in schizophrenics of above-normal verbal intelligence. Research by Cleveland (1960; Cleveland, Fisher, Reitman, and Rothaus, 1962) and by Arnhoff and Damianopoulos (1964) on the clinically well-known body-image anomalies in schizophrenia suggests that this domain yields quantitative departures from the norm of such magnitude that with further instrumental and statistical refinement it might be used as a quasi-pathognomonic sign of the disease. It is interesting to note a certain thread of unity running through this evidence, which perhaps lends support to Rado's hypothesis that a kinesthetic integrative defect is even more characteristic of schizotypy than is the radical anhedonia.

All these kinds of data are capable of a psychodynamic interpretation. 'Soft' neurological signs are admittedly ambiguous, especially when found in the severely decompensated case. The only point I wish to make here is that *since* they exist and are at present unclear in aetiology, an otherwise plausible neurological view cannot be refuted on the ground that there is a *lack* of any sign of neurological dysfunction in schizophrenia; there is no such lack.

Time forces me to leave detailed research strategy for another place, but the main directions are obvious and may be stated briefly: The clinician's Mental Status ratings on anhedonia, ambivalence, and interpersonal aversiveness should be objectified and preferably replaced by psychometric measures. The research findings on cognitive slippage, psychomotor dyscontrol, vestibular malfunction, body image, and other spatial aberrations should be thoroughly replicated and extended into the pseudo-neurotic and semicompensated ranges. If these efforts succeed, it will be possible to set up a multiple sign pattern, using optimal cuts on phenotypically diverse indicators, for identifying compensated schizotypes in the nonclinical population. Statistics used must be appropriate to the theoretical model of a dichotomous latent taxonomy reflecting itself in otherwise independent quantitative indicators. Family concordance studies should then be run relating proband schizophrenia to schizotypy as identified by this multiple indicator pattern. Meanwhile we should carry on an active and varied search for more direct neurological signs of schizotaxia, concentrating our hunches on novel stimulus inputs (e.g., the stabilized retinal image situation) which may provide a better context for basic neural dysfunction to show up instead of being masked by learned compensations or imitated by psychopathology.

In closing, I should like to take this unusual propaganda opportunity to play the prophet. It is my strong personal conviction that such a research strategy will enable psychologists to make a unique contribution in the near future, using psychological techniques to establish that schizophrenia, while its content is learned, is fundamentally a neurological disease of genetic origin.

References

ANGYAL, A. and BLACKMAN, N. (1940), 'Vestibular reactivity in schizophrenia', *Arch. neurol. Psychiat.*, vol. 44, pp. 611–20.

ANGYAL, A. and BLACKMAN, H. (1941), 'Paradoxical reactions in schizophrenia under the influence of alcohol, hyperpnea, and CO_2 inhalation', *Amer. J. Psychiat.*, vol. 97, pp. 893–903.

ANGYAL, A. and SHERMAN, N. (1942), 'Postural reactions to vestibular stimulation in schizophrenic and normal subjects', *Amer. J. Psychiat.*, vol. 98, pp. 857–62.

ARNHOFF, F. and DAMIANOPOULOS, E. (1964), 'Self-body recognition and schizophrenia: an exploratory study', *J. general Psychol.*, vol. 70, pp. 353–61.

BLEULER, E. (1912), *Theory of Schizophrenic Negativism*, Nervous and Mental Disease Publishing.

BLEULER, E. (1950), *Dementia Praecox*, International Universities Press.

CLEVELAND, S. E. (1960), 'Judgment of body size in a schizophrenic and a control group', *Psychol. Rev.*, vol. 7, p. 304.

CLEVELAND, S. E., FISHER, S., REITMAN, E. E. and ROTHAUS, P. (1962), 'Perception of body size in schizophrenia', *Arch. gen. Psychiat.*, vol. 7, pp. 277–85.

COLBERT, G. and KOEGLER, R. (1959), 'Vestibular dysfunction in childhood schizophrenia', *AMA Arch. gen. Psychiat.*, vol. 1, pp. 600–17.

COLLINS, W. E., CRAMPTON, G. H. and POSNER, J. B. (1961), 'The effect of mental set upon vestibular nystagmus and the EEG', *USA Med. Res. Lab. Rep.*, no. 439.

DELAFRESNAYE, J. E. (ed.), (1961), *Brain Mechanisms and Learning*, Charles C. Thomas.

DELGADO, J. M. R., ROBERTS, W. W. and MILLER, N. E. (1954), 'Learning motivated by electrical stimulation of the brain', *Amer. J. Physiol.*, vol. 179, pp. 587–93.

FISH, BARBARA (1961), 'The study of motor development in infancy and its relationship to psychological functioning', *Amer. J. Psychiat.*, vol. 117, pp. 1113–18.

FREEMAN, H. and RODNICK, E. H. (1942), 'Effect of rotation on postural steadiness in normal and schizophrenic subjects', *Arch. neurol. Psychiat.*, vol. 48, pp. 47–53.

FULLER, J. L. and THOMPSON, W. R. (1960), *Behavior Genetics*, Wiley, pp. 272–3.

HOSKINS, R. G. (1946), *The Biology of Schizophrenia*, Norton.

KING, H. E. (1954), *Psychomotor Aspects of Mental Disease*, Harvard University Press.

LEACH, W. W. (1960), 'Nystagmus: an integrative neural deficit in schizophrenia', *J. abnorm. soc. Psychol.*, vol. 60, pp. 305–9.

LIDZ, T., CORNELISON, A., TERRY, D., and FLECK, S. (1958), 'Intra-familial environment of the schizophrenic patient: VI. The transmission of irrationality', *AMA Arch. neurol. Psychiat.*, vol. 79, pp. 305–16.

McCONAGHY, N. (1959), 'The use of an object sorting test in elucidating the hereditary factor in schizophrenia', *J. Neurol. Neurosurg. Psychiat.*, vol. 22, pp. 243–6.

MEYERS, D. and GOLDFARB, W. (1962), 'Psychiatric appraisals of parents and siblings of schizophrenic children', *Amer. J. Psychiat.*, vol. 118, pp. 902–8.

OLDS, J. and MILNER, P. (1954), 'Positive reinforcement produced by electrical stimulation of septal area and other regions of rat brain', *J. comp. physiol. Psychol.*, vol. 47, pp. 419–27.

PAYNE, R. W. (1961), 'Cognitive abnormalities', in H. J. Eysenck (ed.), *Handbook of Abnormal Psychology*, Basic Books, pp. 232–50.

PAYNE, R. S. and HEWLETT, J. H. G. (1960), 'Thought disorder in psychotic patients', in H. J. Eysenck (ed.), *Experiments in Personality*, vol. 2, Routledge & Kegan Paul, pp. 3–106.

POLLOCK, M. and KRIEGER, H. P. (1958), 'Oculomotor and postural patterns in schizophrenic children', *AMA Arch. neurol. Psychiat.*, vol. 79, pp. 720–6.

RADO, S. (1956), *Psychoanalysis of Behavior*, Grune & Stratton.

RADO, S. and DANIELS, G. (1956), *Changing Concepts of Psychoanalytic medicine*, Grune & Stratton.

RAMEY, E. R. and O'DOHERTY, D. S. (1960), *Electrical Studies on the Un-anesthetized Brain*, Hoeber.

ROSENTHAL, D. (1962), 'Problems of sampling and diagnosis in the major twin studies of schizophrenia', *J. psychiat. Res.*, vol. 1, pp. 116–34.

STERN, K. (1960), *Principles of Human Genetics*, Freeman, pp. 581–4.

5 F. Fish

A Neurophysiological Theory of Schizophrenia[1]

F. Fish, 'A neurophysiological theory of schizophrenia', *Journal of Mental Science*, vol. 107, 1961, pp. 828–39.

In the psychiatric literature in English there is a tendency today to deprecate speculative neurophysiological theories of the 'functional' psychiatric disorders, while little is done to halt the flood of far-fetched and untestable hypotheses of the 'dynamic' psychopathologists. The present author believes that it is legitimate to postulate a neurophysiological basis for schizophrenia in the hope that those with a more adequate knowledge of neurophysiology will be obliged to re-examine the problem of schizophrenia more fruitfully. Conrad (1958) has given a very interesting interpretation of acute schizophrenic symptoms, so that his approach to schizophrenia forms a very convenient starting point for further speculation. This worker's views will therefore now be presented in some detail before the present author's theories are discussed.

The Gestalt theory of schizophrenia

Using Gestalt theory, Conrad has put forward the view that in schizophrenia there is a loosening of the coherence of perception and thought which results in the emergence of new gestalts[2] and the fragmentation of psychic activity. He divides the acute schizophrenic shift into five phases, viz.:

1. The trema.
2. The apophanous phase.
3. The apocalyptic phase.

1. Lecture given at the Department of Psychiatry, Upstate Medical Centre, State University of New York, Syracuse, N.Y., by kind invitation of Professor Marc H. Hollender.

2. In order to avoid confusion, the word 'gestalt' will be treated as an English technical word, so that the plural form is gestalts, not gestalten, which is the German plural.

4. The consolidating phase.
5. The residual phase.

We will now consider each of these in turn.

1 The trema

This word comes from the German stage slang for the stage fright which is experienced just before the actor makes his entrance. In this phase the patient feels that he has lost his freedom of action, is somehow shut in and unable to communicate with his environment. Often there is marked anxiety, but depression is also common and usually associated with ideas of guilt and disgust with life. Frequently during the trema the patient carries out rather silly actions which he rationalizes, but which are out of keeping with his personality and the total situation. These senseless actions may lead the patient into difficulties which may then be incorrectly understood as reactive factors in the production of the depressive mood or the schizophrenic symptoms. In many patients there is a general feeling of suspicion which pervades all experiences and leads to the feeling that there is 'something going on'. In the end a delusional mood occurs in which the environment is experienced as being changed in a strange and threatening way. Conrad believes that there is scarcely a case of early schizophrenia in which this phenomenon does not occur. The delusional mood marks the point of transition from the trema to the apophanous phase. The trema itself may last for days, weeks or months and may even subside before the next phase can occur.

2 The apophanous phase

Delusional experiences in which a delusional significance occurs in connection with a psychological event such as a perception or a sudden idea have been considered by most German workers to be the primary irreducible elements of schizophrenic delusions. Since the German technical terms for these phenomena are cumbersome, Conrad has introduced the term apophany to include all these delusional experiences. This word, which is Greek for 'becoming manifest', is a very suitable term for these strange experiences, in which a new meaning becomes manifest in connection with a psychological event. This word also has the advantage that the adjective apophanous can be derived from it, so that it is possible to refer to apophanous ideas, moods, perceptions and so on. Conrad has therefore called the phase in the schizophrenic shift in which delusional experiences occur the apophanous phase.

Before we consider the apophanous phase in detail, we must discuss delusional perception, since this was the first schizophrenic symptom which was subjected to Gestalt analysis (Matussek, 1952, 1953). Delusional perception occurs when an abnormal significance, usually in the sense of self-reference, is attributed to a normal perception in the absence of any rational or emotional reason. The older German investigators all insisted that delusional perception was not due to a disorder of perception itself, but a disorder of thought. However, Matussek has pointed out that there are two varieties of delusional perception, one in which perception is disordered and the other where verbal associations are important. An example of this second variety is a patient of mine who heard a floorboard squeak as a colleague stood on it and looked down to see the linoleum. The word 'Lino' came into his mind and was followed by the thought 'No lie', which he took as an instruction from his colleague that he was not to lie. This resembles the play upon words of the obsessional ruminator who repeatedly finds indications of his obsessional thoughts in his environment. In the other variety of delusional perception, Matussek believes that there is a loosening of the coherence of perception which allows the essential properties of the object to come into undue prominence.

This concept of the essential property comes from Metzger (1954) who considers that percepts may have three types of gestalt property, structural properties, total quality properties and essential properties. Structural properties are those of arrangement and organization, such as figural form, brightness, colour profile and so on. The properties straight, round, closed and constant are examples of structural properties. The total quality properties are material properties which are not simple sensory qualities independent of structure. The properties indicated by the adjectives transparent, rough and soft are examples of total quality properties. Essential properties are expressions of the essence of the object and include all the physiognomic or expressive properties such as character, ethos, habits, mood, emotional value and so on. Solemn, friendly, proud and elegant are examples of these properties. Although they have been called 'subjective impressive qualities' or subjective impressions, Metzger insists that they are perceptually given properties which immediately make an impression on us and affect our own essence.

The apophanous phase can be divided into two subphases, apophany of external space and apophany of internal space. In the first, all external events which are experienced acquire a new significance, while in the latter internal psychic events acquire a special meaning. One can use a more familiar jargon and talk of apophany of perception and apophany of the mediating processes.

Delusional perception is the most common definite external apophanous experience and Conrad has differentiated three stages of this phenomenon, viz.:

Stage 1. The perceived object indicates to the patient that it concerns him, but he cannot say to what extent. This is pure apophany.

Stage 2. The perceived object indicates to the patient that it concerns him and he knows the extent of this immediately. Thus, for example, he may know that it has been put there to test whether he observes it. Thus the patient has the experience that the object or sequence of events has been made for him, or, in other words, he has prefabricated experiences.

Stage 3. The perceived object signifies something quite definite, and the essential properties of the percept have come into prominence because of a change in the total structure of perception. This is delusional perception in the strict sense of the word.

This undue prominence of essential properties explains the mis-identification of persons, which is common in the apophanous phase. Unknown persons may be recognized as friends or acquaintances, while relatives and friends are not recognized as such by the patient. The emerging essential properties can be considered as causing these confusions of identity.

The patient is, of course, in the ptolemaic position in that he experiences himself at the centre of things. This being so, he may attribute a delusional significance to his actions and have the experience of omnipotence. Conrad calls the experience of being the centre of the world 'anastrophe' and regards it as the subjective aspect of apophany or, as he puts it, 'Whenever there is apophanous experience, the ego must, at the same time, be anastrophically changed.'

From Conrad's case material it seems as if there is a barrier which stops the schizophrenic process from passing quickly from the perceptual field to the mediating processes. In some cases apophany only affected external space, while in others it was some time before internal space was affected. Once internal space is affected, there is a loosening of the coherence of the mediating processes. Memory images may lose their connection with the total field and be experienced as delusional inspirations. Thought broadcasting in which the patient's thoughts become manifest to the environment can be regarded as the reverse of delusional perception, where a new significance of a perception becomes manifest to the patient. The loss of adequate figure ground relationships in conceptual thinking naturally leads to the patient hearing his own thoughts spoken aloud, so-called Gedankenlautwerden. As the disorder becomes worse, all personal indication of the thoughts is lost and hallucinatory voices occur. Bodily hallucinations can be understood as the effect of apophany on bodily sensations and the body image.

3 The apocalyptic phase

If the schizophrenic process is very severe, the loosening of the coherence of perception and of the mediating processes may lead to fragmentation of psychic life or the apocalyptic phase. This is another name for catatonia, since the release of the representations of bodily sensations and body movements leads to a gross motor disorder. Sense continuity is destroyed, and this accounts for the fact that frequently only fragments of the total experience can be remembered after an acute catatonic illness. Rarely the gross fragmentation of psychological activity in the apocalyptic phase leads to death. This is the acute, deadly catatonia of Stauder.

4–5 The consolidatory and residual phases

The phase of consolidation begins after a few weeks or months, and a final residual phase occurs. In this phase there may be no active symptoms, but the patient feels less capable intellectually than before the shift, but this change is often more subjective than objective. Conrad suggests that every individual has his own energy potential or his particular ability to direct and apply his energies and that this potential is lower than normal in the residual phase.

Conrad has described seven different types of course of illness in a schizophrenic shift. These are shown in Figure 1. They are:

Type 1. The process does not pass beyond the trema, only abuts on the apophanous phase and usually subsides in a few weeks.

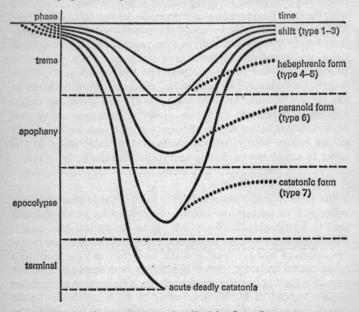

Figure 1 Varieties of acute schizophrenic shifts (after Conrad)

The loss of energy potential is minimal, so that the defect is very slight.

Type 2. The process passes through the trema, enters the apophanous phase and subsides after a few weeks, leaving behind only a slight loss of energy potential.

Type 3. The trema and apophanous phases are quickly passed through, and the apocalyptic phase is briefly touched on before the process subsides: the residual defect is very slight.

Type 4. The trema and the apophanous phase are rapidly passed through without the psychosis being recognized, but a marked loss of energy potential occurs, so that the residual state may make adaptation difficult. This corresponds to the type of schizophrenia called dementia simplex by some authors, but it can also be regarded as a variety of hebephrenia (Fish, 1957).

Type 5. The process does not pass beyond the trema, but there is a severe loss of energy potential. This is another way in which a chronic hebephrenic illness can occur.

Type 6. The process reaches the apophanous phase and is arrested there, so that a chronic paranoid schizophrenia occurs.

Type 7. The process reaches the apocalyptic phase and is arrested there, giving rise to a chronic catatonic clinical picture.

Conrad's theory links together all the phenomena which occur in acute schizophrenia by supposing that they are the result of a loosening of the coherence of psychological activity produced by a neurophysiological disorder. His concept of loss of energy potential in the defect state has nothing to do with Gestalt theory and is merely another term to explain the peculiar psychological disability in this condition. It is difficult to understand why Conrad has not attempted a Gestalt explanation of the defect states. Is it not possible, for example, that the so-called loss of energy potential can be explained as a partial loss of the normal integration of psychological functions or the mediating processes, while the paranoid and catatonic syndromes are abnormal reintegrations of the mediating processes?

This failure to deal with the chronic schizophrenic syndromes can be considered as a product of Gestalt theory itself which dogmatically insists that all psychological phenomena occur in figure-ground relationships which are not learned, but innate and immutable. If this is so, then once the interfering schizophrenic neurophysiological process subsides, the previous figure-ground relationships should reassert themselves. This would lead to the conclusion that in the paranoid and catatonic chronic clinical pictures the process was still active. However, the classical apophanous experiences do not occur in chronic paranoid schizophrenia.

A neurophysiological theory of schizophrenia

There is no doubt that Conrad's views are extremely stimulating, but as they stand it is difficult to use them as in a heuristic way. If we re-interpret his ideas in terms of Hebb's neuropsychological theories, I believe we have a much more useful set of ideas.

Hebb (1949) has summarized his basic theory as follows:

Any frequently repeated particular stimulation will lead to a slow development of a 'cell assembly', a diffuse structure comprising cells in the cortex and diencephalon (and also perhaps in the basal ganglia of the cerebrum), capable of acting briefly as a closed system, delivering facilitation to other such systems and usually having a specific motor facilitation. A series of such events constitutes a 'phase sequence' – the thought process. Each assembly action may be aroused by a preceding assembly, by a sensory event or – normally – by both. The central facilitation from one of these activities on the next is the prototype of 'attention'. The theory proposes that in this central facilitation, and its varied relationship to sensory processes, lies the answer to an issue that is made inescapable by Humphrey's (1940) penetrating review of the problem of the direction of thought.

The kind of cortical organization discussed in the preceding paragraph is what is regarded as essential to adult waking behaviour. It is proposed also that there is an alternate 'intrinsic' organization occurring in sleep and in infancy which consists of hypersynchrony in the firing of critical cells. But besides these two forms of cortical organization there may be disorganization. It is assumed that the assembly depends completely on a very delicate timing which might be disturbed by metabolic changes as well as by sensory events which do not accord with the pre-existent central process. When this is transient, it is called emotional disturbance; when chronic, neurosis or psychosis.

Hebb's views can be partly represented diagrammatically as shown in Figure 2, which is a modification of a diagram by

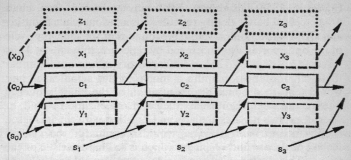

Figure 2 Diagram of the selective process in thinking (after Hebb)

Hebb (1958). C is the central process consisting of simultaneous active assemblies at three successive moments, while S is the corresponding sensory input. X is an assembly subliminally excited by the central process, Y is an assembly subliminally excited by the sensory input, and Z is an assembly which would become subliminally excited if X were excited. In the following discussion these assemblies will be referred to as X, Y and Z assemblies. C consists of assemblies which are active because they receive excitation from both sources, but if one accepts Milner's modification of the cell assembly (Milner, 1957), then priming of X assemblies may lead to the central process deviating to X assemblies and to the sensory input having little influence on the central process for a short time. This diagram does not show the effect of the arousal or reticular system, but this system is, of course, partly responsible for the maintenance of the central process, since it facilitates the firing of cortical neurones.

Let us suppose that in schizophrenia there is an overactivity of the reticular system. This would lead to the X and Y assemblies being nearer their firing thresholds than usual. It could be argued that the Y assemblies would be more likely to fire than the X when the reticular overactivity is relatively mild, since the sensory input would tip the balance. It may also be that the sensory input at the cortical level is enhanced by reticular over-activity, although there is evidence that it is diminished at lowest levels by reticular stimulation. Fuster de Carulla

(Magoun, 1958) has shown that briefly presented visual clues are perceived better during reticular stimulation, while Lindsley and Griffith (Magoun, 1958) have found that the recovery cycle of the optic cortex was shortened by reticular stimulation. Thus it seems reasonable to assume that sensory events would, under these circumstances, acquire a much greater significance and would tend to produce disorganization of the phase sequence much more often than usual. Such a disorganization would, of course, express itself as anxiety, and together with the increased significance of neutral events would account for the general feeling of unease and suspicion which is so characteristic of the trema. This diversion of the central process would initially be sporadic and the central process would be mainly determined in the normal way by the previous cell assembly and the sensory input. However, as the intensity of the reticular overactivity increased, the central process would be diverted and disrupted by the sensory input much more frequently. When this disruption was occurring very often, then a delusional mood would occur. The uncanny, unpleasant nature of this symptom can be explained as due to the repeated disorganization of the central process by the sensory input and the feeling of some unknown significance produced by the increased impressiveness of all perceptions. In the end, some sensory event would dominate the central process for some time and the individual would experience a kind of fascination for this object. It would therefore acquire a new meaning for him, i.e. it would be a delusional perception.

Here we must pause to consider Matussek's concept of the coming into prominence of essential properties in delusional perception. Objects with marked essential properties have a greater tendency to evoke an emotional response, or, to use Hebb's terminology, to produce a cortical disorganization. Such objects would therefore be likely to form the subject of delusional perception. Since human beings have marked essential properties, the perception of others could lead to cortical disorganization and this could give rise to a lack of recognition, since the appropriate phase sequence would not be aroused, because another X or Z assembly takes over the train of thought. Conversely, a similarity of features may lead to a domination of the central process by the sensory input and the evocation of a memory image (phase sequence) of a relative.

However, once the reticular overactivity passed a certain point, sensory over-determination of the central process would not be the only expression of the disorder, since a central process, consisting entirely of Z cell assemblies, could then become active independent of the specific sensory input.

Any central process consisting of X or Z assemblies could either be the sole central process or a central process running parallel with, but interfering with the 'normal' central process which is sensorily over-determined. Such a parallel process seems necessary in order to explain auditory hallucinations which are, of course, experienced as being foreign. It seems legitimate to assume that the sense of self is associated with the central process which is determined by the preceding phase sequences and the sensory input. Normally, the central process gives rise to behaviour leading to environmental modification, which, in turn, leads to a modification in the sensory input which then influences the central process and so on. Thus the interaction of the organism with the environment in which the self is experienced is expressed in the central process. In the trema the sensory over-determination of the central process gives rise to a paranoid attitude. The ability of the central process to detach itself from sensory input, but to be reorganized by impressive sensory input is lost. If a parallel process were set up and constantly interfered with the central process, then these interferences would be experienced as foreign thoughts or voices, since the only continuous influence on the central process which has been previously experienced is a sensory one. Sudden ideas or 'brain waves' can be considered as interference with the central process in normals, but they are, of course, brief and probably have a connection with the on-going central process, which is not conscious, but is expressed by the fact that the idea is not foreign. Since language plays such a great part in human thought, it is easy to understand that the interfering parallel process is often experienced as hallucinatory voices.

This parallel process need not be permanent, so that there could be periods when the sensorily over-determined central process alone was active, other periods when the parallel process was active on its own, and others when the two processes ran parallel. The phenomenon of hearing one's own thoughts spoken aloud could be understood as an activation of the phase assemblies for words which are activated to just below threshold by the reticular system and fully activated by the central process. They would thus occur just before the commencement of the parallel process.

This change from apophany of external space to apophany of internal space could be regarded as the point at which X assemblies become independently active. Thought insertion and thought deprivation can be explained as due to the parallel process.

The acute phenomenon can be explained in one of two ways. Firstly, if the parallel process became entirely autonomous and the normal central process disappeared, then gross behavioural disorder would occur, since behaviour would not be influenced by sensory input. Some acute catatonic illnesses and oneirophrenia could be accounted for in this way. Again rapid switching between two parallel processes, an autonomous central process and a sensorily dominated central process could cause stupor, since neither central process could find motor expression before it was interrupted by the other. Finally, in young people, especially children, disordered thinking expresses itself as disordered behaviour. There is no doubt that catatonia is a disorder of the young. Thus X and Z assemblies in young people are much more likely to have a strong motor element, and it is reasonable to assume that maturity is associated with an increase in X assemblies which are not directly expressed in motor activity. Thus a parallel central process in a young person would be likely to cause non-goal motor activity.

The maintenance of this parallel central process poses a question. Chance factors might lead to the establishment of such a process, but without continuous reinforcement it would tend to link up with the sensorily directed central process. It is possible that a parallel process might be kept going by reverberatory circuits involving the so-called cortical association areas and the subcortical nuclei. It has been shown that in the monkey there are corticofugal projections to the arousal system which are only second in importance to the inflow from the peripheral receptors (French, Hernández-Peón and Livingston, 1955). Segundo, Naquet and Buser (1955) found that the cortical areas which were specially effective in producing arousal were the cingulate, orbital and lateral frontal regions, the para-central and para-occipital areas and, I would like to stress this, particularly the superior gyrus and pole of the temporal lobe. Supposing that this is also true of the human brain, then a parallel process taking place in one of these areas might produce even more reticular overactivity, but this would have no reinforcing effect on the sensorily dominated central process, but would reinforce the parallel central process. It could well be that the ability to form a stable parallel process is the decisive factor in true schizophrenia. All the previous disorders are potentially reversible, but once the parallel central process is firmly established, the further progress of the illness is no longer dependent on the original reticular overactivity, but on this vicious circle which is now firmly established.

I think it is possible to account for the symptoms of the different varieties of paranoid schizophrenia by postulating that the parallel process interferes to a varying degree with the normal central process and the parallel process involves different cortical areas.

I hope to deal with this problem in more detail in a later paper, and I would like now to consider the chronic schizophrenic states. If the reticular overactivity disappears before a stable parallel process has been established, then it is obvious that complete recovery could occur. The chronic states can be accounted for in three ways:

1. The reticular overactivity does not decline. This would account for those paranoid illnesses in which delusions remain affect laden for years and which Leonhard has called affect-laden paraphrenia (Fish, 1957; Leonhard, 1959).

2. The reticular overactivity subsides, but the cortical vicious circle remains. This would account for many paranoid and catatonic clinical pictures with marked affective blunting.

3. The reticular overactivity subsides, but it has caused a cortical reorganization which is less efficient than the premorbid one. Hebb's theory is based on the postulate that some struc-

tural change occurs at synapses which are repeatedly active. In the sensorily dominated central process produced by reticular overactivity all those cell assemblies and phase sequences which were well linked to perception would be reinforced, while the ones mediating more abstract thought would not be. Thus if the reticular overactivity were severe enough or prolonged enough, a reorganization of phase sequences could occur which would make abstract thought more difficult. Thus a mild, prolonged trema could cause a marked defect. This would account for the insidious development of schizophrenic defect in the eccentric and silly hebephrenias (Leonhard, 1959).

The course of the illness would obviously be determined by the duration and severity of the primary reticular overactivity and also by establishment of a stable parallel process. This theory would explain the atypical or schizo-affective psychoses as being due to a reticular overactivity without the formation of a stable central process. It would also explain that strange condition paranoid depression in which there are marked persecutory delusions which go far beyond what can be understood as due to projected guilt feelings. These depressions are always associated with marked anxiety (Bumke, 1948; Janzarik, 1959) and attempts have been made in the past to explain the paranoid delusions psychologically as partly due to the severe anxiety. The theory presented here would suggest that the severe anxiety is associated with marked overactivity of the reticular system. This would produce a sensorily dominated central process which would lead to a paranoid attitude.

We must now come to the evidence in favour of reticular overactivity as the cause of schizophrenia. The most important supporting evidence is the fact that amphetamine overdosage in normal individuals will produce a psychosis which is clinically indistinguishable from paranoid schizophrenia. It is, of course, well known that amphetamine produces an arousal response in the EEG in animals which is similar to that produced by reticular stimulation. Bradley and his associates (1957) have produced evidence to suggest that in animals amphetamine stimulates activity in the reticular system below the level of the midbrain. Now both sodium amylobarbitone and chlorpromazine will produce marked improvement in patients suffering from acute schizophrenic shifts. There is evidence (Bradley, 1957) that chlorpromazine may block the receptors related to afferent collaterals entering the reticular formation at brain stem and mesencephalic levels. Thus it is fair to assume that such general blocking of the afferents to the reticular system would diminish reticular activity. There is evidence that phenobarbitone and other quick-acting barbiturates depress activity within the reticular system. This would account for the effectiveness of sodium amytal in acute schizophrenic clinical pictures. The fact that it often has no effect on chronic patients would again support the theory presented here. One final point about amphetamine is that it has been shown to cause worsening of symptoms in schizophrenia.

An interesting clinical condition which supports our present theory is the paranoid psychosis in clear consciousness which occurs in some epileptics. Some of these patients show a relatively normal electroencephalogram when psychotic and an epileptic electrocephalogram when normal. Landolt (1958, 1960) has suggested that the normal electrocephalogram is a 'forced normalization' produced by overactivity of the arousal system. This worker has also claimed to have found 'forced normalization' in thirty-two non-catatonic schizophrenics. The electroencephalographic investigation of a series of fifty adolescent schizophrenics by Lescable, Lelord and Fardeau gives some support to the theory presented here. There was an immature record in 18 per cent of their patients and in only one patient with such a record was the outcome unfavourable. In 74 per cent the record was normal, but eighteen of the records in this group were rich in fast rhythms and five were hypermature. The outcome in these five patients was unfavourable.

The overactivity of the reticular system which has been suggested as the immediate cause of schizophrenia is, of course, a final common path, and there are many possible morbid processes which could give rise to such overactivity. The following are obvious possibilities:

1. A cortical focus could produce reticular overactivity by stimulating corticofugal pathways to the reticular system. The

electroencephalographic evidence of focal activity might then be masked by the effect of the reticular system on the cerebral cortex. This would be the 'forced normalization' of Landolt, and could account for the schizophrenic clinical pictures seen in epilepsy, brain injury and organic hallucinosis.

2. An irritative lesion of the reticular due to physical trauma, toxins or infection could produce overactivity of the reticular system. This would account for the schizophrenic clinical pictures seen in post-encephalitic states and possibly some post-traumatic schizophrenias.

3. An inherited biochemical disorder of the reticular system such as a lack of mono-amino oxidase or some other enzyme could cause reticular overactivity. Like other enzymatic disorders, e.g. adrenal virilism, this need not manifest itself until puberty and might come to light because of physiological overactivity caused by an adolescent crisis.

4. An excess of adrenaline, nor-adrenaline, or similar substances produced by adrenal disorder could affect the reticular system. Such adrenal dysfunction could be due to primary disease of the adrenal or to a hypothalamic or pituitary disorder, which in turn might be made worse by the adrenal disorder. Thus schizophrenia could be due to a neuroendocrine vicious circle.

Many other combinations of these disorders and other disorders could be postulated as causing the overactivity of the reticular system.

Summary

It is suggested that the trema and early apophanous stage of acute schizophrenia can be explained as due to overactivity of the reticular system producing an undue diversion and disruption of the central process by the sensory input. Internal apophany and catatonic symptoms are explained as due to disruption of the central process with the formation of short-lived parallel central processes. Chronic schizophrenic process clinical pictures are considered to be due to a permanent parallel process which is dependent on a cortical reticular reverberatory system, while defect states without active symptoms are regarded as due to a reorganization of cell assemblies produced by the acute process. Pharmacological and electroencephalographic evidence in support of this theory is discussed. Possible causes of overactivity of the reticular system are briefly outlined.

References

BRADLEY, P. B. (1957), in H. J. Jasper, L. D. Proctor, R. S. Knighton, W. C. Noshay and R. T. Costello (eds.), *Reticular Formation of the Brain*, Churchill.

BUMKE, O. (1948), *Lehrbuch der Geisterskrankheiten*, 7th edn, Bergmann.

CONRAD, K. (1958), *Die beginnende Schizophrenie*, Theime.

FISH, F. J. (1957), 'The classification of schizophrenia: the view of Kleist and his co-workers', *J. ment. Sci.*, vol. 103, pp. 443–63.

FISH, F. J. (1960), A review of *Die beginnende Schizophrenie, J. ment. Sci.*, vol. 106, pp. 34–54.

FRENCH, J. D., HERNÁNDEZ, P. R. and LIVINGSTON, R. B. (1955), *J. Neurophysiol.*, vol. 106, pp. 34–54.

HEBB, D. O. (1949), *The Organization of Behaviour*, Chapman & Hall.

HEBB, D. O. (1958), *A Textbook of Psychology*, W. B. Saunders.

HANSARIK, W. (1959), *Dynamische Grundskonstellationen in Endogenen Psychosen*, Springer.

LANDOLT, H. (1958), in *Lectures on Epilepsy*, Lorente de Haas, (ed.) Elsevier.

LANDOLT, H. (1960), *Die Temporallappenpilepsie und ihre Psychopatholgie*, Karger.

LESCABLE, R., LELORD, G. and FARDEAU, R. (1957), 'Aspects of EEG de la schizophrénie de l'adolescence', *Proceedings of Second International Congress*, vol. 4.

LEONHARD, K. (1959), *Die Aufteilung der Endogenen Psychosen*, Akademie Verlag.

MAGOUN, H. W. (1958), *The Waking Brain*, Thomas.

MATUSSEK, P. (1952), 'Untersuchungen über die Wahnwahrnehmung: 1. Veränderungen der Wahrnehmungswelt bei beginnendem, preimaren Wahn', *Archiv. für Psychiatrie*, vol. 189, pp. 279–319.

MATUSSEK, P. (1953), 'Untersuchungen über die Wahnwahrnehmung: 2. Die auf einem abnormen Vorrang von Wesenseigenschaften beruhenden Eigentümlichkeiter der Wahnwahrnehmung', *Schweitz. Archiv. fur Neurologie und Psychiatrie*, vol. 71, pp. 189–210.

MILNER, P. (1957), 'The cell assembly: mark II', *Psychological Review*, vol. 64, pp. 242–52.

SEGUNDO, J. P., NAQUET, R. and BUSER, P. J. (1955), 'Effects of cortical stimulation on electrocortical activity in monkeys', *J. Neurophysiol.*, vol. 18, pp. 236–45.

6 A. McGhie

Psychological Studies of Schizophrenia

A. McGhie, 'Psychological studies of schizophrenia', *British Journal of Medical Psychology*, 1966, vol. 39, pp. 281–8.

In many recent psychological studies of schizophrenia the term 'overinclusion', or some other semantic equivalent, has been put forward as a central feature of schizophrenic thought disorder. This term was first used by Norman Cameron (1938) to describe the schizophrenic patient's inability to preserve conceptual boundaries, with a resulting tendency for his thinking to be diffuse and overladen with irrelevancies. In a factor-analytical study of the performance of schizophrenic and other psychiatric groups Payne and Hewlett (1960) later demonstrated that the factor of overinclusive thinking was specific to schizophrenic patients. Overinclusiveness as measured by Payne was not, however, found to be a feature of the performance of all schizophrenic patients, roughly 50 per cent of such patients being markedly *retarded* rather than overinclusive in their thinking. Psychomotor retardation was found to be a characteristic feature of the performance of patients with a depressive psychosis and of those schizophrenic patients who were not overinclusive. Using a small battery of three tests yielding a combined score of the overinclusive factor Payne and his colleagues later suggested that overinclusive thinking was more typical of the acute phase of the illness and was clinically associated with the presence of delusional thinking (Payne, Caird and Laverty, 1964). Employing Payne's three-test battery of 'overinclusion' we (McGhie, Chapman and Lawson, 1964) found that the scores obtained could not be related to other measures of 'overinclusive' tendencies. It might be argued of course that such findings merely underline the absence of a precise operational definition of the concept of overinclusion. Of more import was the further finding that the tests did not distinguish the schizophrenic patients from patients in all other diagnostic categories, and finally, that the three tests did not yield any significant intercorrelations. Hawks (1964), in a more systematic replication of Payne's work, also failed to find any significant correlations among Payne's three tests concluding that there was no evidence that they were measuring the same factor.

An entirely different approach to the assessment of schizophrenic thought disorder has been developed by Bannister in his application of Kelly's (1955) Repertory Grid technique to cognitive disorder. The underlying theory upon which the technique is based argues that each individual's experiences cause him to develop a personal complex of interrelated concepts or constructs which subsequently determine his cognitive attitude to any new situation. Thus, if our construct of reliable–unreliable is inter-linked with other constructs such as punctual, trustworthy, loyal, honest and affectionate, then such relationships will cause us to assume certain expectations of a person construed by us as reliable. Bannister's (1960, 1962) initial hypothesis is that schizophrenic thought disorder is a direct result of a process of *serial invalidation* by which construct systems are continually invalidated as the expectations they generate are not fulfilled. To take an illustration, we might normally link together such constructs as loving, kind, sincere, affectionate, reliable, in our relationships with others. If, however, experience invalidates such inter-relationships (that is people do not behave according to such predictions) this would lead to a loosening and weakening of relationships between such constructs. Repeated invalidation of this form leads to a general weakening and general loosening of the subject's conceptual structure with an inability to anticipate events, and thus to a general breakdown in the individual's responses to his environment. Weakened conceptual structure is defined in Bannister's Repertory Grid test as a loss of the substantial correlations between concepts in use which are apparent in the normal integrated personality. Although Bannister's view of the loosening in conceptual structure in schizophrenia has much in common with Payne's concept of overinclusion the Repertory Grid test does offer a method of assessing not only the form but also the content of the individual patient's thinking. Another difference between Bannister's approach and that of most other attempts to measure thought disorder is that Bannister's adherence to Kelly's Construct theory of personality leads him to make implicit assumptions about the aetiology of schizophrenic thinking. Schizophrenic thinking is here seen to emanate from the patient's past interpersonal experiences, particularly within the early family group. In speculating on the genesis of the schizophrenic's disturbed thinking Bannister (1965) refers to predominantly psychogenic theories such as Bateson's 'double-bind' (1964), Lidz's 'teaching of distorted meaning' and Laing's 'family mystification' process (1964). In view of the current tendency of many psychiatrists to look upon the nuclear form of schizophrenia as an organic rather than a functional disorder, it would be interesting to see the results of applying Bannister's technique to patients with a known organic dementia.

In an earlier discussion of his own studies Payne (1960) suggested that the type of thought disorder denoted by the term overinclusion may, in fact, be a disorder in the process of selective attention. He postulated that the primary failure occurred in the hypothetical filter mechanism which normally ensures that only stimuli relevant to the task enter consciousness and are processed. This view, that schizophrenic thought disorder may be one of many secondary consequences of a basic disturbance in the initial phase of selective attention, has been advanced by many other workers. Schilder (1951) refers to the schizophrenic patient's inability to pursue the 'determinative idea' in so far as he is constantly at the mercy of ideas subsidiary to the main stream of his thinking. In Arieti's (1955) apt phrase 'the [schizophrenic] patient strikes not at the bull's eye but at the periphery of the target.' Weckowicz and Blewett (1959) interpreted the changes in perceptual constancy demonstrated in schizophrenic patients as being due to their 'inability to attend selectively or to select relevant information.' Venables and Wing (1962) and Venables (1963) speak of 'a broadened level of attention which causes the patient to be over-loaded by sensory impressions from his environment.' In summarizing his impressions gathered over many years of experimental studies of schizophrenic patients Shakow (1962) concluded 'it is as if in the scanning process which takes place before the response to a stimulus is made the schizophrenic is unable to select out material relevant for optimal response.' A number of clinical studies of young schizophrenic patients have arrived at a similar conclusion regarding the schizophrenic patient's vulnerability to irrelevant stimuli. McGhie and Chapman (1961) found that, when young schizophrenic patients were asked to describe their earliest symptoms, the reports denoted a subjective awareness of their inability to control attention. Recently, Freeman (1965) and Chapman (1966) have made similar points in more detailed clinical surveys of schizophrenic patients.

There would thus seem to be a fair measure of agreement that schizophrenic patients are pathologically distractible in that they are unable to successfully screen out data irrelevant to the task in hand. Within this general area of agreement, however, there is much disagreement on specific issues regarding the nature of this distractibility. Most workers have made the point that the disorder in selective attention is not common to all patients who bear the diagnostic label of schizophrenia. If some schizophrenic patients are distractible the further question arises as to whether this is true in all situations with all types of stimuli and at all times. The purpose of some recent psychological studies of schizophrenia is to 'fractionate' the rather loose concept of distractibility and to examine in a more careful manner its constituent parts. The experimental studies of Dr Venables and his colleagues relating the schizophrenic deficit to changes in arousal level represent one such direction of research of which we shall be hearing more during this symposium. We have, in our own work, attempted to follow up information derived from our earlier clinical studies of schizophrenic patients in a number of experimental studies of the effect of distraction on the schizophrenic performance. I should like, therefore, to briefly summarize the findings of some of these studies which have been completed to date.

As the psychomotor performance of psychotic patients has been fairly fully investigated by a number of previous workers we began by attempting to assess the effects of auditory and visual distraction on the performance of schizophrenic patients in a variety of psychomotor tasks. These studies (Chapman and McGhie, 1962; McGhie, Chapman and Lawson, 1965a) demonstrated that although the basic psychomotor performance of all psychotic patients was poor, distraction in either modality had very little effect on the performance of the schizophrenic patients. This was true, however, only where the psychomotor tests used required a simple motor response to predictable stimuli (e.g. tapping test). Where the task demonstrated a motor response to a variable and uncertain signal (e.g. signal tracking test) distraction did have a considerable effect on the schizophrenic patient's performance. We concluded from these investigations that the psychomotor performance of schizophrenic patients was affected by distraction only where the task involved some degree of uncertainty and decision making, and particularly where the patient was not able to give an immediate response so that the task involved short-term retention. To investigate this latter suggestion further we carried out a number of studies in which the influence of distraction on the short-term retention was examined more directly. An earlier study (Chapman and McGhie, 1962) indicated that schizophrenic patients had considerable difficulty if asked to process information from more than one sensory modality at the same time. The findings of later studies (McGhie, Chapman and Lawson, 1965b, Lawson, McGhie and Chapman, 1966) indicated that the effect of distraction on the short-term retention of schizophrenic patients depended greatly on the nature of the task, particularly the sensory modality in which the information was presented. In a variety of tasks, each involving the perception and immediate recall of sequences of *auditory* information schizophrenic patients compared favourably with other patients and with normal control subjects. In equivalent tasks involving the short-term retention of *visual* information the schizophrenic group performed very poorly compared with the controls. When distracting stimuli were introduced into the situation this had a pronounced effect on the performance of the schizophrenic patients on the *auditory* tasks but little observable effect on their performance on *visual* tasks. In sum, then, it appeared that schizophrenic patients are at a disadvantage when asked to simultaneously assimilate material in more than one modality. In tasks demanding the processing of data in only one modality the schizophrenic patient copes much better in the auditory as compared with the visual modality. However, any type of distraction exerts a marked effect on the patient's performance on auditory tasks.

Many of the schizophrenic patients who were included in these studies commented on their difficulties in expressing their thoughts in speech and in comprehending the speech of others in conversation. A careful examination of such reports suggested that such difficulties arose, not from the patient's inability to deal with individual words, but from an inability to perceive these words in meaningful relationship to each other as part of an organized pattern. Studies of normal speech (Miller, 1963; Goldman-Eisler, 1961) suggest that speech is usually assimilated in phrase units of three or four words. Listening to speech is basically a matter of making decisions about what has been said and our ability to organize incoming speech into small phrase units ensures that the decision rate is reduced to a comfortable level well within our capacity for processing information (approximately one decision per second). In a number of studies of speech comprehension in schizophrenic patients we are able to demonstrate a deficit in their ability to utilize the transitional bonds between words which normally allow us to perceive the passage of speech as an organized whole (Lawson, McGhie and Chapman, 1964; Lawson, 1965). Instead of processing speech in phrases they appear to process separately each single word in a passage thus putting themselves in the impossible position of having to make speech decisions about what is being said at the rate of three to four decisions per second. We have found that if we take a measure of this 'de-patterning' effect in schizophrenic speech comprehension and relate this to our measure of distractibility the two tend to be significantly correlated. Currently we are investigating methods of examining the difficulties in speech production shown by some schizophrenic patients by analysing the ability of a patient to transfer thought into speech in terms of 'phrase decisions'.

At this stage I should like to pause briefly to suggest a crude conceptual model which may serve to bring together the diverse findings of our own and other investigations.

Studies of early development indicate that the first stages of life are characterized by a primitive, undifferentiated state of consciousness in which there is no distinction between the self and the environment. Differentiated ego development proceeds as the infant learns, not only to discriminate between different environmental stimuli, but also to select and organize the incoming flow of sensory stimuli. For this development to take place we must postulate an internal mechanism which allows the organism to select from the diffuse sensory input the information necessary for it to function effectively. A similar type of mechanism has been postulated by psychologists such as Broadbent (1958) who are interested in studies of the human communication process. Broadbent's model of the human attentive process is that of a decision channel with a limited capacity for handling information. In order to overcome this limitation a filter operation is performed at the input level, thus allowing the individual to select and process information in such a way, and at such a rate, as to avoid overloading his limited capacity to deal with it. It has been demonstrated that when information is presented at a rate above the individual's capacity for dealing with it performance breaks down. Studies of the schizophrenic patient indicate that these patients suffer from a marked inability to attend selectively to stimuli in such a way that only relevant information is processed. If they are dealing with a situation which requires responding to simple predictable stimuli overloading is less likely and the patient's deficit thereby less evident. If, however, the task requires the patient to deal with a range of stimuli involving more complex decisions the failure in selective attention leads to overloading and consequent breakdown of performance. The suggestion that the performance of the schizophrenic patient is particularly poor when visually presented information is being processed might be explained by recent findings (Sperling, 1960; Conrad, 1964) that visual data are usually recoded into the auditory modality before storage. This recoding process appears to impose a further strain on the already overburdened capacities of the schizophrenic patient. What we have referred to as the depatterning effect in the speech perception of some schizo-phrenic patients might also be explained within the context of this model. Although the accurate perception of speech requires the processing of a great amount of information the load on short-term retention is normally reduced by our automatic tendency to organize the incoming data into speech units such as phrases. We are also aided here by the use of the transitional bonds in normal language structure which render many words redundant. The schizophrenic patient appears to be less efficient in his ability to organize the incoming verbal stimuli in an economical way and to screen out the redundant words. Whether he is able to overcome these disabilities and deal effectively with verbal communications will depend on such factors as the rate at which verbal data are presented and the amount of information which they contain.

After the foregoing flight into conceptualization it is perhaps salutory that we bring ourselves down to earth again by raising the question as to whether the findings of such psychological studies have a more practical application to the clinical problem of schizophrenia.

I would suggest that such experimentally derived findings may be usefully applied in two main directions, one relating to the classification of schizophrenia, the other to interpersonal contact with the schizophrenic patient. Many clinicians would now agree that we are unlikely to find a single causal factor to explain the wide range of symptoms contained in the 'over-inclusive' diagnostic category of schizophrenia. Etiological studies are unlikely to be productive unless they are firmly based on a more adequate and reliable system of clinical classification. In their comparative study of schizophrenia and epileptic psychoses Slater and Beard (1963) suggest that, with schizophrenia, we might now be approaching the stage of classification reached half a century ago with epilepsy in the crude division into the idiopathic and symptomatic forms. It would certainly appear that, of the many and varied classificatory systems of schizophrenia advanced, one which has attained a fair measure of agreement is that which separates out a 'nuclear' form of the psychosis corresponding closely in symptomatology to Kraepelin's original concept of dementia praecox. Another relatively stable clinical category is to be found in the deluded but non-demented paranoid sub-group whose distinctive pattern of symptoms would encourage some clinicians to isolate as a separate psychosis outside of the schizophrenias. Others would regard the longitudinal division into the acute and chronic categories as an important variable in classification due to apparent differences in the clinical picture between these two phases of the illness. If the application of experimental psychology can aid this process of clinical delineation by the reliable assessment of changes in mental functions occurring in different forms of the psychosis, its efforts would be more than justified. In our own studies of distractibility it has been consistently clear that all our findings are related to schizophrenic patients who display a particular pattern of symptoms. The clinical picture includes insidious onset of the illness, marked thought disorder, and marked flattening of the affect. Clinically these patients had been diagnosed under the hebephrenic subtype of schizophrenia. Patients presenting a predominantly paranoid picture had, in contrast, no difficulty in fixating attention on one of a number of competing stimuli. Indeed, the paranoid patients were on most tests *less* distractible than our normal controls. This contrast in performance of the two subgroups has been reported by many other workers. Shakow (1963) reports that, in a large number of varied experiments, 'the paranoid and hebephrenic subject scores fell on *either* side of the normals.' It might be argued, however, that difference between these two categories may be confounded by the acute-chronic dichotomy, in so far as the hebephrenic patient would be expected to show a longer duration of illness. In the case of our own findings we could find no significant relationship between the hebephrenic-paranoid and acute-chronic dichotomies. Furthermore, we found that chronic patients tended to perform equally badly, as compared with acutely ill patients, on the distraction tests. Indeed, the main difference between the acutely and the chronically ill patients was seen in the patient's affective reaction to changes in selective attention, the former showing, at least initially, a positive fascination in his altered experience. In describing similar differences in the test performances of different schizophrenic patients Shakow (1962) uses the vivid analogy of a person walking through a wood:

If he is of the paranoid persuasion he sticks even more closely than the normal person to the path through the forest, examining each tree along the path, and sometimes even each tree's leaves, with meticulous care ... if, at the other extreme, he follows the hebephrenic pattern, then he acts as though there were no paths, for he strays off the obvious one entirely ... he is attracted ... by any and all trees and even the undergrowth and floor of the forest, in a superficial, flitting way, apparently forgetting in the meantime about the place he wants to get to. ... My impression is that the acute patient in the same forest undergoes a multitude of thrilling new experiences reacting highly affectively, for instance, to new and unusual patterns of light on the leaves, or to novel and subtle patterns of form in the branches.

In considering the various types of schizophrenia some psychiatrists (e.g. Batchelor, 1964; Chapman, 1966) have commented upon the resemblance between the nuclear or hebephrenic type and an organic dementia. With this suggestion in mind we recently repeated much of our previous work with matched groups of schizophrenic patients, non-schizophrenic psychotic patients, normal controls and with a group of patients with an arterio-sclerotic dementia. This study demonstrated a clear affinity in performance between the hebephrenic patients and those with a known organic dementia. The correspondence between these two groups on distraction tests has already been reported by other workers (Feinberg and Mercer, 1960; Weckowicz, 1960).

Our own experimental findings were initially derived from intensive clinical observation of schizophrenic patients in a therapeutic situation (Freeman, Cameron and McGhie, 1958; Chapman, Freeman and McGhie, 1959; McGhie and Chapman, 1961). It would therefore be satisfying and appropriate to consider whether it is possible to feed back the information obtained in the experimental studies to the clinical handling of the schizophrenic patient. It appears to us that many of the schizophrenic patient's psychological reactions to his physical and social environment are secondary to a breakdown in his cognitive functions which progressively alienates him from his environment. We have presented evidence which indicates that the schizophrenic patient is abnormally vulnerable to distraction by environmental stimuli. It would also appear that he has particular difficulty in integrating information simultaneously from different sensory channels. The patient's deficit in selective attention has a direct effect on his immediate memory and this would appear to be a primary cause of the pronounced difficulty in communication which is so characteristic of the schizophrenic patient. As a result of the primary breakdown, the patient, when listening to another person speaking, has to attend consciously with deliberation to each unit of information as it is presented. Because of the time taken to assimilate information in this way, sequences of verbal information are particularly difficult for him to cope with.

It seems probable, therefore, that the actual environmental conditions prevailing at any particular time will have a profound bearing on the patient's current symptomatology and behaviour. From what our patients have told us and from their behaviour in a test situation, it would seem that they are likely to be at a disadvantage in large, noisy wards where there is much irregular activity and where their senses are being bombarded simultaneously by multiple stimuli. In these circumstances, symptoms such as hallucinations, withdrawal, or catatonic behaviour, appear more likely to emerge.

It is perhaps a truism to say that, in the individual treatment of the schizophrenic patient, one of the main aims is to establish better communication with him. It has been argued often that a better understanding of the current transference relationship and other interpersonal factors will facilitate this and lead to an improvement in the patient's perceptual and cognitive performance. While this may be true we would argue that the reverse is equally important, in that an understanding of the basic perceptual and cognitive difficulties with which the schizophrenic patient is faced leads to an establishment of better communication and facilitates the development of a good relationship with the therapist. We have found that many schizophrenic patients who are initially withdrawn and uncommunicative are encouraged to speak more freely and to relate themselves more easily to the interviewer by their realization that the basic difficulties which they experience are appreciated and understood. A more detailed consideration of the specific cognitive factors influencing the communication process with individual schizophrenic patients has been made elsewhere (Chapman and McGhie, 1963; Chapman, 1966).

I have already underlined the fact that most of the hypotheses assessed in our experimental inquiries were generated by the phenomenological descriptions of schizophrenic experiences given to us by the patients themselves. It might be reasonably argued that it was not necessary for us to step out of this purely clinician framework in so far as most of our subsequent findings could well have been arrived at by more painstaking clinical observations of individual patients. Indeed, our proposed 'model' of the schizophrenic deficiency in selective attention and short-term storage might well be restated in the idiom of ego psychology. There is no built-in advantage with the experimental approach which renders its findings more reliable or more valid than systematically gathered clinical observations. However, unfortunately, clinical data are not always collected in a controlled systematic manner. This is equally true of the approach which we have utilized, its main merit being that it does provide some safeguard against over-enthusiastic speculation. Ideally, these two approaches should complement each other, clinical observations suggesting the lines of future experimental investigation and the findings of such studies in turn helping to modify the clinical approach to the schizophrenic patient.

References

ARIETI, S. (1955), *Interpretation of Schizophrenia*, Brunner.

BANNISTER, D. (1960), 'Conceptual studies in thought disordered schizophrenics', *J. ment. Sci.*, vol. 106, pp. 1230–49.

BANNISTER, D. (1962), 'The nature and measurement of schizophrenic thought disorder', *J. ment. Sci.*, vol. 108, pp. 825–42.

BANNISTER, D. (1965), 'The genesis of schizophrenic thought disorder: retest of the serial invalidation hypothesis', *Brit. J. Psychiat.*, vol. 111, pp. 377–82.

BATCHELOR, I. R. C. (1964), 'The diagnosis of schizophrenia', *Proc. Roy. Soc. Med.*, vol. 57, pp. 418.

BATESON, G. (1956), 'Toward a theory of schizophrenia', *Behav. Sci.*, vol. 1, pp. 251–4.

BROADBENT, D. E. (1958), *Perception and Communication*, Pergamon.

CAMERON, N. (1944), 'Experimental analysis of schizophrenic thinking', in Kasanin (ed.) *Language and Thought in Schizophrenia*, California, University Press.

CHAPMAN, J. (1966), 'The early symptoms of schizophrenia', *Brit. J. Psychiat.*, vol. 112, pp. 225–51.

CHAPMAN, J., FREEMAN, T. and MCGHIE, A. (1959), 'Clinical research in schizophrenia', *Br. J. med. Psychol.*, vol. 32, pp. 75–85.

CHAPMAN, J. and MCGHIE, A. (1962), 'A comparative study of disordered attention in schizophrenia', *J. ment. Sci.*, vol. 108, pp. 487–500.

CHAPMAN, J. and MCGHIE, A. (1963), 'An approach to the psychotherapy of cognitive dysfunction in schizophrenia', *Br. J. med. Psychol.*, vol. 36, pp. 253–60.

CONRAD, R. (1964), 'Acoustic confusions in immediate memory', *Brit. J. Psychol.*, vol. 55, p. 75.

FEINBERG, I. and MERCER, M. (1960), 'Studies of thought disorder in schizophrenia', *A.M.A. Archs. gen. Psychiat.*, vol. 2, pp. 504–11.

FREEMAN, T., CAMERON, J. L. and MCGHIE, A. (1958), *Chronic Schizophrenia*, Tavistock.

FREEMAN, T. (1965), *Studies on Psychosis*, Tavistock.

GOLDMAN-EISLER, F. (1961), 'The distribution of pause durations in speech', *Lang. Speech*, vol. 4, pp. 232–7.

HAWKS, D. V. (1964), 'The clinical usefulness of some tests of overinclusive thinking in psychiatric patients', *Brit. J. Soc. clin. Psychol.*, vol. 3, pp. 186–95.

KELLY, G. A. (1955), *The Psychology of Personal Constructs*, vols. I and II, Norton.

LAING, R. D. and ESTERSON, A. (1964), *Sanity, Madness and the Family*, vol. I, Tavistock.

LAWSON, J. S. (1965), 'Disorders in attention and language in schizophrenia', Ph.D. Thesis, University of St Andrews.

LAWSON, J. S., MCGHIE, A. and CHAPMAN, J. (1964), 'Perception of speech in schizophrenia', *Brit. J. Psychiat.*, vol. 110, pp. 375–80.

LAWSON, J. S., MCGHIE, A. and CHAPMAN, J. (1966), 'A comparative study of the effects of distraction on schizophrenic and organic groups' (to be published in *Brit. J. Psychiat.*).

LIDZ, T. (1964), *The Family and Human Adaptation*, no. 60, Hogarth.

MCGHIE, A. and CHAPMAN, J. (1961), 'Disorders of attention and perception in early schizophrenia', *Br. J. med. Psychol.*, vol. 34, pp. 103–16.

MCGHIE, A., CHAPMAN, J. and LAWSON, J. S. (1964), 'Disturbances in selective attention in schizophrenia', *Proc. Roy. Soc. Med.*, vol. 57, pp. 419–22.

MCGHIE, A. CHAPMAN, J. and LAWSON, J. S. (1965a), 'The effect of distraction on schizophrenic performance (1) Perception and immediate memory', *Brit. J. Psychiat.*, vol. 111, pp. 383–90.

McGhie, A., Chapman, J. and Lawson, J. S. (1965b), 'The effect of distraction on schizophrenic performance (2) Psychomotor ability', *Brit. J. Psychiat.*, vol. 111, pp. 391–8.

Miller, G. A. (1963), 'Decision units in the perception of speech', *I.R.E. Trans. on Information Theory*, vol. IT–8, p. 81.

Payne, R. W. and Hewlett, J. H. G. (1960), 'Thought disorder in psychotic patients', in Eysenck (ed.), *Experiments in Personality*, vol. II Routledge & Kegan Paul.

Payne, R. W., Caird, W. K. and Laverty, S. G. (1964) 'Overinclusive thinking and delusions in schizophrenic patients', *J. abnorm. soc. Psychol.*, vol. 68, pp. 562–6.

Payne, R. W., Friedlander, D., Laverty, S. G. and Haden, P. (1963), 'Overinclusive thought disorder in hospitalized chronic schizophrenic patients and its response to "Proketazine"', *Brit. J. Psychiat.*, vol. 109, pp. 523–30.

Schilder, P. (1951), *Brain and Personality*, New York University Press.

Shakow, D. (1962), 'Segmental set: A theory of the formal psychological deficit in schizophrenia', *Archs. gen. Psychiat.*, vol. 6, pp. 1–17.

Shakow, D. (1963), 'Psychological deficit in schizophrenia', *Behav. Science*, vol. 8, pp. 275–305.

Slater, E. O. and Beard, A. W. (1963), 'The schizophrenia-like psychoses of epilepsy', *Brit. J. Psychiat.*, vol. 109, 95–129.

Sperling, G. (1960), 'The information available in brief visual presentations', *Psychol. Monogr.*, vol. 74, no. 11.

Venables, P. H. (1963), 'Selectivity of attention, withdrawal and cortical activation', *A.M.A. Arch. gen. Psychiat.*, vol. 9, pp. 74–8.

Venables, P. H. and Wing, J. K. (1962), 'Level of arousal and the sub-classification of schizophrenia', *A.M.A. Archs. gen. Psychiat.*, vol. 7, pp. 114–19.

Weckowicz, T. E. (1960), 'Perception of hidden figures by schizophrenic patients', *A.M.A. Arch. gen. Psychiat.*, vol. 2, pp. 521–7.

Weckowicz, T. E. and Blewett, D. B. (1959), 'Size constancy and abstract thinking in schizophrenic patients', *J. ment. Sci.*, vol. 105, pp. 909–34.

7 L. L. Heston

Psychiatric Disorders in Foster Home Reared Children of Schizophrenic Mothers[1]

L. L. Heston, 'Psychiatric disorders in foster home reared children of schizophrenic mothers', *British Journal of Psychiatry*, 1966, vol. 112, pp. 819–25.[2]

Introduction

The place of genetic factors in the etiology of schizophrenia remains disputed. Several surveys have demonstrated a significantly higher incidence of the disorder in relatives of schizophrenic persons as compared to the general population. Furthermore, the closer the relationship, the higher the incidence of schizophrenia. The studies of Kallmann (1938) and Slater (1953) are especially significant and the research in this area has been thoroughly reviewed by Alanen (1958).

Although the evidence for a primarily genetic etiology of schizophrenia is impressive, an alternative explanation – that schizophrenia is produced by a distorted family environment –

1. This research was supported by the Medical Research Foundation of Oregon.

2. The author is greatly indebted to Drs Duane D. Denney, Ira B. Pauly, and Arlen Quan who evaluated the case histories and provided invaluable advice and encouragement. Drs Paul Blachly, John Kangas, Harold Osterud, George Saslow, and Richard Thompson provided advice and/or facilities which greatly contributed to the success of the project. All of the above are faculty or staff members of the University of Oregon Medical School.

This research could not have been completed without the splendid cooperation of numerous officials of various agencies who provided indispensable information. I am especially indebted to the following: Dean R. Mathews, Waverly Baby Home; Elda Russell, Albertina Kerr Nurseries; Stuart R. Stimmel and Esther Rankin, Boys' and Girls' Aid Society of Oregon; Reverend Morton E. Park, Catholic Charities; George K. Robbins, Jewish Family and Child Services; Miss Marian Martin, State of Oregon, Department of Vital Statistics, all of Portland, Oregon. Drs Dean K. Brooks, E. I. Silk, Russel M. Guiss, J. M. Pomeroy, Superintendents of Oregon State Hospital, Eastern Oregon State Hospital, Dammasch State Hospital, and Oregon Fairview Home, respectively. David G. Berger, has not been excluded. A close relative who is schizophrenic can be presumed to produce a distorted interpersonal environment and the closer the relationship the greater the distortion.

This study tests the genetic contribution to schizophrenia by separating the effects of an environment made 'schizophrenogenic' by the ambivalence and thinking disorder of a schizophrenic parent from the effect of genes from such a parent. This is done by comparing a group of adults born to schizophrenic mothers where mother and child were permanently separated after the first two postpartum weeks with a group of control subjects.

Selection of subjects

The experimental subjects were born between 1915 and 1945 to schizophrenic mothers confined to an Oregon State psychiatric hospital. Most of the subjects were born in the psychiatric hospital; however, hospital authorities encouraged confinement in a neighbouring general hospital whenever possible, in which case the children were delivered during brief furloughs. All apparently normal children born of such mothers during the above time span were included in the study if the mother's hospital record: (1) specified a diagnosis of schizophrenia, dementia praecox, or psychosis; (2) contained sufficient descriptions of a thinking disorder or bizarre regressed behaviour to substantiate the diagnosis; (3) recorded a negative serologic

Research Coordinator, Oregon State Board of Control; Stewart Adams, Research Director, Los Angeles County Probation Department; Robert Tyler, Research Information Director, California Bureau of Corrections; Evan Iverson, State of Washington, Department of Institutions; Anthony Hordern, Chief of Research, California Department of Mental Hygiene; Captain George Kanz, Oregon State Police; J. S. Gleason, Administrator, Veterans' Administration; and Lt.-General Leonard D. Heaton, Rear-Admiral E. C. Kenney, and Major-General R. L. Bohannon, Chief Medical Officers of the Army, Navy and Air Force respectively.

Renate Whitaker, University of Oregon Medical School, and Eliot Slater and James Shields of the Psychiatric Genetics Research Unit, Maudsley Hospital, London, reviewed the manuscript and made many helpful suggestions.

Finally, I wish gratefully to acknowledge the contribution made by the subjects of this research project, most of whom freely gave of themselves in the interest of furthering medical science.

test for syphilis and contained no evidence of coincident disease with known psychiatric manifestations; and (4) contained presumptive evidence that mother and child had been separated from birth. Such evidence typically consisted of a statement that the mother had yielded the child for adoption, a note that the father was divorcing the mother, the continued hospitalization of the mother for several years, or the death of the mother. In practice these requirements meant that the mothers as a group were biased in the direction of severe, chronic disease. No attempt was made to assess the psychiatric status of the father; however, none were known to be hospital patients. The seventy-four children ascertained as above were retained in the study if subsequent record searches or interviews confirmed that the child had had no contact with its natural mother and never lived with maternal relatives. (The latter restriction was intended to preclude significant exposure to the environment which might have produced the mother's schizophrenia.)

All of the children were discharged from the State hospital within three days of birth (in accordance with a strictly applied hospital policy) to the care of family members or to foundling homes. The records of the child care institutions made it possible to follow many subjects through their early life, including, for some, adoption. The early life of those subjects discharged to relatives was less completely known, although considerable information was developed by methods to be described.

Sixteen subjects were dropped because of information found in foundling home records; six children, four males and two females, died in early infancy. Ten others were discarded, eight because of contact with their natural mother or maternal relatives, one because of multiple gastro-intestinal anomalies, and one because no control subject whose history matched the bizarre series of events that complicated the experimental subject's early life could be found. The remaining fifty-eight subjects comprise the final experimental group.

A like number of control subjects, apparently normal at birth, were selected from the records of the same foundling homes that received some of the experimental subjects. The control subjects were matched for sex, type of eventual placement (adoptive, foster family, or institutional), and for length of time in child care institutions to within ± 10 per cent up to five years. (Oregon State law prohibited keeping a child in an institution more than five years. Subjects in institutions up to this maximum were counted as 'institutionalized' regardless of final placement.) Control subjects for the experimental children who went to foundling homes were selected as follows: When the record of an experimental subject was located, the admission next preceding in time was checked, then the next subsequent, then the second preceding and so on, until a child admitted to the home within a few days of birth and meeting the above criteria was found. Those experimental subjects who were never in child care institutions were matched with children who had spent less than three months in a foundling home. The above method of selection was used with the record search beginning with an experimental child's year of birth. The above restrictions regarding maternal contacts were applied to the control group. Oregon State psychiatric hospital records were searched for the names of the natural parents (where known) of the control subjects. In two cases a psychiatric hospital record was located and the children of these persons were replaced by others. All of the children went to families in which both parental figures were present.

Exact matching was complicated by the subsequent admission of several subjects to other child care institutions and by changes of foster or even adoptive homes. However, these disruptions occurred with equal frequency and intensity in the two groups and are considered random.

Table 1 gives the sex distribution of the subjects and the causes of further losses. Fifteen of the seventy-four experimental

Table 1

| | Experimental | | Control | |
	Male	Female	Male	Female
Number	33	25	33	25
Died, infancy or childhood	3	6		5
Lost to follow-up		2		3
Final groups	30	17	33	17

subjects died before achieving school age. This rate is higher than that experienced by the general population for the ages and years involved, but not significantly so.

Follow-up method

Starting in 1964, it proved possible to locate or account for all of the original subjects except five persons, all females. During this phase of the research, considerable background information of psychiatric import was developed. The records of all subjects known to police agencies and to the Veterans' Administration were examined. Retail credit reports were obtained for most subjects. School records, civil and criminal court actions, and newspaper files were reviewed. The records of all public psychiatric hospitals in the three West Coast States were screened for the names of the subjects and the records located were reviewed. Inquiries were directed to psychiatric facilities serving other areas where subjects were living, and to probation departments, private physicians, and various social service agencies with which the subjects were involved. Finally, relatives, friends and employers of most subjects were contacted.

In addition to information obtained from the above sources, for most subjects the psychiatric assessment included a personal interview, a Minnesota Multiphasic Personality Inventory (MMPI), an I.Q. test score, the social class of the subject's first home, and the subject's current social class. As the subjects were located, they were contacted by letter and asked to participate in a personal interview. The interview was standardized, although all promising leads were followed, and was structured as a general medical and environmental questionnaire which explored all important psycho-social dimensions in considerable depth. Nearly all of the interviews were conducted in the homes of the subjects, which added to the range of possible observations. The short form of the MMPI was given after the interview. The results of an I.Q. test were available from school or other records for nearly all subjects. If a test score was not available, the Information, Similarities, and Vocabulary subtests of the Wechsler Adult Intelligence Scale (WAIS) was administered and the I.Q. derived from the results. Two social class values were assigned according to the occupational classification system of Hollingshead (1958). One value was based on the occupation of the father or surrogate father of the subject's first family at the time of placement, and a second on the subject's present occupational status, or, for married females, the occupation of the husband. The social class values move from one to seven with decreasing social status.

All of the investigations and interviews were conducted by the author in fourteen States and in Canada.

Evaluation of subjects

The dossier compiled on each subject, excluding genetic and institutional information, was evaluated blindly and independently by two psychiatrists. A third evaluation was made by the author. Two evaluative measures were used. A numerical score moving from 100 to 0 with increasing psycho-social disability was assigned for each subject. The scoring was based on the landmarks of the Menninger Mental Health-Sickness Rating Scale (MHSRS) (Luborsky, 1962). Where indicated, the raters also assigned a psychiatric diagnosis from the American Psychiatric Association nomenclature.

Evaluations of ninety-seven persons were done. Seventy-two subjects were interviewed. Of the remaining twenty-five persons, six refused the interview (7·6 per cent of those asked to participate), eight were deceased, seven are inaccessible (active in Armed Forces, abroad, etc.), and four were not approached because of risk of exposure of the subject's adoption. It did not seem reasonable to drop all of these twenty-five persons from the study, since considerable information was available for most of them. For instance, one man was killed in prison after intermittently spending most of his life there. His behavioural and social record was available in prison records plus the results of recent psychological evaluations. A man who refused the interview was a known, overt, practising homosexual who had a recent felony conviction for selling narcotics. All persons in the Armed Forces were known through letters from their Commanding Officers or medical officers to have been serving honourably without psychiatric or serious behavioural problems. One twenty-one-year-old man, the least known of any of the subjects, had been in Europe for the preceding eighteen months in an uncertain capacity. He is known to have graduated from high school and to have no adverse behavioural record. In a conference the raters agreed that it would be misleading to discard any cases, and that all subjects should be rated by forced choice.

The MHSRS proved highly reliable as a measure of degree of incapacity. The Intraclass Correlation Coefficient between the scores assigned by the respective raters was 0·94, indicating a high degree of accuracy. As expected, several differences arose in the assignment of specific diagnoses. In disputed cases a fourth psychiatrist was asked for an opinion and differences were discussed in conference. The only differences not easily resolved involved distinctions such as obsessive-compulsive neurosis versus compulsive personality or mixed neurosis versus emotionally unstable personality. All differences were within three diagnostic categories: psychoneurotic disorders, personality trait or personality pattern disturbances. The raters decided to merge these categories into one: 'neurotic personality disorder'. This category included all persons with MHSRS scores less than seventy-five – the point on the scale where psychiatric symptoms become troublesome – who received various combinations of the above three diagnoses. In this way, complete agreement on four diagnoses was achieved: schizophrenia, mental deficiency, sociopathic personality, and neurotic personality disorder. One mental defective was also diagnosed schizophrenic and another sociopathic. Only one diagnosis was made for all other subjects.

Results

Psychiatric disability was heavily concentrated in the Experimental group. Table 2 summarizes the results.

The MHSRS scores assess the cumulative psycho-social disability in the two groups. The difference is highly significant with the experimental group, the more disabled by this measure. However, the difference is attributable to the low scores achieved by about one half (twenty-six/forty-seven) of the Experimental subjects rather than a general lowering of all scores.

The diagnosis of schizophrenia was based on generally

Table 2

	Control	Experimental	Exact probability
Number	50	47	
Male	33	30	
Age, mean	36·3	35·8	
Adopted	19	22	
MHSRS, mean (total group mean = 72·8, SD = 18·4)	80·1	65·2	0·0006
Schizophrenia (Morbid Risk = 16·6%)	0	5	0·024
Mental deficiency (IQ < 70)	0	4	0·052
Sociopathic personality	2	9	0·017
Neurotic personality disorder	7	13	0·052
Persons spending > 1 year in penal or psychiatric institution	2	11	0·006
Total years institutionalized	15	112	
Felons	2	7	0·054
Armed forces, number serving	17	21	
Armed forces, number discharges, psychiatric or behavioural	1	8	0·021
Social group, first home, mean	4·2	4·5	
Social group, present, mean	4·7	5·4	
IQ, mean	103·7	94·0	
Years school, mean	12·4	11·6	
Children, total	84	71	
Divorces, total	7	6	
Never married, > 30 years age	4	9	

One mental defective was also schizophrenic.
Another was sociopathic.
Considerable duplication occurs in the entries below Neurotic Personality Disorder.
Fisher Exact Probability Test.

accepted standards. In addition to the unanimous opinion of the three raters, all subjects were similarly diagnosed in psychiatric hospitals. One female and four males comprised the schizophrenic group. Three were chronic deteriorated patients who had been hospitalized for several years. The other two had been hospitalized and were taking anti-psychotic drugs. One of the latter persons was also mentally deficient: a brief history of this person follows.

A farm labourer, now 36 years old, was in an institution for mentally retarded children from age 6–16. Several I.Q. tests averaged 62. He was discharged to a family farm, where he worked for the next 16 years. Before his hospitalization at age 32 he was described as a peculiar but harmless person who was interested only in his bank account: he saved $5,500 out of a salary averaging $900 per year. Following a windstorm that did major damage to the farm where he worked he appeared increasingly agitated. Two days later he threatened his employer with a knife and accused him of trying to poison him. A court committed him to a psychiatric hospital. When admitted, he talked to imaginary persons and assumed a posture of prayer for long periods. His responses to questions were incoherent or irrelevant. The hospital diagnosis was schizophrenic reaction. He was treated with phenothiazine drugs, became increasingly rational, and was discharged within a month. After discharge he returned to the same farm, but was less efficient in his work and spent long periods sitting and staring blankly. He has been followed as an out-patient since discharge, has taken phenothiazine drugs continuously, and anti-depressants occasionally. This man exhibited almost no facial expression. His responses to questions, though relevant, were given after a long and variable latency.

The age-corrected rate for schizophrenia is 16·6 per cent, a finding consistent with Kallmann's 16·4 per cent (Weinberg's short method, age of risk fifteen–forty-five years). Hoffman (1921) and Oppler (1932) reported rates of from 7 to 10·8 per cent of schizophrenia in children of schizophrenics. No relationship between the severity and sub-type of the disease in the mother-child pairs was evident.

Mental deficiency was diagnosed when a subject's I.Q. was consistently less than seventy. All of these persons were in homes for mental defectives at some time during their life and one was continuously institutionalized. His I.Q. was thirty-five. The other mentally deficient subjects had I.Q.s between fifty and sixty-five. No history of CNS disease or trauma of possible causal importance was obtained for any of these subjects. The mothers of the mentally defective subjects were not different from the other mothers and none was mentally defective.

Three behavioural traits were found almost exclusively within the Experimental group. These were: (1) significant musical ability, seven persons; (2) expression of unusually strong religious feelings, six persons; and (3) problem drinking, eight persons.

The results with respect to the effects of institutional care, social group, and type of placement will be discussed in a later paper. None of these factors had measurable effects on the outcome.

Discussion

The results of this study support a genetic aetiology of schizophrenia. Schizophrenia was found only in the offspring of schizophrenic mothers. The probability of this segregation being effected by chance is less than 0·025. Furthermore, about one-half of the experimental group exhibited major psychosocial disability. The bulk of these persons had disorders other than schizophrenia which were nearly as malignant in effect as schizophrenia itself. An illustration is provided by the eight of twenty-one experimental males who received psychiatric or behavioural discharges from the armed services. If three subjects who were rejected for service for the same reasons are added, the ratio becomes eleven:twenty-four, or essentially one:two. Only three of these eleven subjects were schizophrenic and one schizophrenic served honourably. Kallmann's (1938) rate for first degree relatives and Slater's (1953) for dizygotic twins of schizophrenic persons who developed significant psycho-social disability not limited to schizophrenia are slightly lower, though in the same range, as those found in the present study.

The association of mental deficiency with schizophrenia has been reported by Hallgren and Sjögren (1959) who noted an incidence of low-grade mental deficiency (I.Q. < 50–55) in schizophrenic subjects of about 10·5 per cent Kallman (1938) found from 5–10 per cent mental defectives among his descendants of schizophrenic persons, but did not consider the finding significant. The association of mental deficiency with schizophrenia – if such an association exists – remains uncertain.

Two sub-groups of persons within the impaired one-half of experimental subjects exhibited roughly delineable symptom-behaviour complexes other than schizophrenia or mental deficiency. The personalities of the persons composing these groups are described in aggregate below.

The first group is composed of subjects who fit the older diagnostic category, 'schizoid psychopath'. This term was used by Kallmann (1938) to describe a significant sub-group of his relatives of schizophrenic persons. Eight males from the present study fall into this group, all of whom received a diagnosis of sociopathic personality. These persons are distinguished by anti-social behaviour of an impulsive, illogical nature. Multiple arrests for assault, battery, poorly planned impulsive thefts dot their police records. Two were homosexual, four alcoholic, and one person, also homosexual, was a narcotics addict. These subjects tended to live alone – only one was married – in deteriorated hotels and rooming houses in large cities, and locating them would have been impossible without the co-operation of the police. They worked at irregular casual jobs such as dishwasher, race-track tout, parking attendants. When interviewed they did not acknowledge or exhibit evidence of anxiety. Usually secretive about their own life and circumstances, they expressed very definite though general opinions regarding social and political ills. In spite of their suggestive life histories, no evidence of schizophrenia was elicited in interviews. No similar personalities were found among the control subjects.

A second sub-group was characterized by emotional lability and may correspond to the neurotic sibs of schizophrenics described by Alanen *et al.* (1963). Six females and two males from the experimental group as opposed to two control subjects were in this category. These persons complained of anxiety or panic attacks, hyper-irritability, and depression. The most frequent complaint was panic when in groups of people as in church or at parties, which was so profoundly uncomfortable that the subject was forced to remove himself abruptly. Most subjects described their problems as occurring episodically; a situation that they might tolerate with ease on one occasion was intolerable on another. The woman reported life-long difficulty with menses, especially hyper-irritability or crying spells, and depressions coincident with pregnancy. These subjects described themselves as 'moody', stating that they usually could not relate their mood swings to temporal events. Four such subjects referred to their strong religious beliefs much more frequently than other respondents. Psychophysiological gastro-intestinal symptoms were prominent in five subjects. The most frequent diagnoses advanced by the raters were emotionally unstable personality and cyclothymic personality, with neurosis a strong third.

Of the nine persons in the control group who were seriously disabled, two were professional criminals, careful and method-ical in their work, two were very similar to the emotionally labile group described above, one was a compulsive phobia-ridden neurotic, and four were inadequate or passive-aggressive personalities.

The twenty-one experimental subjects who exhibited no sig-nificant psycho-social impairment were not only successful adults but in comparison to the control group were more spon-taneous when interviewed and had more colourful life histories. They held the more creative jobs: musician, teacher, home-designer; and followed the more imaginative hobbies: oil painting, music, antique aircraft. Within the experimental group there was much more variability of personality and behaviour in all social dimensions.

Summary

This report compares the psycho-social adjustment of forty-seven adults born to schizophrenic mothers with fifty control adults, where all subjects had been separated from their natural mothers from the first few days of life. The comparison is based on a review of school, police, veterans, and hospital, among several other records, plus a personal interview and MMPI which were administered to seventy-two subjects. An I.Q. and social class determination were also available. Three psychiat-rists independently rated the subjects.

The results were:

1. Schizophrenic and sociopathic personality disorders were found in those persons born to schizophrenic persons in an excess exceeding chance expectation at the 0·05 level of probability. Five of 47 persons born to schizophrenic mothers were schizophrenic. No cases of schizo-phrenia were found in 50 control subjects.

2. Several other comparisons, such as persons given other psychiatric diagnoses, felons, and persons discharged from the Armed Forces for psychiatric or behavioural reasons, demonstrated a significant excess of psycho-social disability in about one-half of the persons born to schizophrenic mothers.

3. The remaining one-half of the persons born to schizophrenic mothers were notably successful adults. They possessed artistic talents and demonstrated imaginative adaptations to life which were uncommon in the control group.

References

ALANEN, Y. O. (1958), 'The mothers of schizophrenic patients', *Acta psychiat. neurol. scand.*, suppl. 1227.

ALANEN, Y. O., REKOLA, J., STAVEN, A., TUOVINEN, M., TAKALA, K. and RUTANEN, E. (1963), 'Mental disorders in the siblings of schizophrenic patients', *Acta psychiat. neurol. scand.*, suppl. 169, vol. 39, p. 167

HALLGREN, B. and SJÖGREN, T. (1959), 'A clinical and genetico-statistical study of schizophrenia and low grade mental deficiency in a large Swedish rural population', *Acta psychiat. neurol. scand.*, suppl. 140, vol. 35.

HOFFMAN, J. (1921), *Studien über Verevung und Entstehung geistiger Störungen. II. Die Nachkommenschaft bei endogenen Psychosen*, Springer.

HOLLINGSHEAD, A. B. and REDLICH, F. C. (1958), *Social Class and Mental Illness: A Community Study*, Wiley.

KALLMANN, F. J. (1938), *The Genetics of Schizophrenia*, J. J. Augustin.

LUBORSKY, L. (1962), 'Clinicians' judgements of mental health: a proposed scale', *Arch. gen. Psychiat.*, vol. 7, p. 407.

OPPLER, W. (1932), 'Zum Problem der Erbprognosebestimmung', *Z. Neurol.*, vol. 141, pp. 549–616.

SLATER, E., and SHIELDS, J. (1953), 'Psychotic and neurotic illnesses in twins', Medical Research Council Special Report Series No. 278, HMSO.

8 A. F. Fontana

Familial Etiology of Schizophrenia: Is a Scientific Methodology Possible?[1]

A. F. Fontana, 'Familial etiology of schizophrenia: is a scientific methodology possible?', *Psychological Bulletin*, vol. 66, 1966, pp. 214–27.

The three major research approaches toward identifying familial etiological factors in schizophrenia are examined from a methodological viewpoint. Both the clinical observational and retrospective recall methods are judged to be inadequate. The third approach, direct observation and recording of family interactions, is concluded to be free of intrinsically disqualifying inadequacies, given the limiting assumption that the variables under investigation are etiological in nature. Although the limitations of this assumption can only be overcome by a longitudinal approach, family interaction studies are considered to be an indispensable, practical precondition to the formulation of longitudinal studies. Results from a subset of methodologically adequate studies are examined and conclusions drawn. Several cautions and recommendations for future research are offered.

The functional role of the family in the development of schizophrenia[2] has been the subject of intensive investigation. Re-

1. The preparation of this paper was supported by Research Grant M H 08050 from the National Institute of Mental Health, United States Public Health Service. The author wishes to thank Edward B. Klein and Carmi Schooler for their critical reading of the manuscript.

2. It is assumed that the term 'schizophrenia' applies to a subset of behaviors or processes which differentiates persons so labeled from others. The reliability of psychiatric diagnosis has been a topic much discussed and argued. It is clear from the extant literature that schizophrenia, as a major category, is the most reliable of the diagnoses. The possibility exists, however, that psychiatric and psychological professionals are inconsistently 'overinclusive' or 'underinclusive' in applying schizophrenia as a concept, and for this reason 'schizophrenics' may be just as different from each other as they are from others. The crucial question is, of course, 'What is schizophrenia?' In attempting to answer this, there seems to be little choice but to study people *called* schizophrenic.

searchers have reported that several personality characteristics differentiate between parents of schizophrenics and nonschizophrenics, and that several aspects of family interaction patterns differ in the families of schizophrenics and nonschizophrenics. However, reviewers (Frank, 1965; Meissner, 1964; Rabkin, 1965; Sanua, 1961) have not shared the optimism and conclusions of the majority of researchers. The recent review by Frank (1965) states that in the last forty years of research, *no* factors have been found which either differentiate between the families of psychopathological and normal members, or among families of pathological members who are classified according to different diagnostic categories. That author's pessimism extends to the more general issue concerning the applicability of the scientific method to the study of human behavior:

Apparently, the factors which play a part in the development of behavior in humans are so complex that they almost defy being investigated scientifically and defy one's attempt to draw meaningful generalizations from the exploration which has already been done (p. 201).

Frank is quite correct in raising the issue of methodology. It is a truism that any body of scientific facts must rest upon a scientifically sound methodology. The conclusions from any study not so based cannot be considered scientific, no matter how scholarly they may be. Some of the previous reviewers have paid insufficient attention to the methodology of individual studies. Rather, their approach has been to tabulate positive and negative results without evaluating the methodological adequacy of individual studies. This approach may have obscured some consistent empirical trends which can be found in well-designed studies.

The purpose of this paper is to examine the scientific status of the three major research approaches, first methodologically and then in terms of empirical results. The sources of data for the approaches to be considered are: (*a*) clinical observations and psychiatric impressions of family members in treatment, (*b*) retrospective accounts of child-rearing practices and attitudes obtained from family members' responses to interviews and questionnaires, and (*c*) current patterns of interaction among family members directly recorded and systematically coded by the investigator. Rabkin (1965) and Sanua (1961) have presented excellent critiques of much of the work in this area, particularly those studies classified under the first two headings above. Their papers provide extensive coverage of inadequacies, such as the lack of control groups and nonspecification of subjects' demographic characteristics, which are not essential to the viability of the methodology itself. The present analysis will focus on issues concerning the scientific appropriateness of the methodology *per se*.

Clinical observational studies

The major limitation inherent in the methodology of clinical observational studies is that the theoretical biases of the therapists tend to become inextricably interwoven with the recording and obtaining of data. Since there is no mechanical recording of the data, the therapist becomes the recording instrument. The therapist typically makes notes after the therapy session has been completed. Thus not only are his perceptions of the moment colored by his biases, but his recollections are subject to primary-recency effects. Acquisition of the data is also likely to be affected by the therapist's preconceptions. Verbal conditioning studies have demonstrated that people's verbal productions can be shaped to a marked degree by the listener's expressions of interest. Therapists are likely to be unaware that they are selectively reinforcing certain aspects of their patient's behavior.

There is some evidence that many of the theoretical concepts that serve as a framework for therapists' descriptions of the familial characteristics of schizophrenics are not accurate (Jackson, Block, Block, and Patterson, 1958). Jackson *et al.* asked twenty well-known psychiatrists, who had had considerable experience with schizophrenics and their families, to perform two Q sorts on 108 statements according to their conceptions of the schizophrenic's mother and father. Factor analysis produced three factors for each parent. The six factors were considered to represent the conceptions of mothers and fathers of schizophrenics most widely held in the field of psychiatry. The conceptions were correlated with descriptions of the parents of twenty autistic and twenty neurotic children which had been made by Q sorts of the same 108 items. None of the conceptions showed even a trend toward differentiating the two groups of parents. The results of the Jackson *et al.* study provide an empirical example and documentation of the inadequacies of this method. Whereas the clinical observational method is valuable as a source of provocative hypotheses and potentially fruitful insights, intrinsic difficulties make it unsuitable as a firm basis for a scientific methodology.

Retrospective studies

The validity of interviews and questionnaires for ascertaining the actual parental child-rearing practices and attitudes during the subject's childhood rests upon several assumptions: (1) that people conceptualize their lives in terms of the language used by the investigator so that their understanding of the questions is similar to that of the investigator; (2) that people can accurately recall events and feelings of many years past with minimal forgetting; (3) that people will report unpleasant events without selective forgetting, defensive distortion, and justification of actions by inaccurate elaboration; and (4) that people will report past events unaffected by social desirability or other response sets. Fortunately, there is a substantial amount of empirical data available for evaluating the tenability of these assumptions. McGraw and Molloy (1941) interviewed mothers twice concerning their retrospective accounts of the developmental history of their children. The first time, they conducted the interviews in the usual manner of an intake interviewer. One month later they interviewed the mothers again with more detailed and specific questioning, including pictorial representations of many of the developmental skills involved in the questions. The accuracy of the reports, when compared to staff examination of the children during their development, increased markedly from first to second interview for many questions, particularly for those accompanied by pictorial representations. These results demonstrate the considerable lack of commonality of meaning between investigator and subject when questions are phrased in their typical, unelaborated form. Moreover, questions dealing with feelings and attitudes are not amenable to the pictorial specificity possible in other areas.

The ability of people to recall past events and feelings reliably has been investigated in wider, longitudinal research projects. Haggard, Brekstad, and Skard (1960), Robbins (1963), and Yarrow, Campbell, and Burton (1964) have compared retrospective parental reports to historical parental reports, and Jayaswal and Stott (1955), McGraw and Molloy (1941), Pyles, Stolz, and Macfarlane (1935), and Yarrow *et al.* (1964) have compared parental recollections to observational material obtained by a research staff during the children's development. All these studies found considerable unreliability in retrospective reports, as well as large intrasubject variability in accuracy across items.

Content of the material to be recalled has an important effect on accuracy of recall. Questions asking for recall of quantitative information and concrete events are answered more reliably than inquiries about attitudes and feelings (Haggard *et al.*, 1960; Yarrow *et al.*, 1964). Haggard *et al.* (1960) have reported further, that the greater the initial anxiety associated with an attitude, the less accurately the attitude is recalled. In fact, recall of attitudes originally associated with great anxiety is almost completely unreliable. Kohn and Carroll (1960) found that the picture of past events varied considerably depending upon the member of the family doing the reporting. Heilbrun (1960) found no difference between the way the mothers of schizophrenic and of normal daughters described their child-rearing attitudes, but did find that schizophrenic daughters described their mothers as more pathological in their attitudes than did normal daughters. On the other hand, Jayaswal and Stott (1955) reported that young adults and their parents showed high agreement in their descriptions of the young adults as children. However, neither set of descriptions bore much relation to teachers' descriptions of the young adults obtained when they were children.

Many empirical studies have shown that social desirability and other response sets affect subjects' responses to questionnaire items. There are some data to indicate that responses to questions in an interview are subject to similar biases. McGraw and Molloy (1941) and Pyles *et al.* (1935) have shown that maternal inaccuracies in recall tended to be made in the direction of precocity in their children, that is, mothers tended to underestimate the age at which their children acquired developmental skills and the time taken to acquire the skills. Robbins (1963) has reported a variation on this finding. Inaccuracies tended to reflect the recommendations of a noted contemporary child-rearing expert.

The results of studies evaluating the reliability of retrospective reports make the assumptions underlying the method untenable. Kasanin, Knight, and Sage (1934), Rabkin (1965), and Sanua (1961) have pointed out additional weaknesses in this method. Two are peculiar to the use of interview material from case history folders. These records vary widely in their completeness, with the result that many are rejected because of missing data. Overprotective mothers give more information about their children's background, so that a selective bias influences the characteristics of the records accepted. Offspring of such mothers are very likely over-represented in samples drawn on the basis of completeness. Another bias derives from the manner in which the case histories are obtained. The intake interviewer asks questions and records the data according to his theoretical biases. This same limitation was discussed in connection with the clinical observational method. There is one reservation peculiar to questionnaire data. A high and consistent relationship between current attitudes and current behavior has not yet been empirically demonstrated. It would seem to be an almost insurmountable task to demonstrate a high and consistent relationship between past attitudes and past behavior. For all the above reasons, the retrospective report method is judged to be an inadequate foundation for a body of scientific facts.

Family interaction studies

A criticism that has been applied to each of the preceding methods of investigation is that, in many cases, the data are not recorded and coded objectively and systematically. Haley (1964) and Rabkin (1965) have extended this criticism to family interaction studies, pointing out that high interjudge reliabilities may occur as a result of two or more judges coding within the framework of the same theoretical biases. Thus, one could not be sure that the data were free of inferences from the observer.

Haley has suggested and used automatic recording and tabulating of interactional indices by electronic instruments (Haley, 1962, 1964). This insures highly reliable coding, but is purchased at a high price. In one study, Haley (1964) used a machine to tabulate automatically the number of times one person followed another in conversation. However, it is impossible to tell from the data whether the second person interrupted, asked a question, answered a question, disagreed, agreed, said something irrelevant, or was even talking to the first person. The meaningfulness of the data is questionable when they are stripped of such categories. It should be possible, however, to make increased use of instrumentation without sacrificing most of the content of the interaction. Even at best, instrumentation would not solve the problem completely, since the investigator must still program his instruments to code selected aspects of the interaction. A balance must be reached between unchecked observer contamination and such rigid control of possible contamination that essential aspects of the phenomenon under investigation are obscured. At the present time, establishment of high interjudge reliabilities seems to be a workable solution to the dilemma.

Family interaction studies that seek to discover factors which are etiologically relevant to the development of schizophrenia necessarily assume that the causal factors lie in the characteristics of the family interaction pattern. Many people have made the opposite assumption that it is the schizophrenia of the child which has caused the family to develop certain interactional characteristics. Thus, if family interaction studies could demonstrate differences between families of schizophrenics and non-schizophrenics, the question would still be moot as to the locus of cause and effect. At the present time, one assumption is as valid as the other. The assumption that the family interaction patterns are the causal factors in the development of schizophrenia is important for present purposes because it implies several other assumptions concerning methodology. The first is that the interaction patterns in the experimental setting are the usual family patterns and the subjects' usual behavior is not altered by the knowledge that they are being studied by professional experts. This assumption is particularly dubious for those studies in which a hospitalized schizophrenic group is compared to a nonhospitalized control group. The two groups of families undoubtedly have different perceptions of the meaning of the experimenter's request for participation. For the families of schizophrenics, participation is probably perceived as a way of helping their children; while for the families of non-hospitalized controls, it may well be seen as a test of their psychological health or normality. Each family's perception of its role in the research program would probably affect its mode of interaction. For example, Cheek (1964) has found that mothers of normals were significantly more ego defensive than mothers of schizophrenics. A similar trend was also obtained for fathers (Cheek, 1965). The problem of differential defensiveness can be largely circumvented by utilizing families of other institutionalized and stigmatized groups as controls so that all are recruited on the same basis and are likely to share the meaning of the request for participation. People could still be expected to react to being studied, but the groups would not be differentially affected. The possibility (and probability) that people's behavior will be affected by the knowledge that they are being observed is present in all areas of psychology.

A second assumption, related to the first, is that current interaction patterns are unchanged from their characteristics before the child became a patient. This means that the way family members interact is unaffected by the hospitalization, and consequent change in status. It is particularly unlikely that this assumption would be valid for chronic patients. If a person has been hospitalized for a long time or for a large number of times, the family is likely to incorporate his status as a mental patient into its image of him. Likewise, the person could be expected to modify his self-concept to include the attributes of the chronic mental patient. Institutionalization effects can be lessened by using only families of acute patients, for whom hospitalization would more likely be perceived as transitory. An even more desirable group would be families of persons on outpatient or trial visit status.

A third assumption is that current interaction patterns are essentially unchanged from their characteristics at the time the child was becoming schizophrenic. In order for this assumption to be valid, there must have been no essential change over time due to aging of the parents and maturation of the child. The crucial aspect of this position revolves around the word 'essential'. The extent to which basic personality and interactional characteristics are modifiable beyond the first few years of life is still an issue of considerable dispute.

A fourth assumption is also made that the task around which the interaction is organized does not alter the pattern in some unique way so that it is specific to that task and a circumscribed group of similar tasks. Rather, it is assumed that the families react to the experimental task as they characteristically react to most tasks.

A fifth assumption is that family interaction patterns are the same when some members are absent as they are when all members are present. This assumption appears of dubious validity, but whether different groups of families are affected differentially by missing members is unknown. Siblings of the patients or control subjects could be included in the interactions in order to investigate this possibility.

Consideration of these five assumptions highlights the tentativeness of etiological conclusions that might be drawn from family interaction studies. Nevertheless, the study of family interaction holds promise for providing valuable guidelines for the design and hypothetical formulations of longitudinal studies, from which appropriate cause and effect statements can be made. If the inconclusiveness of the etiological assumption is granted and accepted, then there are no apparent, intrinsic methodological inadequacies to the study of family interaction which would disqualify it as a scientific endeavor. The possible limitations of method arising from the etiological assumption can be largely circumvented or minimized by careful attention to specific controls. With this in mind, let us proceed to an examination of family interaction studies, first from a methodological viewpoint and then from the perspective of empirical results from the better designed studies.

Difficulties of interpretation and evaluation

Studies employing the direct recording and systematic coding of actual family interactions have been few in number and

Table 1 Methodological summary of family interaction studies

Author	Demographic comparability of control and schizophrenic groups	Sex of subjects[1]	Hospital status of schizophrenic group	Subdivision of schizophrenic group
Baxter et al. (1962)	No control group	m & f	Acute	Poor premorbid[4]
Baxter & Arthur (1964)	No control group	m	Acute	Poor & good premorbid
Behrens & Goldfarb (1958)	Questionable	m & f	Ns	—[5]
Caputo (1963)	Good	m	Chronic	—
Cheek (1964a)	Fair	m & f[2]	Convalescent	—
Cheek (1964b)	Fair	m & f[2]	Convalescent	—
Cheek (1965)	Fair	m & f[2]	Convalescent	—
Farina (1960)	Fair	m	Acute	Poor & good premorbid
Farina & Dunham (1963)	No control group	m	Acute	Poor & good premorbid
Ferreira (1963)	Questionable	m & f	Ns	—
Ferreira & Winter (1965)	Good	m & f	Ns	—
Fisher et al. (1959)	Good	m	Ns	—
Haley (1962)	Fair	m & f	Ns	—
Haley (1964)	Questionable	m & f	Ns	—[5]
Lennard et al. (1965)	Fair	m	Ns	—[5]
Lerner (1965)	Good	m	Ns[3]	High & low genetic level[6]
McCord et al. (1962)	Good	m	Prehospitalization	—[5]
Meyers & Goldfarb (1961)	Fair	m & f	Ns	Organic & non-organic
Morris & Wynne (1965)	Questionable	m & f	Ns	—
Stabenau et al. (1965)	Good	m & f	Ns	—

Note: Ns = not stated, Vs = vaguely stated, Mt = machine tabulated.
[1] m = male, f = female.
[2] Analyzed separately.
[3] Schizophrenic and control groups were equated on length of current hospitalization.
[4] Premorbidity rated according to the Phillips' (1953) scale.
[5] Included unspecified psychotics.
[6] According to Becker's (1956) system of Rorschach analysis.
[7] Hospitalized.
[8] F = father, M = mother, C = child, S = sib, F(u) = family (unspecified).
[9] Patient present but not a verbal contributor.
[10] Modification of the Revealed Difference Technique, after Strodtbeck (1951).

Control group	'Blind' coding of data	Reliability of coding	Members in inter-action[8]	Task characteristics
—	Ns	Good	F, M, C	Joint interview
—	Ns	Good	F, M	Joint interview
Maladjusted persons	No	Fair	F(u)	Home interactions
Normals[7]	Ns	Vs	F, M	RDT[10]
Normals	Ns	Vs	F, M, C	RDT
Normals	Ns	Vs	F, M, C	RDT
Normals	Ns	Vs	F, M, C	RDT
Tubercular patients[7]	Ns	High	F, M	RDT
—	Ns	High	F, M, C	RDT
Normals, maladjusted persons	Ns	Ns	F, M, C	RDT
Normals, delinquents, maladjusted persons	Ns	Ns	F, M, C	RDT
Neurotics,[7] normals,[7] normals	Yes	High	F, M	Family discussion, TAT story construction
Normals	Mt	High	F, M, C	Game
Normals	Mt	High	F, M, C	RDT, TAT story construction
Normals	Ns	Ns	F, M, C	Family discussion
Normals[7]	Ns	High	F, M	RDT
Maladjusted persons	Yes	Good	F, M, C	Home interactions
Normals	No	Ns	F(u)	Home interactions
Neurotics[7]	Yes	Unobtained	F, M[9]	Joint therapy
Delinquents, normals	Ns	Ns	F, M, C, S	RDT

recent in origin. This reviewer is aware of only twenty reports subsequent to the year 1950 which fall into this category, with the earliest published in 1958. The paucity of such studies is primarily due to two factors: (a) the recent interest in the study of interpersonal relations, and (b) the difficulty in conducting such studies. In view of the latter factor, it is unfortunate that the results of the labor and effort invested in the majority of studies have been negated by insufficient attention to essential controls. On the basis of considerations arising from the etiological assumption and from date demonstrating the possible confounding effects of certain variables, nine criteria were selected for evaluating the methodological adequacy of studies in this area. This reviewer's judgements of the methodological status of family interaction studies are summarized in Table 1. It is apparent from the table that there is great variability among the studies, and that much-desired information is unavailable from the published reports. It is important that control and experimental groups be comparable on as many demographic variables as possible, but particularly on ages of parents and children, sex and birth order of the children, family size, and social class of the family.

Different rates of interaction and patterns of participation could be expected between parents and offspring, depending on the ages of both. All parents might plausibly be expected to be more indulgent of a small child than of a young or middle-aged adult. Similarly, adult patients and control subjects could be expected to relate somewhat differently to their parents if the latter were middle-aged than if they were close to retirement age.

The importance of keeping the sexes separate in the data analysis has been demonstrated in a number of studies. Cheek (1964) found that schizophrenic women were more active in family interactions than were normal women, and schizophrenic men were less active than normal men. In addition, women were higher than men in acknowledgements, tension release, giving opinions, and asking for opinions. Ferreira (1963) reported a difference in frequency of coalitions with each parent in normal families, depending on the sex of the child. Same-sex coalitions were more frequent than opposite-sex coalitions. This same relationship was found in a subsequent study (Ferreira and Winter, 1965) in terms of the initial private agreement between parents and children, and observed to increase with increasing age of the children. Again, this relationship only occurred in normal families. Baxter, Arthur, Flood, and Hedgepeth (1962) found that families of male and female schizophrenics differed in amount of conflict, depending on whether conflict was coded from the extent of initial, private agreement among members or from disagreements arising during family interaction. Also, families of male patients tended to have more mother-father conflict, while mother-patient conflict tended to be greater in the families of female patients. Investigators in most studies using the families of both male and female subjects have not equated their experimental and control groups for the number of each sex, while, at the same time, they have summed their interaction indices across sex. It is impossible to tell how much confounding this procedure may have introduced into the data analysis.

A control related to sex effects, which no study has considered, concerns the possible effects of birth order on interaction behavior. Schooler has used birth order as an independent variable in several studies of schizophrenia. He found that female schizophrenics disproportionately come from the last half of the birth order regardless of social class, while lastborn male schizophrenics disproportionately come from middle-class families and firstborns from lower-class families (Schooler, 1961, 1964). In two other studies, female schizophrenics born in the first half of the birth order were found to be more sociable than those born in the last half (Schooler and Scarr, 1962), and firstborn male schizophrenics were observed to perform better than middleborns who in turn performed better than lastborn patients on a task where their performance was seen as helpful to another person (Schooler and Long, 1963). These findings parallel those of Schachter (1959), obtained with normal women.

Closely allied with birth order is the issue of family size. It seems reasonable to expect that parents might have more contact with each of their children, the fewer of them there are. Also, the number of children in the family might reflect differences in parental attitudes and behavior toward their offspring.

Schooler (1964) and Cheek (1964) have identified an important qualification which must be applied to all studies using hospitalized persons as subjects. It is most appropriate to generalize only to hospitalized schizophrenics and not to all schizophrenics. Schooler noted that latter-born female schizophrenics manifested more noticeable symptomatology, such as hallucinations and suicidal tendencies, than did their counterparts born in the first half of the birth order. He has suggested that the florid character of their symptoms might lead to latterborns being hospitalized more readily, therefore being disproportionately represented in hospitals. In a similar vein, Cheek has suggested that overactive females and underactive males manifest interaction patterns deviant from societal norms, which may result in their being hospitalized more readily than those whose activity patterns are congruent with socially normative behavior. If many symptom characteristics turn out to be epiphenomena of a more basic, common schizophrenic process, the search for schizophrenic-specific factors will be somewhat confounded by society's attitudes toward different symptoms.

Social class embodies many attitude, value, knowledge, and social skill differences between people and, for this reason, is an extremely important variable to keep comparable among groups. Baxter and Arthur (1964) have provided striking evidence of how social class can interact with an independent variable to confound the results of the unwary investigator. These authors found that social class interacted with the premorbid adjustment of their male schizophrenic patients, so that middle-class parents of patients who had made a relatively adequate premorbid adjustment showed more conflict in interaction than did middle-class parents of patients who had made an inadequate premorbid adjustment, with the reverse results obtaining for lower-class groups of parents. All differences disappeared when the data were analysed by social class or premorbidity alone. These results also argue for a subdivision of the schizophrenic sample according to some criteria such as good-poor premorbid adjustment or the process-reactive distinction. Both of these subdivisions have been empirically demonstrated to have prognostic validity (Becker, 1959; Phillips, 1953), to reduce the heterogeneity of schizophrenic performance (Garmezy and Rodnick, 1959; Herron, 1962), and to be highly interrelated (Solomon and Zlotowski, 1964). Thus, either subdivision makes an empirically meaningful distinction within schizophrenia, and holds promise of indicating a fruitful theoretical distinction as well.

Religion and ethnicity are two interrelated variables which have rarely been controlled. Sanua (1961) has argued that reports of contradictory results in the literature might be reconciled by closer consideration of differences in the subjects' religion and ethnicity. In an exploratory study, he (Sanua, 1963) found that parental characteristics differed widely according to the religion and social class of the families. These data are only suggestive, however, since some essential methodological controls were not employed. A well-controlled study in this area has been reported by McClelland, de Charms, and Rindlisbacher (1955). These investigators questioned Protestant, Jewish, Irish-Catholic, and Italian-Catholic parents about their expectations concerning their children's mastery of several independence skills. In addition to main effects for sex of parent, level of parental education, and religion, they found a complex triple interaction of these variables with the expected age of mastery. There also tended to be a difference within religion between the expectations of Irish and Italian parents. The available evidence is sufficiently strong to warrant attention to the religious and ethnic composition of the subject sample. Certainly, it would be hazardous to ignore sizable religious and ethnic differences between experimental and control groups by assuming on an *a priori* basis that such differences are irrelevant to the style of family interaction.

A minority of studies specify the characteristics of their hospitalized samples in terms of the acuteness-chronicity dimension. In view of one of the assumptions of the method and the unknown effects of institutionalization on relatives and patients, it would seem to be a highly relevant variable.

Most studies have utilized some mechanical means of recording data, yet some have relied on an interviewer to manually record the interaction as it occurs or even after it has occurred. Most reports do not state whether the data were coded in a 'blind' fashion or not, that is, with the coder unable to identify the group membership of the families. In many cases, the reliability of the coding procedure is not stated or is so vaguely stated as to be of unknown value.

Difficulties of comparison

Aside from differing degrees of methodological adequacy among studies, there are two factors which complicate direct comparison of results. One is the differing group membership comprising the 'family'. In some cases only parental interaction has been measured, while in other cases, interaction has included the contributions from the parents and the patient or control child, and in one case assessment was made of the interaction among parents, patient or control child, and another child of the family. It is difficult to assess the possible differential effects of group size, role diversity, and other factors which accompany variation in the number of members in interaction.

A second factor is the difference in task characteristics utilized in the studies. The majority have used modifications of the revealed difference technique (RDT) initially developed by Strodtbeck (1951). The RDT essentially consists of having each member of the family privately state his solutions to a number of problem situations. Then the experimenter asks the family to discuss each problem and to arrive at a group solution. The family discussion is recorded and coded for interaction indices such as agreement, yielding, interruption, and compromise. In studies employing the RDT, however, the range of problem situations extends from highly loaded interpersonal situations involving parent-child conflict to rather trivial, neutral situations. The focus of attention on the structure of family inter-action has led to a neglect of the content, around which the interaction is organized, as a factor worthy of systematic study itself. It is not readily apparent that family reactions to situations involving parent-child conflict are structurally indistin-guishable from reactions to differences among members concerning trivial preferences, such as choice of colors for an automobile or choice of food from a restaurant menu.

Instead of the RDT, other investigators have used joint interviews, family discussions, joint construction of TAT stories, home interactions, game playing, and joint therapy sessions. Haley (1964), using both the RDT and the construc-tion of stories in the TAT, found that each task yielded some-what different results, though each individually was inferior to the two combined in differentiating families of normals from those of psychiatric subjects. One must conclude that task characteristics do affect results, but that the extent of influence is currently undetermined.

Empirical results

The methodology of most family interaction studies leaves much to be desired. Several controls which are either essential or desirable have been suggested. The five most essential controls have been selected as the bases for determining the subset of studies with sufficiently sound methodology to permit comparison of results and evaluation of conclusions. Four studies have (*a*) utilized only schizophrenics in an experimental group, (*b*) analysed the data separately by sex, (*c*) made some statement indicating attention to reliability of coding, (*d*) specified adequate comparability of control and experimental groups on demographic variables, and (*e*) included at least one hospitalized control group (Caputo, 1963; Farina, 1960; Fisher, Boyd, Walker and Sheer, 1959; Lerner, 1965). The Baxter and Arthur (1964) and Farina and Dunham (1963) studies did not include control groups, but are reviewed here because they were designed to test specific points concerning premorbidity differences in Farina's (1960) study. In addition, Cheek's (1964a, 1964b, 1965) reports of her study will be reviewed. Since neither the experimental nor the control group was hospitalized at the time of data collection, the extent to which this difference may have affected her data in comparison to the data of the other studies is unknown.

One of the most widespread and persistent notions concerning schizophrenic aetiology is that of the 'schizophrenogenic' mother (Fromm-Reichmann, 1948). According to this notion, the family pattern of a strong, dominant mother and a weak, passive father deprives the son of an adequate model of identification. The son reacts to the stresses of this culturally atypical pattern by becoming schizophrenic. As a result of the popularity of this notion, the most frequently coded aspects of family interaction have been maternal and paternal dominance. Fisher *et al.* (1959) have reported that mothers of normals talked more than did mothers of neurotics or schizophrenics.[3] The latter two groups did not differ. There were no differences among the fathers of the three groups in amount of talking or initiation of conversation. Caputo (1963) found that the fathers of schizophrenics were generally more dominant than the mothers, with the fathers winning more disagreements than mothers. The parents of normals did not differ in the number of disagreements

3. All differences reported in this review have been found to be statistically significant at the ·05 level or less, unless they are otherwise stated herein as tending to be the case, as trends, or as not significant.

won. Lerner (1965) obtained no differences for mothers and fathers of normals and of two groups of schizophrenics in yielding to the other's position. Cheek (1964a, 1964b, 1965) found no support for the notion of the domineering 'schizophrenogenic' mother. In the families of males, each member of the normal's family interacted in a more dominant way than each corresponding member of the schizophrenic's family. Thus *all* members of the schizophrenic's family were more passive than members of the normal's family when the offspring were males. The reverse tended to be true for fathers and offspring in the families of females: each of these members of the schizophrenic's family acted in a more dominant way than each corresponding member of the normal's family. On the other hand, mothers of both male and female normals were more dominant than mothers of schizophrenics. When pairs of means for indices relating to dominance are compared for mothers and fathers, the largest discrepancies between parents occur most often for the parents of normals. In other words, there tended to be a greater imbalance in dominance between parents in the families of normals than in the families of schizophrenics. The most notable exception to this trend was for the index, Total Interaction, for which fathers of both male and female schizophrenics tended to be more active relative to their wives, than fathers of normals. All of these findings are counter to what would be expected according to the schizophrenogenic mother notion.

Rodnick and Garmezy (1957; Garmezy and Rodnick, 1959) have proposed a theory which essentially states that the pattern of the schizophrenogenic mother can be found in the families of patients with a poor premorbid adjustment (Poors), while the reverse pattern can be observed in the families of schizophrenics with a relatively good premorbid adjustment (Goods). The adequacy of premorbid adjustment and degree of pathology are presumed to be causally related to the sex of the dominant parent, with the Poors being 'sicker' because of the cultural atypicality of their family pattern. Discrepancy in parental dominance is held to be one of the pathognomonic factors predisposing to schizophrenia. One of the keystone studies testing the theory was conducted by Farina (1960). He found that the parents of Poors and Goods were different on all seven of his dominance indices, with Poors being mother dominated and Goods father dominated. However, enthusiasm for this finding as support for the theory must be tempered by consideration of other aspects of these and subsequent data. The parents of Poors were not different from the normals on any of the dominance indices. Goods differed from normals on four of the seven indices. However, two of the nonsignificant indices involved the extent of yielding of one parent to the other. Thus, although the parental dominance pattern for Poors is quite different from that of Goods, neither is strikingly different from the pattern for normals. It is particularly puzzling that the lesser difference from normals was found where the greater difference could have been expected from the theory, that is, in the families of Poors.

Farina also coded the interactions for conflict. It seems reasonable that initiation of conflict could be another way of viewing dominance. Inspection of the index means for conflict reveals that, in all groups, mothers tended to interrupt more and to disagree and aggress more than did fathers. The parental differences are not significant, but the data indicate that the mothers in all groups initiated conflict at least as much as fathers did. A later study by Farina and Dunham (1963) investigated the interactions of mother, father, and patient for groups of Poors and Goods. Although some differences exist, this study can be considered an approximate replication of the Poor-Good comparisons in Farina's study. In the replication, the parental differences for the means of the dominance indices were not as consistent in direction as in the initial study, nor were any of the differences statistically significant. These studies neither support the proposition that the schizophrenogenic pattern is uniquely characteristic of the families of poor premorbid schizophrenics, nor do they offer strong or consistent support for the proposed interaction between parental dominance pattern and adequacy of the patients' social and sexual premorbid adjustment.

Another popular conception is that the schizophrenic's family, in many cases, is characterized by high levels of parental hostility and conflict (Lidz, Cornelison, Fleck, and Terry, 1957). Fisher et al. (1959) found that the parents of schizophrenics and neurotics disagreed more than the parents of normals when they were discussing their sons. The parents of schizophrenics and neurotics did not differ in amount of disagreement. When parents worked jointly on constructing a TAT story, the parents of schizophrenics were higher in disagreement than parents of neurotics who were higher than parents of normals. Caputo (1963) reported that parents of schizophrenics disagreed more and displayed more hostility toward one another than did parents of normals. In Lerner's (1965) study, parents of normals compromised their differences more than either schizophrenic group did, although there were no significant differences among groups in lack of agreement without distortion. However, when lack of agreement with distortion was coded from the interaction, parents of the low genetic level schizophrenic group scored higher than parents of the high genetic level and normal groups. The theoretical significance of this distinction will be elaborated in the next section dealing with clarity of communication. Farina (1960) coded parental interactions on ten indices of conflict. Parents of Poors manifested more conflict than parents of normals on seven of the indices, while parents of Goods and normals did not differ on any of the indices. Three indices showed differences within schizophrenia, with parents of Poors consistently higher than parents of Goods. The Farina and Dunham (1963) replication provided some support for the differences within schizophrenia obtained by Farina. It will be recalled that Baxter and Arthur (1964) found an interaction between social class and premorbidity affecting parental conflict scores. They suggested that Farina's Poor-Good differences in conflict may have resulted from the particular social-class characteristics of his groups and may not be attributable to premorbidity alone. In brief, the evidence consistently favors support of the contention that there is more conflict in the families of schizophrenics (particularly in the families of the more pathological patients, poor premorbids, and those with a low genetic level of development) than in the families of normals. Whether there is more conflict in the families of schizophrenics than in those of other psychiatric groups is less clear. Systematic variation of social class in this area is necessary for clarification and generalization of present trends.

A fourth theoretical position which can be evaluated in terms of the present data is that the etiological family factor pathognomonic for schizophrenia is lack of clarity in parental communication patterns. This idea has been most systematically developed by Wynne and Singer (1963a, 1963b). They have proposed that the unique characteristic of schizophrenia is disorder of the thought processes, particularly inability to focus attention on thematic material in a consistent and prolonged manner. The thought disorder is learned by imitation of parental patterns of communication, in which meanings are blurred by subtle shifts in attention to progressively tangential material. These authors have reported several successful attempts at differentiating the parents of schizophrenics from the parents of other groups on the basis of their projective test protocols (Singer and Wynne, 1963, 1965a, 1965b). Morris and Wynne (1965) have reported similar success using excerpts from joint therapy sessions. It is evident that these authors have engaged in a systematic research approach. However, before their results can be considered to be scientifically demonstrated, their research needs the introduction of some basic methodological controls such as specification of an objective coding system and establishment of acceptable interjudge reliabilities. Fortunately, the studies of Fisher *et al.* (1959) and Lerner (1965) provide more scientifically established evidence relevant to this theoretical position. Fisher *et al.* (1959) found that parents of normals were less ambiguous in their communication with each other than were the parents of neurotics and schizophrenics when they were discussing their sons, and were less ambiguous than parents of schizophrenics when jointly constructing a TAT story. It will be recalled that in the Lerner (1965) study there were no differences among parental groups of high and low genetic level schizophrenics and normals in extent of agreement without distortion of communication. When interactions were coded for lack of agreement *with* distortion, parents of the low genetic level group scored higher than parents of the high genetic level and normal groups. The latter two groups did not differ significantly. In addition, parents of the low genetic level group yielded more often than parents of the other two groups by 'masking', that is, by claiming that they held a position different from the one which they had previously endorsed privately. These data lend support to Wynne and Singer's position that communication between parents of schizophrenics is less clear and comprehensible than it is between parents of normals.

Conclusions and recommendations

Studies obtaining data by clinical observation or by retrospective recall are unsuitable bases for a scientific body of etiological facts since the data are confounded by intrinsic methodological inadequacies. Interpretation of data acquired from direct recording and systematic coding of family interactions is subject to the cautions and tentativeness necessitated by the etiological assumption. *If the etiological assumption is granted and if the behavior sample is characteristic of the families' usual behavioral repertoire*, there are no apparent, intrinsic methodological inadequacies which disqualify this approach as unscientific. The greatest value of current studies of family interaction seems to lie in the guidelines the findings might provide for longitudinal research. Truly appropriate etiological conclusions can only be drawn from careful longitudinal studies. This reviewer doubts that sufficient knowledge is currently available to warrant the great expenditure involved in longitudinal research at the present time.

Four general findings are consistently supported by the few methodologically adequate research studies reviewed here: (*a*) there is no evidence for the proposed 'schizophrenogenic' pattern of dominant mother-passive father, (*b*) there is little support for the proposed interaction between parental dominance pattern and premorbid adjustment of patients, (*c*) there is more conflict between the parents of schizophrenics (or a schizophrenic subgroup) than between the parents of normals, and (*d*) communication between parents of schizophrenics (or a schizophrenogenic subgroup) is less clear than it is between the parents of normals. These generalizations apply mainly to hospitalized white males. Future research on family interaction and schizophrenia would seem to require (*a*) use of families of recently institutionalized persons only; (*b*) comparability of control and experimental groups on social class, religion and ethnicity of the family, and sex, birth order, and premorbidity of the patients and control subjects; (c) inclusion of other institutionalized and stigmatized groups as controls, for example, nonschizophrenic psychiatric patients, tubercular patients, and prisoners; (d) investigation of the interaction of parents of schizophrenics with their nonschizophrenic children as a control condition; and (e) objective data recording, 'blind' coding, and attainment of high interjudge reliabilities.

Handel (1965) and Haley (1962) have argued that it is premature to attempt to differentiate between the families of normal and pathological subjects or to attempt to differentiate among the families of pathological individuals. In their opinion, before such differentiation is attempted, a typology of families according to dimensions and characteristics peculiar to intimate groups is needed. This reviewer believes that the most fruitful approach would direct attention to the two goals concurrently. Certainly the typology and classification of individuals according to traits and motives, independent of theoretical concerns, has not been very effective in the more traditional realms of psychology. A similar approach to family psychology could not reasonably be expected to have a different history.

References

BAXTER, J. C. and ARTHUR, S. C. (1964), 'Conflict in families of schizophrenics as a function of premorbid adjustment and social class', *Family Process*, vol. 3, pp. 273–9.

BAXTER, J. C., ARTHUR, S. C., FLOOD, C. G. and HEDGEPETH, B. (1962), 'Conflict patterns in the families of schizophrenics', *J. nerv. and ment. Disease*, vol. 135, pp. 419–24.

BECKER, W. C. (1956), 'A genetic approach to the interpretation and evaluation of the process-reactive distinction in schizophrenia', *J. ab. soc. Psych.*, vol. 53, pp. 229–36.

BECKER, W. C. (1959), 'The process-reactive distinction: A key to the problem of schizophrenia?', *J. nerv. ment. Disease*, vol. 129, pp. 442–9.

BEHRENS, M. L. and GOLDFARB, W. (1958), 'A study of patterns of interaction of families of schizophrenic children in residential treatment,' *Amer. J. Orthopsychol.*, vol. 28, pp. 300–312.

CAPUTO, D. (1963), 'The parents of the schizophrenic', *Family Process*, vol. 2, pp. 339–56.

CHEEK, F. E. (1964a), 'The "schizophrenic mother" in word and deed', *Family Process*, vol. 3, pp. 155–77.

CHEEK, F. E. (1964b), 'A serendipitous finding: sex roles and schizophrenia', *J. ab. soc. Psych.*, vol. 69, pp. 392–400.

CHEEK, F. E. (1965), 'The father of the schizophrenic', *Arch. gen. Psychol.*, vol. 13, pp. 336–45.

FARINA, A. (1960), 'Patterns of role dominance and conflict in parents of schizophrenic patients', *J. ab. soc. Psychol.*, vol. 61, pp. 31–8.

FARINA, A. and DUNHAM, R. M. (1963), 'Measurements of family relationships and their effects', *Arch. gen. Psych.*, vol. 9, pp. 64–73.

FERREIRA, A. J. (1963), 'Decision-making in normal and pathologic families', *Arch. gen. Psychol.*, vol. 8, pp. 68–73.

FERREIRA, A. J. and WINTER, W. D. (1965), 'Family interaction and decision making', *Arch. gen. Psych.*, vol. 13, pp. 214–23.

FISHER, S., BOYD, I., WALKER, D. and SHEER, D. (1959), 'Parents of schizophrenics, neurotics and normals', *Arch. gen. Psych.*, vol. 1, pp. 149–66

FRANK, G. H. (1965), 'The role of the family in the development of psychopathology', *Psychological Bulletin*, vol. 64, pp. 191–205.

FROMM-REICHMANN, F. (1948), 'Notes on the development of treatment of schizophrenics by psychoanalytic psychotherapy', *Psychiatry*, vol. 11, pp. 263–73.

GARMEZY, N. and RODNICK, E. H. (1959), 'Premorbid adjustment and performance in schizophrenia: implications for interpreting heterogeneity in schizophrenia', *J. nerv. ment. Disease*, vol. 129, pp. 450–66.

HAGGARD, E. A., BREKSTAD, A. and SKARD, A. (1960), 'On the reliability of the anamnestic interview', *J. ab. soc. Psychol.*, vol. 61, pp. 311–18.

HALEY, J. (1962), 'Family experiments: a new type of experimentation', *Family Process*, vol. 1, pp. 265–93.

HALEY, J. (1964), 'Research on family patterns: an instrument measurement, *Family Process*, vol. 3, pp. 41–64.

HANDEL, G. (1965), 'Psychological study of whole families', *Psychol. Bull.*, vol. 63, pp. 19–41.

HEILBRUN, A. B. (1960), 'Perception of maternal child rearing attitudes in schzophrenia', *J. cons. Psychiat.*, vol. 24, pp. 169–73.

HERRON, W. G. (1962), 'The process-reactive classification of schiziophrenia', *Psychol. Bull.*, vol. 59, pp. 329–43.

JACKSON, D. D., BLOCK, J., BLOCK, J. and PATTERSON, V. (1958), 'Psychiatrists' conceptions of the schizophrenogenic parent', *Arch. Neur. and Psychol.*, vol. 79, pp. 448–59.

JAYASWAL, S. R. and STOTT, L. H. (1955), 'Persistence and change in personality from childhood to adulthood', *Merrill-Palmer Q.*, vol. 1, pp. 47–56.

KASANIN, J., KNIGHT, E. and SAGE, P. (1934), 'The parent-child relationship in schizophrenia. I. Overprotection-rejection', *J. nerv. and ment. Disease*, vol. 72, pp. 249–63.

KOHN, M. L. and CARROLL, E. E. (1960), 'Social class and the allocation of parental responsibilities', *Sociometry*, vol. 23, pp. 372–92.

Lennard, H. L., Beaulieu, M. R. and Embry, N. G. (1965), 'Interaction in families with a schizophrenic child', *Arch. gen. Psychiat.*, vol. 12, pp. 166–83.

Lerner, P. M. (1965), 'Resolution of intrafamilial role conflict in families of schizophrenic patients. I. Thought disturbance', *J. nerv. ment. Disease*, vol. 141, pp. 342–51.

Lidz, T., Cornelison, A. R., Fleck, S. and Terry, D. (1957), 'The intrafamilial environment of schizophrenic patients: II. Marital schism and marital skew', *Amer. J. Psychol.*, vol. 114, pp. 241–8.

McClelland, D. C., de Charms, R. and Rindlisbacher, A. (1955), 'Religious and other sources of parental attitudes toward independence training', in D. McClelland (ed.), *Studies in Motivation*, Appleton-Century-Crofts, pp. 389–97.

McCord, W., Porta, J. and McCord, J. (1962), 'The familial genesis of psychoses', *Psychiatry*, vol. 25, pp. 60–71.

McGraw, M. B. and Molloy, L. B. (1941), 'The pediatric anamnesis: Inaccuracies in eliciting developmental data', *Child Devel.*, vol. 12, pp. 255–65.

Meissner, W. W. (1964), 'Thinking about the family-psychiatric aspects', *Family Process*, vol. 3, pp. 1–40.

Meyers, D. F. and Goldfarb, W. (1961), 'Studies of perplexity in mothers of schizophrenic children', *Amer. J. Orthopsychiat.*, vol. 31, pp. 551–64.

Morris, G. O. and Wynne, L. C. (1965), 'Schizophrenic offspring and parental styles of communication', *Psychiatry*, vol. 28, pp. 19–44.

Phillips, L. (1953), 'Case history data and prognosis in schizophrenia', *J. nerv. and ment. Disease*, vol. 117, pp. 515–25.

Pyles, M. K., Stolz, H. R. and Macfarlane, J. W. (1935), 'The accuracy of mothers' reports on birth and developmental data', *Child Devel.*, vol. 6, pp. 165–76.

Rabkin, L. Y. (1965), 'The patient's family: research methods', *Family Process*, vol. 4, pp. 105–32.

Robbins, L. C. (1963), 'The accuracy of parental recall of aspects of child development and of child rearing practices', *J. ab. soc. Psychol.*, vol. 66, pp. 261–70.

Rodnick, E. H. and Garmezy, N. (1957), 'An experimental approach to the study of motivation in schizophrenia', in M. R. Jones (ed.) *Nebraska Symposium on Motivation: 1957*, University of Nebraska Press, pp. 109–84.

Sanua, V. D. (1961), 'Sociocultural factors in families of schizophrenics', *Psychiatry*, vol. 24, pp. 246–65.

Sanua, V. D. (1963), 'The sociocultural aspects of schizophrenia: a comparison of Protestant and Jewish schizophrenics', *Int. J. soc. Psychiat.*, vol. 9, pp. 27–36.

Schacter, S. (1959), *The Psychology of Affiliation*, Stanford University Press.

Schooler, C. (1961), 'Birth order and schizophrenia', *Arch. gen. Psychiat.*, vol. 4, pp. 117–23.

Schooler, C. (1964), 'Birth order and hospitalization for schizophrenia', *J. ab. soc. Psychol.*, vol. 69, pp. 574–79.

Schooler, C. and Long, J. (1963), 'Affiliation among chronic schizophrenics: Factors affecting acceptance of responsibility for the fate of another', *J. nerv. and ment. Disease*, vol. 137, pp. 173–9.

Schooler, C. and Scarr, S. (1962), 'Affiliation among chronic schizophrenics: relation to intrapersonal and birth order factors', *J. of Person.*, vol. 30, pp. 178–92.

Singer, M. T. and Wynne, L. C. (1963), 'Differentiating characteristics of parents of childhood schizophrenics, childhood neurotics and young adult schizophrenics', *Amer. J. Psychiat.*, vol. 120, pp. 234–43.

Singer, M. T. and Wynne, L. C. (1965a), 'Thought disorder and family relations of schizophrenics. III. Methodology using projective techniques', *Arch. of gen. Psych.*, vol. 12, pp. 187–200.

Singer, M. T. and Wynne, L. C. (1965b), 'Thought disorder and family relations of schizophrenics. IV. Results and implications,' *Arch. gen. Psychiat.*, vol. 12, pp. 201–12.

Solomon, L. and Zlotowski, M. (1964), 'The relationship between the Elgin and Phillips measures of process-reactive schizophrenia', *J. nerv. and ment. Disease*, vol. 138, pp. 32–7.

Stabenau, J. R., Tupin, J., Werner, M. and Pollin, W. (1965), 'A comparative study of families of schizophrenics, delinquents and normals', *Psychiatry*, vol. 28, pp. 45–95.

Strodtbeck, F. (1951), 'Husband-wife interaction over revealed differences', *Amer. soc. Rev.*, vol. 16, pp. 648, 473.

Wynne, L. C. and Singer, M. T. (1963a), 'Thought disorder and family relations of schizophrenics. I. A research strategy', *Arch. gen. Psychiat.*, vol. 9, pp. 191–8.

Wynne, L. C. and Singer, M. T. (1963b), 'Thought disorder and the family relations of schizophrenics. II. Classification of forms of thinking', *Arch. gen. Psychiat.*, vol. 9, pp. 199–206.

Yarrow, M. R., Campbell, J. D. and Burton, R. V. (1964), 'Reliability of maternal retrospection: a preliminary report', *Family Process*, vol. 3, pp. 207–18.

9 N. Garmezy

Vulnerability Research and the Issue
of Primary Prevention

N. Garmezy, 'Vulnerability Research and the Issue of Primary
Prevention', *American Journal of Orthopsychiatry*, vol. 41, 1971,
pp. 101–16.

For psychiatry, primary prevention is aimed at 'modifying the
environment and strengthening individual capacities to cope
with situations' in order to reduce 'the incidence of new cases of
mental disorder and diability in a population', Kaplan and
Grunebaum (1967). Such a goal is a laudatory one for any
discipline. To a nation beset with problems, citing mental illness
statistics to log still another crisis of our times seems almost
gratuitous. But a crisis exists and the number of our emotionally wounded suggests the magnitude of this problem: nineteen
million citizens suffering from diverse forms of mental or
emotional illness that require professional intervention; a rising
tide of criminality, delinquency, suicide, drug addiction, alcoholism and assault; a half-million severely mentally ill children
joined by four million more whose emotional difficulties can
only foster a pattern of social and economic incompetence that
will fetter them in adulthood. One can cite endless statistics of
despair such as these to justify the need for knowledge that will
provide the basis for programs of primary, secondary and
tertiary prevention.

   Unfortunately, empirical data that would buttress such programs are in small supply. We lack fundamental knowledge for
determining and, in many instances, identifying early in development those among our citizens who will, in time, constitute
the most vulnerable members of our population. Who will fall
to the ravaging effects of mental disorder or who will, despite
stress and adversity, remain inviolate to psychopathology remains a problem of mystery and challenge. One can, of course,
cite numerous case histories to substantiate many factors that
may contribute to breakdown; but a simple declaration of

physical, psychosocial or sociocultural resources cannot explain divergent paths to adaptation or to deviance.

High-risk research

The complexity of this problem is evident in the literature of high-risk studies. We can begin with a question. What are the consequences in adulthood for children born to schizophrenic mothers (or fathers, since the data tend to be comparable)? Mednick and Schuslinger (1968) suggest that by end of the risk period of age forty-five, perhaps 12 per cent–14 per cent of a sample of such children will themselves have suffered some form of schizophrenic disorder, while an additional 35 per cent or so will likely manifest some alternate form of deviant, atypical behavior. On the other hand, expressed, too, in terms of overt behavior, some 50 per cent can be expected to be functioning adequately and to be symptom-free. And of this latter group a small subset (and this is extrapolated from the work of Heston and Denny in 1968 and Karlsson in 1966), may even reveal elements of creative expressiveness in their makeup. This last point deserves elaboration, for it reveals the variability in outcomes so characteristic of psychiatric study.

In his follow-up study of infants born to schizophrenic women and placed away from their mothers shortly after birth, Heston (1968), in collaboration with Denny, has reported an interesting finding within this experimental (risk) group:

One further result deserves special emphasis. The twenty-one Experimental subjects who exhibited no significant psychosocial impairment were not only successful adults but in comparison to the Control group were more spontaneous when interviewed and had more colorful life histories. They held the more creative jobs: musician, teacher, home-designer; and followed the more imaginative hobbies: oil painting, music, antique aircraft. It must be emphasized that the finding of what may be especially adaptive personality traits among persons in the Experimental groups was noticed only in retrospect as the material compiled on each person was being reviewed. Such traits were not systematically investigated: Most psychiatric studies focus on pathology, not on the delineation of degrees of normal psychological health, and this study was not an exception. Also it is uncertain what influence the known greater variability in intelligence among the relatives of schizophrenics might have had. We wish to report a strong *impression* [authors' italics] that within the Experimental group there was much more variability of personality and behavior but more evidence is required before this can be regarded as confirmed (p. 371).

Karlsson (1966), referring to his genetic study of schizo-phrenia in Iceland, also alludes to individuals who are 'genetic carriers . . . with thought disorders' and who

seem not infrequently to be persons of unusual ability, such as leaders in society or creative persons with performance records suggestive of a superior capacity for associative thinking (p. 61).

And elsewhere he asks:

Could it be that some highly creative individuals are nonpenetrant schizophrenics and that society is thus dependent in terms of social and scientific progress on persons with a schizophrenic constitution? This suggestion is compatible with the observation that on certain psychologic tests the same type of response is seen with highly creative persons and schizophrenic patients. . . . It is impressive that lists of the most creative contributors to the various fields of art and science are generally found to include individuals who developed psychotic dis-orders. This is true in the fields of philosophy, mathematics, physics, music, prose literature, poetry, sculpture, painting, etc.

Recently McNeil (1969), using the Adoption Registry for the Copenhagen metropolitan area in Denmark, reported pre-liminary evidence related to mental illness in adoptees working in creative (e.g. performing and graphic arts, literary) occupa-tions as contrasted with non-creative ones (bookkeeper, bank clerk, factory foreman, etc.). Histories of mental disorder in the adoptees, their biological and adoptive parents and siblings, were subsequently checked through the Danish national psy-chiatric register. Despite the small number of cases, creative ability level was found to be related to mental illness rates among the adoptees and their biological relatives but not to the rates for the adoptive relatives.

These citations are not offered as determinate evidence for a correlation between genius and madness or creativity and emo-tional disorder. That elusive relationship will demand a more stringent, empirical test. What is suggested, however, is that even in the presence of a markedly deleterious family environ-ment – which some consider to be the most central psychosocial factor determining dysfunction (Karlsson 1966) – the outcomes for children born into such families are not invariant. Of course, one can suggest in rebuttal that the presence of a psychotic mother does not *per se* guarantee a deleterious environment; but certainly even the most conservative of clinicians would be loath to point to such a maternal state as a source of strength for the child.

Poverty and the etiology of mental disorder

Perhaps attention to another area of concern in matters of primary prevention may provide additional support for the point I seek to make. With regard to the different social structures that characterize communities and subcultures, Kaplan and Grunebaum (1967) have written:

If a person happens to be born into an advantaged group in a stable society, his social roles and their expected changes over a lifetime will tend to provide him with adequate opportunities for healthy personality development. If, on the other hand, he belongs to a disadvantaged minority, suffers from economic deprivation ... he may find his progress blocked and he may be deprived of opportunity and challenge. This may have an adverse effect on his mental health (p. 333).

These authors are appropriately cautious in expressing this hypothesis. But other professionals have not adopted a comparable restraint in considering the role of slums and poverty as potential aetiologic agents for mental disorder. The view that slums induce mental disorder is, as I have noted elsewhere (Garmezy, 1970) rooted in American social science. It is the product of a long-term concern for the social welfare of disadvantaged citizens as well as a derivative of a political ideology that sees environmental influences as the most powerful forces shaping behavior.

But the hypothesized powerful negative effect of slum life on personal adaptation remains an assumption and not a given. Slums, like other environments, seem to produce individuals who vary markedly in their ability to cope. It is demeaning to suggest that for those reared in our festering slums the prognosis for successful adaptation is inevitably bleak. Such a position ignores the history of an urbanized nation that has been built by a succession of ethnic groups each of which, in turn, has cast off disadvantaged economic status and pestilent neighbourhoods without assuming the burdens of psycho-pathology.

A more sophisticated sociological view of the socially inte-grative power of a highly disadvantaged environment is found in Suttles' fascinating volume, *The Social Order of the Slum* (1968) in which he details three years of participant observation in one of Chicago's more malignant neighbourhoods. Dun-ham's (1965) summary of his epidemiological study of schizo-phrenia in two subcommunities of Detroit is also congruent with the shift away from viewing a disordered ecology *per se* as an etiologic agent in mental disorder. Dunham challenges and then rejects the prior interpretation of the classical investigation that he conducted in conjunction with Faris (Faris and Dunham 1939) of the differential rates of prevalence of mental disorder in Chicago and its environs. Earlier he had assigned conditions of social isolation, culture conflict, social deprivation and stress to the high prevalence rates of psychopathology found in the central city. Dunham now focuses on the 'extreme competitive-ness' of an open class society and 'the personality character-istics of the pre-schizophrenic' that constrict his quest for education and employment.

We can further examine this issue of variation of outcomes in disadvantaged social settings by turning to the significant study by Robins (1966) detailed in her superb volume, *Deviant Children Grown Up*. Robins sought to follow up, some thirty years later, a group of children who had been diagnosed and treated in a small child guidance clinic in St Louis. For controls she selected children from the same lower social class milieu who met the following criteria: they had never been seen in a psychi-atric clinic; they had never repeated a full year of elementary school; and they had not left school for reasons of expulsion or transfer to a correctional institution.

Although the slum environment in which the experimental and control children had been reared was extremely similar in terms of the degree of manifest physical deprivation, the con-trols, when examined in adulthood, were found to be 'extra-ordinarily well adjusted'. Some 60 per cent had moved to the

suburbs, possessed good jobs, had a high rate of home owner-
ship, a relatively low divorce rate, and an absence of incarcerations, indigence or mental disorder. In Norman Podhoretz's
words, they were 'making it'. Within the clinic group, too, outcomes were found to be variable; anti-social children more
typically revealed maladaptive adult behavior, while the prognosis for neurotic problem cases proved to be relatively favorable.

Retrospection, continuity, and prediction

What, then, shall we say about primary prevention when the
major variables of family and social structure produce such
highly diverse outcomes? It would seem more appropriate if
we did not presume to use the word 'prevention' (for it holds
greater promise than our mental health disciplines can fulfill). It
also suggests a historical basis for our assumption that we know
the variables that produce disorder and can stay their action.
What is the source of this complacent belief that the factors for
programming primary prevention efforts are known to us?

I believe we in psychiatry have become ensnared by restrictions in our traditional method of gathering information. The
focus of past efforts at understanding patients has been the case
study. As with many medical specialties, the method has served
its discipline well. For psychiatry, it has been the instrument for
bringing order to a bewildering array of symptoms and psychopathologies; it has provided a basis for the taxonomy of psychiatric disorders, and has stimulated insights into developmental
events that may help produce a vulnerability to mental illness
Rosenthal *et al* (1968). The case method has led to many studies of
prognosis that provide evidence for a continuity of pathological
development extending from premorbid adjustment through
morbid symptom formation to postmorbid outcome. Furthermore, the case history has generated hypotheses for experimental studies of a psychological, biological and genetic cast.

Given these many virtues, it is difficult to be disparaging of
the case history method. And yet we must, for it has served to
disfigure our formulations of personality development. Studies
of normal families (Mednick and Shaffer, 1964; Robbins, 1963;
Wenar, 1961) have revealed the unreliability of the case history,

with its exclusive reliance on retrospective reconstruction of an earlier time period. These investigations conducted with normal mothers of primary school age (and younger) children provide evidence that not only do mothers suffer deficits in recalling events in the early years of their children's lives but that the deficiency is particularly acute in those very spheres of behavior, such as emotions and affectively-tinged attitudes, that are presumed to be potentially significant for the formation of maladjustment in children. The central issue, then, is this: If 'normal' mothers engaged in the act of recall of 'normal' events related to the growth and development of their own 'normal' children are found to have defective memory for such events, then with what confidence can we view the reliability of recall provided by disordered mothers of disordered children? Yet this has not deterred us from creating a substantial edifice for a science of psychopathology (with its attendant view of prevention) using as the structure's foundation data gathered by just such unreliable retrospective procedures.

Why should such retrospective elaborations provide us with this unwarranted degree of comfort regarding the antecedents of behavior disorder? Looking backward, the behavioral scientist can always find support for his belief in the developmental continuities he believes to be evident in personality formation. The scientist is not alone in his belief system. I recently presented 185 competent undergraduates enrolled in an Abnormal Psychology course at a distinguished university with this hypothetical situation:

Imagine [I told them] that I am capable of dropping a potion into your drink which will, in the brief passage of time, induce a marked psychosis (surely not an outlandish fantasy in these days). You, however, have neither memory nor awareness of this intervening event. Within a day your worried parents take you to a psychiatric center where you and they are interviewed at intake by a social worker followed in turn by a psychiatrist. You are asked to detail the background of your life. Consider this situation tonight and at the next class session let me know whether or not a rational reconstruction of your psychotic state could be inferred from your previous life experiences.

All but two students in this class of 185 indicated that they believed their 'fantasy' psychoses would be justified by a recital of events in their lives, despite the evident competencies most of them possessed.

Looking backward from an end point of a developmental sequence, we can construct justification for an outcome marked by either competence or incompetence. Provide us with a slum child who is forging a pattern of strength and we will cast about for environmental surrogates who *must* have served as inoculators against despair, for events that *must* have encouraged hope rather than hopelessness, for inner resources that *must* have proclaimed vitality rather than helplessness. However, were we to convert this same slum child into someone prone to violence or aberration, our focus would be turned with equal efficiency and perhaps even greater facility to alternate figures and facets that would buttress our perception of deviance. Thus do we become victimized by our self-fulfilling clinical prophecies, ignoring the insightful observation of Freud, for whom the case history was the royal road into theory.

In his *Psychogenesis of a Case of Homosexuality in a Woman*, (1955) Freud wrote:

So long as we trace the development from its final outcome backwards, the chain of events appears continuous, and we feel we have gained an insight which is completely satisfactory or even exhaustive. But if we proceed the reverse way, if we start from the premises inferred from the analysis and try to follow these up to the final result, then we no longer get the impression of an inevitable sequence of events which could not have been otherwise determined. We notice at once that there might have been another result, and that we might have been just as well able to understand and explain the latter. The synthesis is thus not so satisfactory as the analysis; in other words, from a knowledge of the premises we could not have foretold the nature of the result.

It is very easy to account for this disturbing state of affairs. Even supposing that we have a complete knowledge of the etiological factors that decide a given result, nevertheless what we know about them is only their quality, and not their relative strength. Some of them are suppressed by others because they are too weak, and they therefore do not affect the final result. But we never know beforehand which of the determining factors will prove the weaker or the stronger. We can only say at the end that those which succeeded must have been the stronger. Hence the chain of causation can always be recognized with certainty if we follow the line of analysis, whereas to predict it along the line of synthesis is impossible (pp. 167, 168).

I believe too that we are biased in our interpretation of events by those ardently cathected theories that form the base for programs of primary prevention. Let me illustrate this point with reference to a serious contemporary social problem – the threat of bombings from militants of the radical left and the radical right. In an astute analysis of the problem, Thomas R. Brooks in *The New York Times* March 15, 1970, searched for the roots of the violence espoused by the Weathermen, the most radical fringe of SDS. Indicating that these persons typically tend to be the educated children of middle-class and often wealthy parents, Brooks inquired:

What prompts them to live the life of terrorists? Are they sensitive idealists, turned off by the wrongs of our society and by the greater violence of the Vietnam war?

He cites, on the one hand, the view of Dr John Spiegel of the Lemberg Center for the Study of Violence at Brandeis University that the motives underlying the violent behavior can be comprehended within a normal context.

The young people have had protests and riots and disorders – they've done everything one can do in the way of peaceful and unplanned protest, and not much has changed. To that degree there is an increasing sense of desperation, and a sense of vengefulness.

Yet, as Brooks points out, other militants have not chosen the path of violence. I have an able, young SDS inconclast in one of my seminars who will bow to no man in his distaste for the Establishment, yet who terms the Weathermen 'action freaks'. He is prone to define their behavior in the context of pathology, as is Mr Brooks when he writes:

Nonetheless, it is difficult to escape the feeling that these youngsters are demented. How else explain the admiration for Sirhan Sirhan, the murderer of Senator Robert F. Kennedy, or for Charles Manson, group leader of a band of alleged murderers. Among these youngsters, there are open jokes about assassinations, and a salivating over violence. Witness Bernadine Dohrn: 'Dig it, first they killed those pigs [actress Sharon Tate and her friends], then they ate dinner in the same room with them, then they even shoved a fork into a victim's stomach! Wild!'

This is, perhaps, a dramatic, overblown instance of how different our orientations can be when viewing behavior in terms of the presence or absence of manifest pathological content. If we perceive the Weathermen's behavior as the representation of altruism and humanitarian concern, we are quite unlikely to introduce such acts into our concepts of primary prevention. On the other hand, if we view the same behavior as bordering on madness, then the behavior, the instigator and his background will be factors of concern in action programs. The tale of the Weathermen merely demonstrates our lack of clarity regarding the nature of deviance and normality. But, lacking such clarity, is it not premature for the mental health disciplines to assert a readiness to set forth on programs of primary prevention?

The place of action programs

Those concerned with the overwhelming problem of mental disorder nevertheless have every reason to ask: 'All right, then, what do we do – wait until we can collect a core of hard data and in the meantime mount no programs at all? Do we turn away from efforts to prevent the onset of disorder and direct our energies solely to the treatment of deviance when it appears?'

I would suggest two replies to these questions; one is pragmatic, the other strategic. No, we cannot sit still and by so doing add to the nation's festering crisis. We will initiate programs as best we can, hoping that through a juncture of heart and mind we can set up efforts at intervention that will restrict disorder, or at worst will do little to enhance its expression. The view seems an appropriate one since much intervention presumably will center on those programs that good government and a responsible society should maintain anyway: adequate prenatal, postnatal and infant care and nutrition; prevention of birth defect; economic security for citizens to insure family stability; extended support for education, including development of pre-school and school programs devoted to the enhancement of social and cognitive competence; a more adequately financed and more sophisticated network of social agencies dedicated to meeting the emotional and economic needs of citizens; a plan for the eradication of slums; the pledge of freedom from contaminants and pollutants, etc. Securing these goals is a worthy direction for any society to take. I would urge, however, that we do not oversell our power to reduce the numbers of mentally ill and that we do not proclaim to the nation that we stand on the threshold of a preventive break-through in psychiatry. Such a promise, emulating the unful-filled pledge of the mental health community clinic movement that it can provide the base for secondary and tertiary preven-tion, could bring us well-deserved condemnation from those who take our pledges and promises seriously. There is only one way to strengthen such a pledge, and that is to develop our knowledge of the phenomenon of deviance and its roots. And yet the entire governmental health apparatus is now being turned rapidly toward the delivery of health care services, while neglecting programs of research that in time might provide wiser methods for intervening in the cycle of pathology than those suggested by traditionalists.

A strategy for research

This brings me to my central concern, namely the strategies for research in psychopathology that may ultimately provide us with a more adequate return. Roberts (1968) has expressed the problem in this manner:

The development of programmes for primary prevention will require a clear recognition of the inadequacies as well as the possibilities of our present knowledge. Developments in this area must not be deferred because of the inadequacy of present knowledge, rather efforts must be made to prevent disorders and promote mental health. To the maximum extent possible, these efforts should be accompanied by research programmes which will, at this stage, be as much con-cerned with the development of methodology for such research as they will be with the monitoring of efforts in the field (p. 37).

One direction in research now being undertaken by investi-gators here and abroad centers on studies of 'high-risk groups' in what can be called generically *vulnerability research*. Vulner-ability research involves the selection of those children in a community who are at high risk for the later onset (typically in late adolescence and adulthood) of severe psychopathology. Selection criteria may be based on genetic loading within the family (as revealed by the psychiatric status of parents or relatives), evidence of excessive family disorganization or the undesirable effects generated by a disordered environment. In essence, the status of a child as 'vulnerable' or at 'high-risk' (as in the case of a genetic predisposition) typically is derived from the three basic models that characterize our speculations about the etiology of mental disorder: (1) genetic transmission of the predisposition or the diathesis; (2) pathological disorganization within the near environment (the family), or (3) within the molar (sociocultural) environment of the child. We can also identify a fourth model that is coming to prominence, although its applicability to adult psychopathology is not yet clear – one stressing deprivation within the prenatal and neonatal period in which faulty maternal care and inadequate nutrition can serve to render the infant vulnerable to subsequent stressors Pasamanick and Knobloch (1961) and Stabenau and Pollin (1967).

Once these children are selected, the study of their adaptation or maladaptation, compared with appropriate control groups, becomes the focus of investigation. To evaluate such adaptation, programs of research have used a long-term longitudinal focus (Mednick and Schulsinger, 1968), a relatively short-term prospective format (Anthony, 1968), or a cross-sectional design (Garmezy, 1970; Goldstein *et al.*, 1968).

Investigators of vulnerability in childhood have been concerned with a number of critical issues: the defining of vulnerable groups and attendant controls; the selection of variables to be studied; and the implications for intervention prior to the onset of disordered behavior in risk cases.

Defining high-risk groups and controls

As I have indicated, the determination of what constitutes a high-risk group is a function of one's etiological model. Thus, in the study of schizophrenia, the dominant models have included emphasis on genogenic, psychogenic and sociogenic factors. Of these three major orientations, selection on the basis of genetic disposition has clearly assumed the ascendant position in vulnerability research. To Mednick and Schulsinger (1968) must go the credit for initiating the study of high-risk children in a manner that stresses genetic loading: their method utilizes a schizophrenic-mother group as the cohort while their biological children serve as the probands. The expectation that, by this method of selection, the frequency of anticipated schizophrenic outcomes in such children would approximate 14 per cent clearly indicates its base in psychiatric genetics. Since then other projects have followed similar selection procedures, including those of Anthony (1968), Beisser, Glasser and Grant (1967), Rolf (1969) and Garmezy (1970). More recently Dr Erlenmeyer-Kimling (1968) has suggested that true high-risk would be more likely to be observed in offspring of marriages in which both parents are schizophrenic, since the prediction of ultimate schizophrenia for such a sample of children would range approximately between 40 and 50 per cent (Rosenthal, in press). Initial efforts by Erlenmeyer-Kimling to locate such children in New York State have convinced her of the viability of selecting for risk in this fashion, despite the manifold methodological difficulties that are involved.

The psychogenic orientation to schizophrenia finds its expression in the study of disordered families and disturbed modes of family interaction. To approach the study of vulnerability in this manner requires the identification of such families either through the medium of survey research, the selection of parents who are themselves being seen for treatment or diagnosis, or be centering on already disturbed children who are known to some clinical resource. The latter method makes two assumptions: that such severely disturbed children typically reflect a disordered or disorganized family; that such children, in time, also contribute heavily to the pool of adult behaviour pathology.

An example of subject selection based on a criterion of disturbed children within disordered families can be seen in the research program currently being conducted at UCLA by Rodnick, Goldstein and Judd (1968). This group is studying, through departmental clinic intake, groups of children whose differing behavioral modes (withdrawn, social isolation, acting out, passive aggression) may have certain components in common with the coping patterns of the schizophrenic patient. It is the expectation of these investigators that specific family patterns may relate to the form of symptom expression in the offspring, and, in time, may be shown to bear a patterning similar to that observed in families with a schizophrenic offspring. As a strategy for obtaining a high-risk sample, their method appears to have some solid virtues, for the subjects in the UCLA project have already slipped into schizophrenia at a rate not appreciably different from the rates observed by Mednick and Schulsinger in their Denmark project, in which selection is based on mothers' schizophrenia status. Wynne (1969) and Singer (1969), having in common an orientation to disorder espoused by the UCLA investigators, have recently suggested that a program of risk research be initiated with groups selected on the basis of deviant modes of parental communication, on the assumption that the preschizophrenic will more often be found among offspring within such family constellations. Thus one can start from a base of disordered families or disordered offspring with the common thread to be found in the importance assigned to faulty parent-child and parent-parent relationships. The search for disturbance is given a locus in the investigation of communication networks, role structure and transactional patterns within the family – an orientation far more sophisticated than that of the earlier studies that examined child-rearing patterns against such simplistic attributes as parental 'dominance', 'overprotection', 'rejection', etc.

A third source of vulnerability to schizophrenia is to be found in studies of the sociology of mental disorder and the inverse relationship that has been consistently found to exist between prevalence rates for schizophrenia and social status (Kohn, 1968). Whether one believes that such a correlation reflects the role of diathesis or stressor, the evidence of studies cast in a sociological context remains a challenge for high-risk researchers and a guide to the importance of social class variables in the design of their studies.

Controls

An examination of risk studies now underway reveals considerable diversity in the choice of controls. Many factors contribute to the heterogeneity that is evident in subject selection: theoretical views regarding aetiology, availability of various subject pools, beliefs about demographic variables that may contribute to later psychopathology, etc.

Most ongoing risk programs employ normal control subjects; the UCLA project does not, however, since it perceives controls to be present in the several constituent adolescent experimental groups that differ largely in the mode of symptom expression. Several projects have used other psychopathological groups as controls, although the reasons for the choice of the specific forms of disorder selected are not always evident.

In the first study of our own Minnesota high-risk project, Dr Jon Rolf (1969), now at the University of Vermont, measured the social and academic competence of a variety of high-risk, vulnerable and control groups. Rolf's cohorts included not only children born to schizophrenic mothers but those born to neurotic depressive mothers as well. Use of a third group of acting-out character disordered mothers was contemplated and then postponed when the logistical demands of Rolf's design became apparent.

The rationale behind the selection of these groups was not happenstance. Data drawn from a number of recent genetic studies of schizophrenia (Heston and Denny, 1968, Kety *et al.*, 1968) have suggested that there exists a *spectrum of schizophrenia* in which pathologic outcomes appear to cohere around schizophrenia, sociopathic personality and impulse disorders; tending to fall outside the spectrum are the depressions and anxiety neurosis. These data are congruent with symptom linkages suggested by Zigler and Phillips (1960) and by Phillips (1968). On these grounds the selection of groups of mothers whose disorders may be schizophrenia-linked together with representation of other non-linked psychopathologies (e.g. depression) would appear to be warranted in high-risk research. Such a method of selection would provide for manifest disturbance in mothers who varied in the adequacy of their premorbid and postmorbid adaptation.

Since the basis for selecting these cohorts does bear a strong genetic emphasis, efforts must also be made to tap groups that would reflect psychogenic speculations about schizophrenic outcomes. Here Rolf chose to focus on two types of disordered children who had already come to psychiatric attention. One group, termed *externalizers* Achenbach (1966) and Weintraub (1968), had been referred to clinics for destructive, acting-out behavior in the community; the second group comprised an internalizer set of children whose symptomatology included fearfulness, excessive inhibition, phobic and avoidance behaviors. Since there is strong evidence that anti-social behavior frequently eventuates in malignant outcomes including sociopathy and schizophrenia (Kohlberg, LaCrosse and Ricks, in press and Robins, 1966), whereas neurotic behaviors of children do not, the stage was set for the inclusion of these two groups in Rolf's study. This decision was given more meaning as a possible road into psychogenic hypothesizing by the empirical evidence of characteristically marked disorganization in the families of externalizing children – a situation that does not obtain to the same degree with children prone to internalizing symptomatology (Achenbach, 1966, and Weintraub, 1968).

An indirect test of the sociogenic hypothesis (although not a very adequate one) was attempted by Rolf, who chose a matched (for age, academic and intellectual ability, intactness of the family and occupation of the breadwinning parent) and a random control child within the same classroon in which each target child was finally located. Thus, for each child in the four vulnerable groups (schizophrenic and depressive mothers; externalizing and internalizing children), there were two controls who shared a comparable neighborhood setting with the child who was at high risk. Since many of these triads came from the more depressed and often less stable areas of the city, while others were drawn from stable, middle-class neighborhoods, it is possible to relate degrees of effectance in these children to area of residence.

Of course, a more adequate test of a sociogenic hypothesis will have to involve, among other things, an extended knowledge of community disorganization including incidence and prevalence rates for mental disorder, incarcerations, indigence, quality of adaptation of families selected randomly from high as well as low prevalence areas, a more extended study of the adjustment of children born within such families, etc. Nevertheless, Rolf's design suggests the complexity of a model necessary for testing the multiple hypotheses that have been posited regarding the aetiology of schizophrenia. Certainly, it seems likely at this point that the decision as to what kinds of groups evaluate in vulnerability research will prove to be far more complex than is evident in most projects now underway.

The choice of variables

What aspects of behavior may be most fruitfully studied in the high-risk child? Typically what one observes in reviewing risk research is that the researcher's decision may be based on a variety of considerations. Choices may be theoretically-based, as in the case of Mednick and Schulsinger's (1968) Denmark projects. Several of the most central dependent variables of this program involve measures of autonomic responsivity, latency of arousal and decay of the autonomic response, generalization and habituation. The source for such measures is to be found in Mednick's theory of the etiology of schizophrenia, in which he has placed great emphasis on these factors: (1) a biological predisposition for rapid arousal; (2) an attendant pattern of excessive generalization induced by the heightened anxiety state; (3) the reinforcement of deviant thought as an escape from anxiety arousal. But one need not be bound by the constraints of theory. The significance of variables to be studied may arise serendipitously, as can be perceived in Mednick's (1970) current preoccupation with prenatal and perinatal complications. Such complications appear to be present in the pregnancy and birth histories of those high-risk adolescents who are now beginning to show signs of significant mental aberration but are absent in comparison with high-risk healthy and normal control subjects.

Unfortunately, theoretical models for the origins of schizophrenia tend not to be circumscribed constructions. Thus, the choice of variables is a complex task for those who bear allegiance to the rather vague doctrine of diathesis-stress theory, since one cannot specify either the nature of the predisposition or the stress. As subscribers to such a view, David Rosenthal (1968) and his colleagues have faced this difficulty in trying to determine what factors to study in Danish adoptees who have been born to schizophrenic parents but reared in adoptive homes. Their selection of tasks to use in a two-day study of these adoptees, in which time considerations precluded their doing many things they had wished to do, was made on three bases: (1) tasks and procedures that had been shown consistently to distinguish schizophrenics from others; (2) assessment procedures to provide measures of more fundamental trait dispositions; and (3) the choice of other methods that had proved to be successful discriminators for other investigators.

My own view is this: I believe it best that we turn away from a premature fixation on global theorizing about the etiology of schizophrenia and engage in the search for relevant behavioral parameters that can differentiate high-risk-maladaptive from high-risk-adaptive children as well as risk from non-risk subjects. Until we have such a strong empirical predictive base, a long-term longitudinal project seems inadvisable. The ideal design compromise could well entail replicated cross-sectional studies employing Bell's (1963) convergence technique with short-term follow-up of different groups of children ranging in age from infancy to late adolescence. Unfortunately, the pattern of subject attrition we have observed within our own project may render such an idealized design difficult to achieve. Furthermore, the competencies of individual investigators will preclude attention to all age segments of the developmental sequence.

As for specific areas of investigation, perhaps some of the parameters we now deem most significant for programs of primary intervention could be tested within high-risk and vulnerability programs: studies of pregnancy and birth difficulties, investigations of stress and frustration tolerance, interaction studies of disordered parents and children, exploration of patterns of attachment and of socialization and dyssocialization, laboratory studies of social competence, peer acceptance, and of cognitive, motivational and perceptual adequacy. More specific studies of processes we know to be deficient in the disordered adult psychotic patient would also be warranted, such as measuring of attention and set, particular forms of cognitive styles (e.g., scanning), associative thought processes, psychophysiological responsivity in relation to arousal and feedback mechanisms, etc.

190 Schizophrenia

Goldstein (1969) has suggested that a focus on *behavioral continuities* (as exemplified by stimulus processing, deviant thinking, social isolation and withdrawal) be joined with investigations of *developmental continuities* initiated by those socio-environmental conditions that may shape pathology (family structure, family communication, child-rearing practices, etc.). Certainly at this point diversity appears to characterize the focus of high-risk projects, but Erlenmeyer-Kimling's (1968) suggestion that an effort be made to standardize some measures across studies of comparable high-risk *S*s seems worth implementing.

The issue of intervention

Finally, what can be said about the issue of intervention? A conservative viewpoint would hold that intervention, in the absence of knowledge about the process of pathological development, would be premature. And yet the ethical demands placed upon those who study high-risk children can be a powerful force that compels one to look, perhaps with hesitancy, upon the necessity of intervening irrespective of one's confidence in the tools that are available for efforts at prevention and containment. The needs may well be pressing. E. James Anthony (1968), who has underway a major program of risk research at Washington University in St Louis, testing the biological children of schizophrenic mothers or fathers, has found such striking instances of early pathology that he has established a special clinic in which these children can be treated.

We shall undoubtedly be called upon to intervene, but hopefully we can do so in a manner that will free us from the formalisms of contemporary therapeutics. By so doing, we may be able to learn more about these vulnerable children in a therapeutic framework that provides a rich source for observations about their adaptation.

In an earlier article (1970), I noted that:

At the turn of the century, Binet moved into the Paris school system to identify and to cope with those children who appeared unable to profit from instruction. Today there are a larger number of children in our schools whose emotional burdens prevent them from profiting from the one major institution of society that can liberate them from incompetence. Identifying and intervening in such situations requires the collaboration of researchers and practitioners in schools, communities, and clinics. Cognitive compensatory educational efforts for the disadvantaged low-risk child deserve to be matched with compensatory stress training efforts with the disadvantaged high-risk child (p. 234).

Perhaps in setting forth such compensatory programs we can adopt paradigms and models that in other contexts have been used to induce behavior change: the model of immunization against efforts at attitude change or models designed to foster such changes; the model of learned helplessness suggested by Seligman, Maier, Mowrer, Masserman and others; and the model of behavior change through the use of operant techniques. The questions for study are these: Can we adapt such methods for use with our high-risk children? Can we use our schools and clinics as centers for training these children in more adaptive techniques for coping? Can we use participation in successful play to increase the flexibility of the response repertoires of these children? Can we stimulate adaptive behavior by introducing into such training centers healthy children who can serve as models for the vulnerable child?

Perhaps the mediators of such change should be drawn not from the ranks of middle-class therapists and teachers but rather from mothers who, by attitude, value, and act, have proved capable of producing healthy children. Perhaps, too, we can select mothers drawn from inner-city families who have ably defended their children from the disorganizing consequences of high-risk environments. Such mothers, in many instances, may well be the major factor in the predisposition of their children toward health. Perhaps they can also be agents for helping other less fortunate children.

Invulnerability

In the study of high-risk and vulnerable children, we have come across another group of children whose prognosis could be viewed as unfavorable on the basis of familial or ecological factors but who upset our prediction tables and in childhood bear the visible indices that are hallmarks of competence: good peer relations, academic achievement, commitment to education and to purposive life goals, early and successful work histories. We have seen such children in our inner-city schools. Mary Engel (1967) has described them in her study, 'Children Who Work'. To these children I have assigned the term 'invulnerables'. School principals not only believe they can identify such children but they resonate to the hopefulness suggested by the concept of an 'invulnerable' child. They can produce instances from within their own school settings of children whose intellectual and social skills are not destroyed by the misfortunes they encounter in home and street.

Thus vulnerability research is also concerned with the children of the inner city, their predisposition to competence (or, in less fortunate circumstances, incompetence) and the various factors within the disadvantaged group that lead some toward disorder while others are seemingly immunized against disorganization. These are the 'vulnerables' and the 'invulnerables' of a society. 'Vulnerables' have long been the province of our mental health disciplines; but prolonged neglect of the 'invulnerable' child – the healthy child in an unhealthy setting – has provided us with a false sense of security in erecting prevention models that are founded more on values than on facts.

With our nation torn by strife between races and between social classes, these 'invulnerable' children remain the 'keepers of the dream'. Were we to study the forces that move such children to survival and to adaptation, the long-range benefits to our society might be far more significant than our many efforts to construct models of primary prevention designed to curtail the incidence of vulnerability.

References

ACHENBACH, T. M. (1966), 'The classification of children's psychiatric symptoms: a factor analytic study', *Psychol. Monogr.*, vol. 80, p. 37.

ANTHONY, E. J. (1968), 'The developmental precursors of adult schizophrenia', in D. Rosenthal and S. S. Kety (eds.), *The Transmission of Schizophrenia*, Pergamon.

BEISSER, A. R., GLASSER, N. and GRANT, M. (1967), 'Psychosocial adjustment in children of schizophrenic mothers', *J. nerv. ment. Dis.*, vol. 145, pp. 429–550.

BELL, R. Q. (1963), 'Convergence: An accelerated longitudinal approach', *Child Devel.*, vol. 24, pp. 145–52.

DUNHAM, H. W. (1965), *Community and Schizophrenia*, Wayne State University Press.

ENGEL, M. (1967), 'Children who work', *Arch. gen. Psychiat.*, vol. 17, pp. 291–7.

ERLENMEYER-KIMLING, L. (1968), 'Studies of the children of schizophrenic parents: Pointers for the analysis of gene-environment interaction', paper presented at the 124th annual meeting of the American Psychiatric Association.

FARIS, R. and DUNHAM, H. W. (1939), *Mental Disorders in Urban Areas*, University of Chicago Press.

FREUD, S. (1955), 'The psychogenesis of a case of homosexuality in a woman', in *The Standard Edition of the Complete Psychological Works of Sigmund Freud*, vol. 18, pp. 146–72, Hogarth Press and The Institute of Psycho-Analysis.

GARMEZY, N. (1970), 'Vulnerable children: implications derived from studies of an internalizing-externalizing symptom dimension', J. Zubin and A. M. Freedman, (eds.), in *Psychopathy of Adolescence*, Grune & Stratton.

GOLDSTEIN, M. (1969), 'Studies of high risk children: what to measure?' position statement, Workshop on Methodological Issues on Research with Groups at High Risk for the Development of Schizophrenia, Center for Studies of Schizophrenia, National Institute of Mental Health.

GOLDSTEIN, M. J. *et al.* (1968), 'A method for studying social influence and coping patterns within families of disturbed adolescents', *J. nerv. ment. Dis.*, vol. 147, pp. 233–51.

HAGGARD, E. A., BREKSTAD, A. and SKARD, A. (1960), 'On the reliability of the anamnesic interview', *J. ab. soc. Psychol.*, vol. 61, pp. 311–18.

HESTON, L. and DENNY, D. (1968), 'Interactions between early life experience and the biological factors in schizophrenia', in D. Rosenthal and S. S. Kety, (eds.), *The Transmission of Schizophrenia*, Pergamon.

KAPLAN, G. and GRUNEBAUM, H. (1967), 'Perspectives on primary prevention', *Arch. gen. Psychiat.*, vol. 17, pp. 331–46.

KARLSSON, J. L. (1966), *The Biologic Basis for Schizophrenia*, Charles C. Thomas.

KETY, S. S. *et al.* (1968), 'The types and prevalence of mental illness in the biological and adoptive families of adopted schizophrenics', in D. Rosenthal and S. S. Kety, (eds.), *The Transmission of Schizophrenia*, Pergamon.

KOHLBERG, L., LACROSSE, J. and RICKS, D. (in press), 'The predictability of adult mental health from childhood behavior', in B. B. Wolman, (ed.), *Handbook of Childhood Psychopathology*, McGraw-Hill.

KOHN, M. L. (1968), 'Social class and schizophrenia: a critical review', in D. Rosenthal and S. S. Kety, (eds.), *The Transmission of Schizophrenia*, Pergamon.

McNEIL, T. F. (1969), 'The relationship between creative ability and recorded mental illness', paper presented at Southeastern Psychological Association.

MEDNICK, S. A. (1970), 'Breakdown in individuals at high risk for schizophrenia: possible predispositional perinatal factors', *Ment. Hygiene*, vol. 54, pp. 50–63.

MEDNICK, S. A. and SHAFFER, J. (1964), 'Mothers' retrospective reports in child rearing research', *Amer. J. Orthopsychiat.*, vol. 33, pp. 461–547.

MEDNICK, S. A. and SCHULSINGER, F. (1968), 'Some premorbid characteristics related to breakdown in children with schizophrenic mothers', in D. Rosenthal and S. S. Kety, (eds.), *The Transmission of Schizophrenia*, Pergamon.

NOVEY, S. (1968), *The Second Look*, Johns Hopkins Press.

PASAMANICK, B. and KNOBLOCH, H. (1961), 'Epidemiologic studies on the complications of pregnancy and the birth process', in G. Kaplan, (ed.), *Prevention of Mental Disorders in Children*, Basic Books.

PHILLIPS, L. (1968), *Human Adaptation and Its Failures*, Academic Press.

ROBBINS, L. C. (1963), 'The accuracy of parental recall of aspects of child development and of child rearing practices'. *J. ab. soc. Psychol.*, vol. 66, pp. 261–70.

ROBERTS, C. A. (1968), F. C. R. CHALKE and J. J. DAY, (eds.), *Primary Prevention of Psychiatric Disorders*, University of Toronto Press.

ROBINS, L. N. (1966), *Deviant Children Grown Up*, Williams and Wilkins.

ROLF, J. E. (1969), 'The academic and social competence of school children vulnerable to behavior pathology', unpublished Ph.D. dissertation, University of Minnesota.

ROSENTHAL, D. (in press), *The Genetics of Psychopathology*, McGraw-Hill.

ROSENTHAL, D. *et al.* (1968), 'Schizophrenics' offspring reared in adoptive homes', in D. Rosenthal and S. S. Kety, (eds.), *The Transmission of Schizophrenia*, Pergamon.

ROSENTHAL, D. (1963), *The Genain Quadruplets*, Basic Books.

SINGER, M. T. (1969), 'Measuring verbal behavior in groups at high risk for schizophrenia: reasoning, roles, and scoring rationale', Workshop Position Statement: Worskhop on Methodological Issues on Research with Groups at High Risk for the Development of Schizophrenia, Center for Studies of Schizophrenia, National Institute of Mental Health.

STABENAU, J. R. and POLLIN, W. (1967), 'Early characteristics of monozygotic twins discordant for schizophrenia', *Arch. gen. Psychiat.*, vol. 17, pp. 723–34.

SUTTLES, G. D. (1968), *The Social Order of the Slum*, University of Chicago Press.

VISOTSKY, H. M. (1967), 'Primary prevention', in A. M. Freedman and H. I. Kaplan, (eds.), *Comprehensive Textbook of Psychiatry*, Williams and Wilkins.

WEINTRAUB, S. A. (1968), 'Cognitive and behavioral impulsivity in internalizing, externalizing and normal children', unpublished Ph.D. dissertation, University of Minnesota.

WEINAR, C. (1961), 'The reliability of mothers' histories', *Child Devel.*, vol. 32, pp. 491–500.

WYNNE, L. C. (1969), 'Strategies for sampling groups at high risk for the development of schizophrenia', Worskhop Position Statement, Workshop on Methodological Issues on Research with Groups at High Risk for the Development of Schizophrenia, Center for Studies of Schizophrenia, National Institute of Mental Health.

ZIGLER, E. and PHILLIPS, L. (1960), 'Social effectiveness and symptomatic behaviors', *J. ab. soc. Psychol.*, vol. 2, pp. 231–8.

Part Three
Psychopathy

Dr Cleckley's book, *The Mask of Sanity*, has been the stimulus for most of the experimental research that has been conducted into the problem of psychopathy. It is one of the best examples available of careful clinical observation leading to hypotheses (not conclusions) which can then be put to controlled test. The wealth of clinical anecdote with which each point is illustrated renders it difficult to find any one sequential extract from the book that might serve to present his hypotheses in a systematic fashion. The extract in this volume consists of several portions of the text selected and assembled to be maximally coherent, while letting Cleckley's own views be presented in his own words.

From Cleckley's hypothesis there has developed naturally a major interest in the psychobiology of the psychopath's emotional experience – or lack of it. A *prima facie* credence must be given to the possibility that the psychopath is deficient in those bodily responses that give rise to the emotional experiences of anxiety, pity and the like. Hare, one of the major investigators of the present time, examines this explanation and presents the pertinent data in his paper here. The paper is not previously published elsewhere and it provides a new synthesis of findings from several related lines of research on the topic.

10 H. Cleckley

Psychopathy: A Basic Hypothesis and Description

Excerpted from H. Cleckley, *The Mask of Sanity*, Mosby, 4th edn, 1964, pp. 404–54.

In the attempt to arrive at an applicable conception, one consistent with the facts of our observation, I find it necessary first of all to postulate that the psychopath has a genuine and very serious disability, or disorder, or deviation. To say that he is merely queer or perverse or in some borderline state between health and illness does little or nothing to account for the sort of behavior he demonstrates objectively and obviously. The practice, quite popular until recent years, of classifying the disorder of these patients, no matter how plain their incapacity to lead normal lives, as (1) no nervous or mental disease and (2) psychopathic personality, whatever the sanctions afforded by tradition, emerges not only as an error but also as an absurdity when we honestly examine the material to which such terms are applied.

Let us for a moment consider the essential evidence brought out in staff meetings on which experienced psychiatrists establish in an obvious case the diagnosis of schizophrenia and on which legal action is taken to declare the patient psychotic and incompetent (insane) and commit him for treatment. In the brief summarizing statement to support such opinions we often find such words as these:

The history shows that he has failed repeatedly to make a satisfactory adjustment in the social group. His actions indicate serious impairment of judgment and show that he cannot be relied upon to conduct himself with ordinary regard for the safety of himself or of others. His irrational and unacceptable behavior has, furthermore, occurred without normal or adequate motivation. He shows no real insight into his condition and tends often to project the sources of his troubles to the environment. His emotional reactions are grossly impaired and he has repeatedly shown inappropriate or inadequate affect. We may say, then, that he is psychotic, incompetent, incapable of carrying on the usual activities of life, and in need of close supervision.

Such facts have often constituted more convincing evidence for the diagnosis of schizophrenia than the delusions and hallucinations also frequently present but sometimes not demonstrable in that psychosis. All of these statements just recorded (excepting only the one word 'psychotic') may be applied with full validity to the psychopath. This, of course, does not make him a patient with schizophrenia but it does, I maintain, afford grounds for saying he has a grave psychiatric disorder, and grounds that cannot be dismissed lightly. Although I insist on the gravity of his disorder, I frankly admit that it is a different kind of disorder from all those now recognized as seriously impairing competency. It is a disorder that differs more widely in its general features from any of those than they differ from one another.[1]

1. After some years of experience with them, I was forced to conclude that, theoretical technicalities notwithstanding, severe psychopaths showed a disorder more like the disorder of those classed as psychotic than the mild or questionable deviation presumed by official psychiatric standards. It was therefore interesting in 1938 to encounter an opinion expressed by Karl Menninger about patients of this type.

After stating that in his earlier psychiatric experience he regarded alcohol addiction as a bad habit and a little later as a neurotic manifestation, Menninger adds, 'Now I regard it as near a psychosis.' He also states, 'I would be inclined, if one of my young relatives had to have either schizophrenia or addiction to alcohol, to believe that his chances for getting back into normal life would be greater if he had schizophrenia.' (Discussion of Knight, 1938.)

Although the term psychopathic personality was not used to designate the patients of whom Menninger speaks, it is plain that he is referring to the underlying personality disorder and not to the direct effects of drinking. I feel that this personality disorder is the one discussed here. This term is, in fact, used by the author of the paper Menninger is discussing, and there seems no reason to doubt that it is the psychopath to whom these statements apply and not reactive or neurotic drinkers.

In view of our current practice of calling persons diagnosed as sociopathic personality legally sane and, in many institutions, of judging them ineligible for treatment, an opinion of such disorders expressed in 1804 by John Cox is significant. Dr Cox wrote, 'Persons of this description might appear actuated by a bad heart, but the experienced physician knows that it is the head and not the heart which is defective.' (Cited in Henderson, D. K., 1939.)

The first and most striking difference is this: In all the ortho-dox psychoses, in addition to the criteria just mentioned, or to some of these criteria, there is a more or less obvious alteration of reasoning processes or of some other demonstrable person-ality feature. In the psychopath this is not seen. The observer is confronted with a convincing mask of sanity. All the outward features of this mask are intact; it cannot be displaced or pene-trated by questions directed toward deeper personality levels. The examiner never hits upon the chaos sometimes found on searching beneath the outer surface of a paranoid schizophrenic. The thought processes retain their normal aspect under psychia-tric investigation and in technical tests designed to bring out obscure evidence of derangement. Examination reveals not merely an ordinary two-dimensional mask but what seems to be a solid and substantial structural image of the sane and rational personality. He is then, in the full literal sense, an example of Trélat's expressive term, *la folie lucide*. Furthermore, this per-sonality structure in all theoretical situations functions in a manner apparently identical with that of normal, sane func-tioning. Logical thought processes may be seen in perfect opera-tion no matter how they are stimulated or treated under experi-mental conditions. Furthermore, the observer finds verbal and facial expressions, tones of voice, and all the other signs we have come to regard as implying conviction and emotion and the normal experiencing of life as we know it ourselves and as we assume it to be in others. All judgements of value and emotional appraisals are sane and appropriate when the psychopath is tested in verbal examinations.

Only very slowly and by a complex estimation or judgement based on multitudinous small impressions does the conviction come upon us that, despite these intact rational processes, these normal emotional affirmations, and their consistent application in all directions, we are dealing here not with a complete man at all but with something that suggests a subtly constructed reflex machine which can mimic the human personality perfectly. This smoothly operating psychic apparatus reproduces consistently not only specimens of good human reasoning but also appro-priate simulations of normal human emotion in response to nearly all the varied stimuli of life. So perfect is this reproduction of a whole and normal man that no one who examines him in a clinical setting can point out in scientific or objective terms why, or how, he is not real. And yet we know or feel we know that reality, in the sense of full, healthy experiencing of life, is not here.

Fortunately for the purpose of this discussion, but unfortunately indeed in any other light, an objective demonstration is available which coincides perfectly with our slowly emerging impression. The psychopath, however perfectly he mimics man theoretically, that is to say, when he speaks for himself in words, fails altogether when he is put into the practice of actual living. His failure is so complete and so dramatic that it is difficult to see how such a failure could be achieved by anything less than a downright *madman*[2] or by a person totally or almost totally unable to grasp emotionally the major components of meaning or feeling implicit in the thoughts that he expresses or the experiences he appears to go through. In the actions of his living, then, he confirms our subjective impression, or it might be said that our surmise coincides with the objective and demonstrable facts.

Let us then assume, as a hypothesis, that the psychopath's disorder or his difference from the whole or normal or integrated personality consists of an unawareness and a persistent lack of ability to become aware of what the most important experiences of life mean to others. By this is not meant an acceptance of the arbitrarily postulated values of any particular theology, ethics, aesthetics, or philosophic system, or any special set of mores or ideologies, but rather the common substance of emotion or purpose, or whatever else one chooses to call it, from which the various loyalties, goals, fidelities, commitments, and concepts of honor and responsibility of various groups and various people are formed.[3] Let us assume that this dimension of

2. This violent and unfortunate term I use with apology but cannot spare here because of its clear-cut emphasis.

3. A vast difference exists, of course, between what various persons regard as good or beautiful or desirable. John Locke observed that 'those who are canonized as saints among the Turks lead lives that we cannot with modesty there relate.' 'An apple by Paul Cézanne is of more consequence artistically than the head of a Madonna by Raphael,' is the initial sentence in a work on painting. In contrast with all the various diversities of view-

experience which gives to all experience its substance or reality is one into which the psychopath does not enter. Or, to be more accurate, let us say that he enters, but only so superficially that his reality is thin or unsubstantial to the point of being insignificant. Let us say that, despite his otherwise perfect functioning, the major emotional accompaniments are absent or so attenuated as to count for little. Of course he is unaware of this, just as everyone is bound, except theoretically, to be unaware of that which is out of his scale or order or mode of experience. If we grant the experience of a far-reaching and persistent blocking, absence, deficit, or dissociation of this sort, we have all that is needed, at the present level of our inquiry, to account for the psychopath.

The effort to express what is meant by experiencing life in a full sense, or by awareness of a solid emotional contact, runs through the psychoanalytic literature, which so often stresses the difference between an actual, or emotionally participating, understanding of some important situation and a mere verbal or academic understanding, however complete in that dimension. (Alexander, 1948; Lorand, 1944.)

This point is also implicit in the concepts of psychobiology, which, by its very definition of terms, shows that it is striving to emphasize the wholeness of experience or the full meaning of reactions. (Billings, 1939; Diethelm, 1936; Muncie, 1948). . . . Without suffering or enjoying in significant degree the integrated emotional consequences of experience, the psychopath will not learn from it to modify and direct his activities as other men whom we call sane modify and direct theirs. He will lack the real driving impulses which sustain and impel others toward their various widely differing but at least subjectively important goals. He will naturally lack insight into how he differs from other men, for of course he does not differ from other men as he sees them. It is entirely impossible for him to see another person from the aspect of major affective experience, since he is blind to this order of things or blind in this mode of awareness.

---

point and degrees of conviction found among ordinary people, the so-called psychopath holds no real viewpoint at all and is free of any sincere conviction in what might be called either good or evil.

It must be granted of course that the psychopath has some affect. Affect is, perhaps, a component in the sum of life reactions even in the unicellular protoplasmic entity. Certainly in all mammals it is obvious. The relatively petty states of pleasure, vexation, animosity, etc., experienced by the psychopath have been mentioned. The opinion here maintained is that he fails to know all those more serious and deeply moving affective states which make up the tragedy and triumph of ordinary life, of life at the level of important human experience. Such capacities vary widely, of course, among normal people and are perhaps proportionate to the general personality development, or, in a far-reaching sense, to true cultural level. The scope or the substantiality of such reactions, if they could be accurately and objectively estimated, would, perhaps more than any other criteria, make it possible to judge how successful and how complete an experiment in nature (Meyer, 1938) a particular person has proved to be. A Beethoven, a Dante, or an Aeschylus, if his real inner life is faithfully represented in his works, would probably present no less a contrast in this aspect with the illiterate peasant or the successful criminal than in objective accomplishments. Nevertheless, no normal person is so unevolved and no ordinary criminal so generally unresponsive and distorted, that he does not seem to experience satisfaction, love, hate, grief, and a general participation in life at human personality levels much more intense and more substantial than the affective reactions of the psychopath. Our concept of the psychopath's functioning postulates a selective defect or elimination which prevents important components of normal experience from being integrated into the whole human reaction, particularly an elimination or attenuation of those strong affective components that ordinarily arise in major personal and social issues.

However intelligent, he only assumes that other persons are moved by and experience the ghostly facsimiles of emotion or pseudoemotion known to him. However quick and rational a person may be and however subtle and articulate his teacher, he cannot be taught awareness of significance which he fails to feel.[4] He can learn to use the ordinary words and, if he is very clever,

4. 'Intellect is invisible to the man who has none.' (From Schopenhauer's *Essays*, 'Our Relation to Others'.)

even extraordinarily vivid and eloquent words which signify these matters to other people. He will also learn to reproduce appropriately all the pantomime of feeling; but, as Sherrington said of the decerebrated animal (Sherrington, 1923), the feeling itself does not come to pass.

Even his splendid logical faculties will, in real life situations, produce not actual reasoning but that imitation of reasoning known as rationalization, for in the synthesis by which reasoning contributes to sound judgement, the sense of value, that is, the value of truth and feeling, cannot be missing. When this is missing, the process is only rationalization, something which, however technically brilliant, does not satisfactorily guide and shape action. And no difference between the two is more fundamental. (Clutton-Brock, 1923).

When we conceive of the thought, the emotional responses, the general psychic processes, and the behavior of a person in whom is postulated a defect of this sort, we have arrived at something identical or all but identical with the psychopath as he appears in actual life.

When we say that a disorder at deep levels of personality integration prevents experience from becoming adequately meaningful to the subject, we become vulnerable to the accusation of talking nonsense. It is easy indeed to become unclear, if not to appear actually ridiculous, in attempting to express a point, however tentatively, on these fundamental matters. One commentator says of the concept here advanced:

If that [understanding of the meaning of life] is the disease from which the psychopathic inferior suffers, this term can be applied to most of us and certainly to the reviewer, since, so far as he knows, no one has yet given us an insight into the meaning of life.[5]

Such a comment is appealing and not without humor, but it scarcely meets the issue in a responsible manner. We need not assume that a normal man understands the ultimate purpose of life or even that he is remotely near final accuracy in his evaluations of his own bits of experience in order to believe that the psychopath is, in comparison, seriously disabled by the specific deficiency we are attempting to formulate.

5. From book review: *The New England Journal of Medicine*: 349, 1941.

Although 'meaning' or 'the meaning of life' can be applied to a philosophic or religious system that attempts to explain man and the universe, it must be obvious that such an application is not intended here. By saying that a good deal of the affective substance which people find in life experiences is lacking in the psychopath's responses, we seek only to point out that he is not adequately moved and that he does not find subjective stimuli to make the major issues of life matter sufficiently to promote consistent striving. Furthermore, he cannot achieve true and abiding loyalty to any principle or any person. It is difficult, perhaps, to express anything about such a matter without inviting misunderstanding. Such an affective alteration of fundamental experience is generally granted in the schizophrenic, who shows superficial indications of it. In the psychopath, although it is so strongly indicated by his conduct, this alteration is well masked by his misleading surface. It should not be said that such an estimate can be scientifically proved in either case, or that any subjective state in another can be so established.

There are other theories that attempt to explain the disorder without taking into consideration the question of such a defect. Alexander has assumed that the psychopath's behavior arises from forces similar to those which in the psychoneurotic are by many believed to be the fundamental cause of his distressing symptoms. (Alexander, 1930, 1948). Postulating unconscious conflict and repressed impulses also in the psychopath, he was led to believe that the asocial, unprofitable, and self-damaging acts of the psychopath are purposive and unconsciously motivated expressions of the conflict. In the classic neurosis, subjective symptoms develop and the patient complains of weakness, headache, or obsessions or develops compulsive rituals, conversion paralysis, blindness, etc. As these manifestations are thought to be reactions of the organism to inner stress, reactions that serve the purpose of protection, relief of anxiety, and gratification (by substitution or displacement, etc.) of rejected or frustrated impulses, so, too, according to Alexander, the pathologic behavior of the other type of patient is an acting out of impulses similarly neurotic. Thus interpreted, the psychopath has, in a sense, genuine and adequate reasons (like the neurotic for his symptoms) for the apparently foolish and uncalled-for things he does that damage himself and others. He himself does not know the reasons or clearly recognize his aims or the real nature of the impulses, and his acts do not constitute a wise solution for his problem; but the acts, according to Alexander, are purposive. This concept of the psychopath as acting out the neurotic problem (in contrast with the more passive development of ordinary symptoms) has been generally accepted by psychoanalysts (Fenichel, 1945; Levin, 1940; Lorand, 1944; Menninger, 1938). It is an interesting concept but it rests chiefly on psychoanalytic theories and assumptions about the unconscious and not upon regularly demonstrable evidence.

Some interpretations of schizophrenia (Fenichel, 1945) assume that it is largely through the relatively undamaged remnants of the personality that the positive features of the psychosis emerge. If the process is complete, if the personality has, so to speak, entirely dissolved in the underlying id, the machinery to express most of the usual symptoms will be lacking. In response to stress and conflict, what remains of the personality produces, by familiar mechanisms, most of what is generally regarded as characteristic of the disorder. The more fundamental feature, and the one that particularly distinguishes schizophrenia from the psychoneuroses, is the disintegration of the personality (Freud, 1942). In the psychopath we maintain there is also a generalized disorder of the personality that can be compared with schizophrenia and contrasted with ordinary psychoneurosis (in which the personality is 'intact' and the organism maintains 'sane' social relations, etc.). It cannot be said that the disorder is that of schizophrenia, but in the whole of the patient's life we find such inadequacy of response, such failure of adaptation, that it seems plausible to postulate alterations more fundamental and more extensive than in classic psychoneurosis.

Beyond the symptomatic acts of the psychopath, we must bear in mind his reaction to his situations, his general experiencing of life. Typical of psychoneurosis are anxiety, recognition that one is in trouble, and efforts to alter the bad situation. These are natural ('normal') whole personality reactions to localized symptoms. In contrast, the severe psychopath, like those so long called psychotic, does not show normal responses to the situation. It is offered as an opinion that a less obvious but nonetheless real pathology is general, and that in this he is more closely allied with the psychotic than with the psycho-neurotic patient. The pathology might be regarded not as gross fragmentation of the personality but as a more subtle alteration. Let us say that instead of macroscopic disintegration our (hypothetical) change might be conceived of as one that seriously curtails function without obliterating form.

In addition to outwardly visible demolition or shattering in material structures, other changes may occur. These may be intracellular and leave the appearance unchanged but greatly alter the substance. Colloidal variations in concrete may rob it of its essential properties although the appearance of the material remains unaltered. Steel under certain conditions is said to crystallize and lose much of its strength. The steel so affected looks the same as any other and no outer evidence of the molecular rearrangement which has so greatly altered the substance can be detected. For the purpose of analogy, one can consider not only intracellular or molecular but also intra-molecular changes. Let us think of the personality in the psycho-path as changed in some such way. The form is perfect and the outlines are undistorted. But being subtly and profoundly altered, it can successfully perform only superficial activities or pseudofunctions. It cannot maintain important or meaningful interpersonal relations. It cannot fulfill its purpose of adjusting adequately to social reality. Its performance can only mimic these genuine functions.

Karl Menninger in *Man Against Himself* (1938), pictures-quely developed the argument that antisocial behavior some-times represents an indirect search for punishment, a veiled but essentially self-destructive activity. The hypothesis of an active 'death instinct' advanced by Freud is, in this dramatic study, applied to many types of disorder (Alexander, 1929; Freud, 1942). In localized symptoms as well as in broad maladjust-ments, self-damaging impulses are interpreted as fulfilling their negative purpose.

In the patients presented here the general pattern of life seems to be more complex. Although thefts are sometimes committed, checks forged, and fraud perpetrated under circumstances that invite or even assure detection, similar deeds are also frequently carried out with shrewdness and foresight that are difficult to account for by such an interpretation. It is also characteristic for the real psychopath to resent punishment and protest indignantly against all efforts to curtail his activities by jail sentences or hospitalization. He is much less willing than the ordinary person to accept such penalties. In the more circumscribed symptoms of acting out, in many of the disorders referred to by Fenichel (1945) as impulse neuroses, the unconscious but purposive quest for punishment might more plausibly be conceived of as a major or regular influence (Roche, 1942). The validity of such an assumption, however, whether or not it is plausible, must be determined by what actual evidence can be produced to establish it, and not by mere surmises and inferences about what may or may not be in the unconscious. . . .

If, in the so-called psychopath, we have a patient profoundly limited in ability to participate seriously in the major aims of life, how, we might inquire, did he get that way? Reference has been made to the traditional viewpoint from which it was assumed that an inborn organic defect left these people 'constitutionally inferior' or 'moral imbeciles', etc. Such a congenital defect, it must be readily admitted, may exist and may account for the failure to experience life normally and hence to react sanely.

During the earlier decades of the twentieth century this concept of the psychopath prevailed. It was widely believed that these patients, often called 'constitutional inferiors', came almost exclusively from families loaded with *stigmata of degeneration* and *signs of neuropathic taint* (Healy, 1915). As time passed it was noted that typical psychopaths were also seen in families of very respectable, ethical, and successful people and were entirely free from all physical *stigmata of degeneration*. Many pointed out that some of the statistical studies giving evidence of hereditary factors are not as reliable as they were once thought. Even the famous studies of the Jukes and the Jonathan Edwards families have been severely criticized and called fallible by some (Sutherland, 1939).

As already mentioned, Healy (1936; Healy and Bronner,

1926) long ago pointed out that antisocial behavior often seemed to occur as a response to unhappy life situations, and Alexander formulated such disorder in psychoanalytic terms as a purposive acting out of unconscious pathologic conflicts (Alexander, 1930, 1948).

The concept of acting out, in lightly disguised symbolic deeds, might be vividly illustrated in a case reported in which a man responded to what is often spoken of as being in the doghouse by putting on his dog's collar and spectacularly caricaturing canine behavior. Another response to a similar situation can be found in a patient who literally got into a kennel at the veterinarian's and so exhibited himself. Although these incidents picturesquely illustrate Alexander's concept of acting out, they do not in themselves constitute evidence of an unconscious conflict which he has assumed causes the behavior. Neither patient showed any reaction that would support belief in the presence of inner, unconscious feelings of guilt or of the type of conflict attributed to sociopaths in such interpretations. The assumption of such guilt in these two patients must be made purely on faith in the theory.[6]

Many other psychiatrists have attempted to explain the psychopath in terms of psychogenic causation. The studies of Greenacre (1945) led her to conclude that the confusing influence of a stern, authoritarian father and an indulgent or frivolous mother is common in the early background of the psychopath. It is plausible to feel that such an influence might contribute to rebellious reactions and to a defective development of conscience and of ordinary social and personal evaluations. Karpman (1940, 1941a, 1941b, 1946) in his extensive work with character and behavior disorders, offers the opinion that in most cases a psychogenic etiology can be established if adequate investigation is made. A relatively small percentage of those we call psychopaths, he believes, are not so motivated. These, presumably disordered because of inborn or constitutional defect, he distinguishes from the majority and calls anethopaths (Karpman, 1941a).

Knight's studies (1937, 1938) of severe alcoholics, many of

6. *Editor's footnote:* Here the author is referring to individual case histories reported in detail earlier in the book.

whom were considered psychopaths, led him to believe that they often had a 'parental background characterized by inconsistency and lack of unanimity in parental discipline resulting in conflicting unstable identifications in the son'. A weak, pampering mother in combination with a domineering father whose severity was fitful and inconsistent appeared frequently in the background of Knight's cases. He feels that important casual relations between this early situation and the subsequent disorder are likely. Knight says:

Innumerable personality shadings and accents are possible from a son's reaction to such parental management, but one regular result seems to be the fostering of excessive passive demands and expectations in the son, such passive, childish, feminine wishes being in marked conflict with masculine strivings inculcated by the father and by the cultural ideology absorbed from schooling and from contacts with other males (from Knight, 1938).

Adelaide Johnson (Johnson, 1949, 1959; Johnson and Szurek, 1954) has expressed a strong conviction that the delinquency of a child or teen-ager is sometimes caused by the parents' own *unconscious* impulses toward antisocial conduct. The child or teen-ager, she tells us, is craftily used as a pawn and unconsciously encouraged in theft, arson, sexual promiscuity, violence, or sexual perversion in order to fulfill the parents' unconscious emotional needs to carry out such conduct themselves. According to this formulation, the child, even after he has become an adult, remains unconscious of the parents' adverse influence and of his real motives for antisocial conduct. Furthermore, Johnson reports that the parents are often unwilling to give up their vicarious criminal satisfactions and that they may actively block the psychiatrist's attempts at therapy. Such an explanation has been accepted as a common cause for the sociopath's disorder by a number of prominent psychiatrists (Noyes and Kolb, 1963).

Perhaps there are delinquents and sociopaths in whom such influences play an important part. Let us remember, however, that some methods of trying to determine what is in the unconscious may allow us unwittingly to project items from our theories into the assumed motivation of the patient and also of his parents. If persistent but unconscious antisocial impulses are really active in the parents, we might also ask ourselves if such tendencies might have been conveyed to the offspring by hereditary factors. I think it very unlikely that the parents of the patients presented here and of the others studied by me found satisfaction, unconsciously or otherwise, in the persistent misconduct of their sons and daughters.

Lindner (1944) devoted almost an entire volume, *Rebel Without a Cause*, to the detailed report of one psychopath studied by hypnoanalytic methods. He believed that through processes of preverbal memory he was able to obtain from the patient a true report of significant and traumatic experiences which he dated as occurring at six or eight months of age. Lindner gives a detailed and ingenious explanation of how he believes these experiences caused the patient to develop seriously disturbed relations with his parents and eventually to adopt the typical role of the sociopath. Despite the strong convictions of Lindner, his excellent presentation, and the superb title of his book, there is much that makes me skeptical about the significance of experiences reported as having occurred at such an early age and about the validity of what may be recalled through preverbal memory or established chiefly by the interpretation of symbols and dreams.

One reason for my skepticism is derived from startling and at times fantastic accounts of events in infancy or very early childhood occasionally given to me by my own patients. Let us consider briefly two examples:

One man, thirty-five years of age, told in vivid detail, under repeated hypnotic investigations, of having been brutally snatched away from the mother's lactating breast by the father, who replaced him and nursed her – forcibly, brusquely, but thoroughly – meanwhile immobilizing her despite her struggles, protests, and screams. Conscious and very overt incestuous impulses toward the mother during his early years and frank and bitter murderous wishes toward the father were spontaneously expressed and with vehemence. Vivid conscious desires to 'crawl up into my mother's womb' were enthusiastically voiced. Much more material equally impressive was elicited, including particularly traumatic details about his reactions to sexual relations between the parents which he claimed to have witnessed frequently during the first year of his life and which he described in spectacular detail. Almost any of his dreams could be interpreted by popular methods to confirm the presence of persistent oedipal problems, as well as problems often ascribed to oral and anal phases of development.

A seventeen-year-old boy claimed similarly unusual experiences. Many details emerged suggesting profound bewilderment, hate, fear, maximal insecurity and subtly and grossly incestuous drives that arose from experiences reported as occurring at the age of three years. These centered about a partial and mystified sensing of major unhappiness in the mother, who sometimes shrieked, wept, or appeared to be at the point of death because of something she complained of to the father, whom she called vile, merciless, a fraud, and a fiend. No clear understanding arose from his repeatedly being taken along by the father (apparently as a screen against the mother's suspicion) on adulterous ventures. He offered details of the scene in which, left to play on the floor of an adjoining room, he overheard much that puzzled him. He described very convincingly a grandfather's clock in the place of rendezvous behind which he sometimes hid so that he could obtain a view of the copulating couple. He claimed that stresses and confusions of the most drastic nature affected him during this period.

Some, but by no means all, of this material impressed me from the first as probably representing fabrication or fantasy confused with memory rather than accurately recalled facts. In the two cases just mentioned, as investigation proceeded, so many implausible events were recounted that it became evident none could be accepted as necessarily factual. Anything the examiner chose to seek was readily produced by the patient and elaborated with marvelous conviction. This proclivity in some patients may play a significant part in explaining how conscientious therapists find confirmation for widely differing and sometimes contradictory theories during prolonged investigations of a patient's infantile experiences and unconscious attitudes. It has tended to make me increasingly cautious about accepting as necessarily true historical data even from much later periods of life from patients of this type. It has often been noted that the psychopath will very convincingly report entirely false incidents and attitudes in others, particularly in parents, that tend to put responsibility for his difficulties upon them.

It is also true that experiences ordinarily withheld or deeply repressed in other people are often quickly and readily divulged by these patients. Disgraceful and extremely uninviting deeds are sometimes reported with a relish that suggests pride in them. Although shame and terrible conflict are sometimes claimed in such matters and superficial indications of such claims may be impressive, I am unable to feel that I regularly get at any level with the patient in which such affects are major or even quite real. This is a factor deserving constant attention, for it can enter very subtly into material obtained from patients of this sort. The point most difficult to corroborate, in my own experience, is the actual or innermost personal reaction of these patients to the events they report. It is more difficult than with others to tell what the events mean to them.

Some comments made by Jenkins are pertinent, it seems to me, to the question of whether or not psychopaths are acting out a conflict based upon unconscious feelings of guilt.

Effective challenge to a basic faith always causes pain and a reaction ridden with emotion in which the issues can easily become clouded. . . . This challenge has been felt by some of the defenders of the modern psychodynamic faith which, at least initially, tended to a narrow conception that functional mental disorders and maladjustments are always due to conflicts within the personality. To enlarge this concept with a realization that morbid conditions and gross maladjustments may be due primarily to a *lack* of conflict within the personality represents a readjustment of thinking which is apparently beyond the flexibility of many professional persons. There is of course, a semantic problem involved. It was not difficult for mankind to understand poisoning, for it is easy to grasp the proposition, 'what he ate made him sick'. The understanding of the vitamin deficiency disease was more difficult because of the greater semantic difficulty of the proposition, 'what he did not eat made him sick' Hardin (1957). Yet this second proposition is as true and as necessary to any adequate consideration of illness as is the first. In the same way many of our dynamically oriented colleagues have great difficulty with the proposition, 'The conflict he does not have makes him a psychopath.' This concept is true and necessary, but requires at least a flexible application of classical psychodynamic theory.

Theories are advantageous when they stimulate some resourceful new attack on a problem. They are handicapping when they make it difficult for us to recognize important facts. . . .

. . . If indeed we must get into the area of theory – and this is not entirely avoidable – I should like to propose that psychopaths differ from psychoneurotics and indeed contrast with them in their most important characteristics. The typical psychopath and the typical psychoneurotic are, in some important regards, on opposite sides of the normal. Where the psychoneurotic suffers from excessive inner conflict, the psychopath makes others suffer from his lack of inner conflict. Only the person who does not come in contact with serious cases of this sort, or whose mind is literally imprisoned by his faith in a theory, can brush aside this fundamental difference (from Jenkins, 1960).

I have become increasingly convinced that some of the popular methods presumed to discover what is in the unconscious cannot be counted upon as reliable methods of obtaining evidence. They often involve the use of symbolism and analogy in such a way that the interpreter can find virtually anything that he is looking for. Freud, for instance, from a simple dream reported by a man in his middle twenties as having occurred at four years of age, drew remarkable conclusions. The four-year-old boy dreamed of seeing six or seven white wolves sitting in a tree. Freud interpreted the dream in such a way as to convince himself that the patient at eighteen months of age had been shocked by seeing his parents have intercourse three times in succession and that this played a major part in the extreme fear of being castrated by his father which Freud ascribes to him at four years of age. No objective evidence was ever offered to support this conclusion. Nor was actual fear of castration ever made to emerge into the light of consciousness despite years of analysis (Cleckley, 1957; Freud, 1943).

In dwelling on the pitfalls and possibilities of error that we face in attempts to explain the sociopath's disorder on a psychogenic basis, I do not mean to discount sober efforts to accomplish this by realistic methods. Let us, however, be cautious and tentative and try always to distinguish surmise from evidence.

I have noted incidents in the early life of some sociopaths that might serve as factors likely to promote rebellion against society, distort the normal aims of life, interfere with the development of basic values, and go far, perhaps, toward accounting for much of the behavior so familiar to all who know them well. Some of these early experiences might indeed go far toward explaining their emotional status that has been so effectively and succinctly summarized by William and Joan McCord in their excellent book. They say:

The psychopath feels little, if any, guilt. He can commit the most appalling acts, yet view them without remorse. The psychopath has a warped capacity for love. His emotional relationships, when they exist, are meager, fleeting, and designed to satisfy his own desires. These last two traits, guiltlessness and lovelessness, conspicuously mark the psychopath as different from other men (McCord and McCord, 1956).

But similar experiences also can be demonstrated in the background of many well-adjusted, happy, and successful adults. In a few of the cases reported here an impressive account was given of incidents and reported reactions (with indications of emotion) that could theoretically be said to explain emotional withdrawal (despite maintenance of excellent rational contact) from the areas or levels of living in which severe hurt, deep joy, genuine pride, shame, dignity, and love are encountered and experienced. Protest reactions, loss of insight, an acting out of unconscious impulses, a behavioral caricature, or a diatribe against life and its (for the psychopath) subjective emptiness could be interpreted as major causal factors in the disorder we encounter clinically. Such interpretations may be correct, but usually there are more elements of assumption or speculation than of evidence in what is offered in support of the argument.

A very large percentage of the psychopaths I have studied show backgrounds that appear condusive to happy development and excellent adjustment. Whatever part psychogenic factors may play, I am inclined to believe that there may be an important relationship between the abstruse, paradoxically compounded, and ambivalent nature of the influences and the complex and deeply masked nature of the disorder such factors may shape. If such a relationship exists, it may to some degree explain the special difficulties we have encountered in obtaining from the psychopath convincing subjective information about what has happened and about how he was affected by it.

In the patients presented here, social service reports and all ordinary information usually indicated normal and helpful family attitudes and general environments. The families themselves often impressed the examiner as good, healthy, wise, and eminently well-adjusted people whose children were particularly fortunate because of what they could offer as parents. When opportunities arose, as they sometimes did, to learn more of matters inward, subtle, and deeply personal, the observer was sometimes led to suspect that even in these apparently superior parents there were attitudes, frustrations, emotional confusions, and deficiencies that might have played a masked but crucially adverse role in the infinite complexities and paradoxes of parent-child relationships.

This is not to say that the parents were wrongly judged as conscientious or as superior people or that in many important respects they were not well adjusted. Despite conscientiousness and a good deal of wisdom and success, characteristics may exist which could subtly but trenchantly distort the milieu of an infant or a child (Ribble, 1944).

People may be fair, kind, and genial, may hold entirely normal or even admirable attitudes about all important matters and yet unknowingly lack a simple warmth, a capacity for true intimacy that seems to be essential for biologic soundness (substantiality) in some basic relationships. There are men and women of whom it might correctly be said that it is impossible for them ever to become really personal. This aspect (or ingredient) of human experience is difficult to describe or to signify accurately. We do not encounter it squarely in thinking but feel it in perceptive modes or at reactive levels not readily translatable into speech (Goldfarb, 1945). Let us remember, however, that such qualities may be found in parents of those who are not sociopaths.

Some who show only superior qualities in all their activities as citizens, in their work, and in all definable responsibilities feel little need for the sort of specific attachment and affective closeness which perhaps constitute the core of deep and genuine love. They also seem to have little perception of such a need in others. There are people who show in changeless formality, poise, and cool 'sensible attitudes' outer indications of what is being discussed, but it is not they who concern us at present. In others, genial informality and manifestations of more than ordinary warmth may prevail in relatively superficial friendships and routine social contacts, in professional and business associations, at dinner parties, and at club meetings. Where intimacy is normally limited they may be spontaneous and show cordiality as real as anything appropriate for such occasions. Their inner formality and remoteness is not encountered until the observer approaches areas of privacy, deep levels of personal affect that ordinarily are only reached in relations between mates, between parent and child, or in the few other very intimate and cherished friendships or sharings of personal understanding and feeling that man never achieves in wholesale lot. Parents of this sort may give an impression of affording each other and the child all that is ideal, and affording it in abundance. One such parent will, however, leave the other (if normal) so deprived in essential needs that the child may be turned to for the exclusive and possessive intimacy normal between mates but full of pathologic potentialities in the other relationship.

The observations reported by Kanner (1949) in his study of infantile autism illustrate some of the points that are being discussed here. In the brilliant and outstandingly successful parents of these seriously disabled infants a complex and profound emotional deficiency was regularly encountered. During all my years of experience with hundreds of psychopaths, however, no type of parent or of parental influence, overt or subtle, has been regularly demonstrable.

Both hereditary factors and influences of the frustrating, or antisocial, environment seem evident in the development of delinquency in many of the patients described long ago by Healy (1915). In the background of the intelligent, charming psychopath who appears in a family of prominent, ethical, and successful citizens, it is often far more difficult to find convincing evidence to account for his disorder on either basis. If an inborn biologic defect exists and plays an important part in such a psychopath's disorder, it is not necessary to assume that the defect is hereditary. Perhaps it may be the result of a subtle failure in maturation, an agenesis of unknown aetiology. A much simpler and more grossly manifested defect of this sort is familiar in the pathology of congenital cerebral palsy. It is well known that encephalitis may be followed by changes in behavior and personality that cause some who have suffered from it to become indistinguishable from the psychopaths we have been discussing and that these changes may occur without any physical signs of neurologic damage.

Many psychiatrists (Campbell, 1945; Mangun, 1942; Thompson, 1953) have continued to express the conviction that some organic injury or deficiency underlies the psychopath's dysfunction. Although no neurologic lesion has been regularly demonstrated in the typical psychopath, it is also true, as Thompson reminds us, that no satisfactory proof of psychogenic factors as the cause of his disorder has been established. Referring to formulations of the psychopathology in terms of environmental influences, he says: 'Here too much is missing that might give us a rational explanation which would be subject to scientific scrutiny, and which would meet the postulates of science necessary for validity.'

Numerous observers (Gottlieb, Ashby and Knott, 1947; Knott and Gottlieb, 1943; Silverman, 1944) have reported records of electroencephalographic abnormality in psychopaths. Others (Gibbs and Bagchi, 1945; Simon, O'Leary and Ryan, 1946) have failed to confirm these findings of a specific abnormality. At present many believe there are non-specific but definitely abnormal electroencephalographic findings in a significant percentage of psychopaths (Ehrlich and Keogh, 1956; Hill, 1952; Hill and Pond, 1952; Thompson, 1953).

If a neurologic defect does exist in the psychopath, it is also quite possible that influences in the milieu may play an important part also in shaping his pattern of life. It seems to me likely that such a defect, if present, must be one that affects complex mechanisms of integration in a subtle and abstruse manner. Some of the superior capacities encountered so often in psychopaths suggest that their difficulties might arise not only from deficiencies but possibly, even if rarely, by misused assets.

It seems reasonable to believe that in differences lie varying susceptibilities to failure or to psychiatric disorder. Such susceptibilities may not necessarily be defects or intrinsically negative qualities. May not superior emotional responses contribute to a boy's developing maternal attachments that can prove crippling in the degree to which he has capacity for loyalty? May not the precociously brilliant child, because of his advancement, encounter deep personal and social problems earlier than the average? And, will he, perhaps, sustain trauma that he might have avoided with additional experience? Such experience may be available to the mediocre child who, in his slower progress, meets the confusing situation a little later. Those whose feelings are highly developed may be more susceptible to hurt than others. The goals of the superior person often demand of him complicated choices and sacrifices that the average person never has to face. Disillusion and suffering because of frustrations escaped by most of his fellows might, it seems reasonable to think, in the child of great talent and potentiality, stimulate attitudes of withdrawal and cynical rejection or other pathologic reactions. Exceptional talent or capacity seems almost regularly to call for exceptional achievement or fulfillment and to put the subject under extraordinary responsibility and into situations peculiarly complex. Courage and initiative lead man not only to take physical risks, but sometimes also into subjective ventures of many sorts with many dangers.

What we value in some as steadfastness may arise from potentialities that, through different shaping, emerge in others as incorrigibility, inelasticity, or perhaps as those elements which may make a psychiatric disorder irreversible. Granting the likelihood of great variation in the basic potentialities of the organism, let us not forget that in so complex a matter as personality maturation and social adjustment not only defects but talents also may contribute to conflict, to confusion, to distortion of the life pattern, and perhaps, to serious clinical disorder.

If what is good or wise or sound comes, or appears to come, mixed, so to speak, with what is untrue or deleterious and is identified in a single concept, and designated by the same term, peculiar difficulties may be promoted. Such difficulties, it seems reasonable to think, might be especially disturbing to the superior child. Conscientious acceptance of what is most necessary for normal growth and development may, under these circumstances, sometimes necessitate commitments to what must later be rejected if the organism is to survive. The deeper the capacity for loyalty, the more profound may be the stress, confusion, and eventual disillusionment.

The psychopath's inner deviation from the normal impresses me as one subtly masked and abstruse. So, too, it has often seemed that interpersonal and environmental factors, if they contribute to the development of his disorder, are likely to be ones so disguised superficially as to appear of an opposite nature. Something pertinent to this concept may be conveyed by the words that follow:

Everything spiritual and valuable has a gross and undesirable malady very similar to it and possessing the same name. Only the very wise can distinguish between them.[7]

I do not believe that the cause of the psychopath's disorder has yet been discovered and demonstrated. Until we have more and better evidence than is at present available, let us admit the incompleteness of our knowledge and modestly pursue our inquiry.

7. From Thompson, D. L.: Address at banquet, meeting of the American Psychiatric Association, Montreal, 1949.

References

ALEXANDER, F. (1929), 'The need for punishment and the death instinct', *Int. J. Psychiat.*, vol. 10, p. 260.

ALEXANDER, F. (1930), 'The neurotic character', *Int. J. Psychoanal.*, vol. 2, pp. 292–311.

ALEXANDER, F. (1948), *Fundamentals of Psychoanalysis*, W. W. Norton.

BILLINGS, E. G. (1939), *A Handbook of Elementary Psychobiology and psychiatry*, Macmillan.

CAMPBELL, J. (1945), *Everyday Psychiatry*, Lippincott.

CLECKLEY, H. (1957), *The Caricature of Love*, Ronald Press.

CLUTTON-BROCK, A. (1923), 'Evil and the new psychology', *Atlantic Monthly*, March, pp. 298–308.

DIETHELM, O. (1936), *Treatment in Psychiatry*, Macmillan.

EHRLICH, S. K. and KEOGH, R. P. (1956), 'The psychopath in a mental institution', *Arch. neurol. Psychiat.*, vol. 76, pp. 286–95.

FENICHEL, O. (1945), *The Psychoanalytic Theory of Neurosis*, Norton.

FREUD, S. (1942), *The Ego and the Id*, Hogarth Press.

FREUD, S. (1943), *Collected Papers: Volume III*, Hogarth Press.

GIBBS, F. and BAGCHI, G. (1945), 'Electroencephalographic study of criminals', *Amer. J. Psychiat.*, vol. 102, pp. 294–8.

GOLDFARB, W. (1945), 'Effects of psychological deprivation in infancy and subsequent stimulation', *Amer. J. Psychiat.*, vol. 102, pp. 18–33.

GOTTLIEB, J., ASHBY, M. and KNOTT, J. (1947), 'Studies in primary behavior disorders and psychopathic personality. Part II. The inheritance of electrocortical activity', *Amer. J. Psychiat.*, vol. 103, pp. 823–7.

GREENACRE, P. (1945), 'Conscience in the psychopath', *Amer. J. Orthopsychiat.*, vol. 15, pp. 495–509.

HARDIN, G. (1957), 'The threat of clarity', *Amer. J. Psychiat.*, vol. 114, pp. 392–6.

HEALY, W. (1915), *The Individual Delinquent*, Little, Brown.

HEALY, W. (1936), *New Light on Delinquency and its Treatment*, Yale University Press.

HEALY, W. and BRONNER, A. F. (1926), *Delinquents and Criminals*, Macmillan.

HENDERSON, D. K. (1939), *Psychopathic States*, W. W. Norton.

HILL, D. (1952), 'EEG in episodic psychotic and psychopathic behavior', *EEG. clin. Neurophysiol.*, vol. 4, pp. 419–42.

HILL, D. and POND, D. (1952), 'Reflections on one hundred capital cases submitted to electroencephalography', *J. ment. Sci.*, vol. 98, pp. 23–43.

JENKINS, R. (1960), 'The psychopathic or antisocial personality', *J. nerv. ment. Disease*, vol. 131, pp. 318–32.

JOHNSON, A. (1949), 'Sanctions for superego lacunae of adolescents', in K. R. Eissler (ed.), *Searchlights on Delinquency: New Psychoanalytic Studies*, International Universities Press.

JOHNSON, A. (1959), 'Juvenile delinquency', in S. Arieti (ed.), *American Handbook of Psychiatry*, Basic Books.

JOHNSON, A. and SZUREK, S. (1945), 'Etiology of the antisocial behavior in delinquents and psychopaths', *J. Amer. med. Assoc.*, vol. 154, pp. 814–17.

KANNER, L. (1949), 'Problems of nosology and psychodynamics of early infantile autism', *Amer. J. Orthopsychiat.*, vol. 19, pp. 416–26.

KARPMAN, B. (1940), 'The principles and aims of criminal psychopathology', *J. crim. Psychopathol.*, vol. 1, pp. 187–218.

KARPMAN, B. (1941a), 'On the need for separating psychopathy into two distinct types: the symptomatic and the idiopathic', *J. crim. Psychopathol.*, vol. 3, pp. 112–37.

KARPMAN, B. (1941b), 'Perversions as neuroses', *J. crim. Psychopathol.*, vol. 3, p. 180.

KARPMAN, B. (1946), 'A yardstick for measuring psychopathy', *Federal Probation*, vol. 10, pp. 26–31.

KNIGHT, R. (1937), 'The psychodynamics of chronic alcoholism', *J. nerv. ment. Disease*, vol. 86, pp. 538–48.

KNIGHT, R. (1938), 'The psychoanalytic treatment in a sanitorium of chronic addiction to alcohol', *J. Amer. Med. Assoc.*, vol. 111, pp. 1443–8.

KNOTT, J. and GOTTLIEB, J. (1943), 'The electroencephalogram in psychopathic personality', *Psychosom. Medicine*, vol. 5, pp. 139–42.

LEVIN, M. (1940), 'The dynamic conception of psychopathic personality', *Ohio State Med. J.*, vol. 36, pp. 848–50.

LINDNER, R. (1944), *Rebel Without a Cause*, Grune & Stratton.

LORAND, S. (1944), *Psychoanalysis Today*, International Universities Press.

MANGUN, C. (1942), 'The psychopathic criminal', *J. crim. Psychopathol.* vol. 4, pp. 117–27.

McCORD, W. and McCORD, J. (1956), *Psychopathy and Delinquency*, Grune & Stratton.

MENNINGER, K. (1938), *Man against Himself*, Harcourt, Brace & World.

MEYER, A. (1938), 'Leading concepts in psychobiology (ergasiology) and psychiatry (ergasiatry)', *Proceedings of the Fourth Conference on Psychiatric Education*, National Committee for Mental Hygiene.

MUNCIE, W. (1948), *Psychobiology and Psychiatry*, Mosby.

NOYES, A. and KOLB, L. (1963), *Modern Clinical Psychiatry*, sixth edn., Saunders.

RIBBLE, M. (1944), 'Infantile experience in relation to personality disorder', in J. McV. Hunt (ed.), *Personality and the Behavior Disorders: Vol. II*, Ronald Press.

ROCHE, P. Q. (1942), 'Masochistic motivations in criminal behaviour', *J. crim. Psychopathol.*, vol. 4, pp. 431–44.

SHERRINGTON, C. (1923), *The Integrative Action of the Nervous System*, Yale University Press.

SILVERMAN, D. (1944), 'The electroencephalogram of criminals', *Arch. neurol. Psychiat.*, vol. 52, pp. 38–42.

SIMON, B., O'LEARY, J. and RYAN, J. (1946), 'Ceberal dysrhythmia and psychopathic personalities', *Arch. neurol. Psychiat.*, vol. 56, pp. 677–85.

SUTHERLAND, E. H. (1939), *Principles of Criminology*, Lippincott.

THOMPSON, G. (1953), *The Psychopathic Delinquent and Criminal*, Charles C. Thomas.

11 R. D. Hare

Autonomic Activity and Conditioning in Psychopaths

R. D. Hare, 'Autonomic activity and conditioning in psychopaths',
paper given at the Symposium on Psychophysiological Responses in
Sociopaths, Society for Psychophysiological Research, New Orleans.

Before discussing the recent research on autonomic activity and
conditioning in psychopaths, some preliminary comments on
the concept of psychopathy are given. To a large extent, these
comments are based upon a paper presented at the 1969 Georgia
Symposium on Experimental Clinical Psychology and published in H. Adams and W. Boardman (eds.) *Advances in
Experimental Clinical Psychology*, vol. 1, New York: Pergamon,
1970, in press.

Although the term psychopathy has been used in a variety of
contexts, there is a growing tendency to restrict its use to the
clinical and behavioral syndrome so vividly described by
Cleckley (1964) and Karpman (1961). This tendency is particularly noticeable among those involved in experimental clinical
psychology – in this case psychopathy is often defined in terms
of the criteria outlined by Cleckley (1964). Although a subjective element is certainly involved in these criteria, their use provides a useful starting point for research.

The main features of psychopathy, according to Cleckley, are
as follows: (1) superficial charm and good intelligence; (2)
absence of delusions and other signs of irrational thinking; (3)
absence of nervousness or other neurotic manifestations; (4)
unreliability; (5) untruthfulness and insincerity; (6) lack of
remorse or shame; (7) antisocial behavior without apparent com-
punction; (8) poor judgement and failure to learn from experience; (9) pathologic egocentricity and incapacity for love;
(10) general poverty in major affective reactions; (11) specific
loss of insight; (12) unresponsiveness in general interpersonal
relations; (13) fantastic and uninviting behavior with alcohol
and sometimes without; (14) suicide rarely carried out; (15) sex

life impersonal, trivial, and poorly integrated; (16) failure to follow any life plan.

Both Cleckley (1964) and Karpman (1961) describe the psychopath as a callous, emotionally immature, two-dimensional person who lacks the ability to experience the emotional components of personal and interpersonal behavior. He is able to *simulate* emotional reactions and affectional attachments when it will help him to obtain what he wants; however, he doesn't really *feel*. He experiences neither the psychological nor the physiological aspects of guilt and anxiety, although he may react with something like fear when his immediate comfort is threatened. His social and sexual relations with others are superficial but demanding and manipulative. Future rewards and punishments do not exist, except in a very abstract and unreal way, with the result that they have little effect on his immediate behavior. His judgement is poor and often his behavior is guided entirely by impulse and current needs. His attempts to extricate himself from difficulty often result in an intricate and contradictory web of blatant lies, coupled with theatrical and sometimes convincing explanations and promises to change. Since the psychopath is egocentric, lacks empathy, and is unable to form warm, emotional relationships with others, he tends to treat people as objects rather than as persons, and he experiences no guilt or remorse for having used them to satisfy his own needs.

Until recently, the American Psychiatric Association (APA) classification for the syndrome described by Cleckley was *Sociopathic personality disturbance: Antisocial reaction* (APA, 1952). In practice, the term *sociopath* was, and is often, used. In 1968, in an attempt to co-ordinate their classification system with that of the WHO, the APA suggested that the classification *Personality disorder: Antisocial personality* be used.

The antisocial personality refers to people who are basically unsocialized and whose behavior pattern brings them repeatedly into conflict with society. They are incapable of significant loyalty to individuals, groups or social values. They are grossly selfish, callous, irresponsible, impulsive, and unable to feel guilt or to learn from experience and punishment. Frustration tolerance is low. They tend to blame others or offer plausible rationalizations for their behavior . . . (p. 43).

R. D. Hare 225

When dealing with children, the Group for the Advancement of Psychiatry (GAP) has proposed that the terms *tension-discharge disorder*, *impulse-ridden personality* be used in place of psychopathy or sociopathy, since the latter terms imply a personality pattern that is perhaps too fixed to apply to children. The impulse-ridden personality is described as follows:

These children show shallow relationships with adults or other children, having very low frustration tolerance. They exhibit great difficulty in control of their impulses, both aggressive and sexual, which are discharged immediately and impulsively, without delay or inhibition, and often with little regard for the consequences. Little anxiety, internalized conflict, or guilt is experienced by most of these children, as the conflict remains largely external, between society and their impulses. . . . The basic defect in impulse controls appears to be reinforced by a deficit in conscience or superego formation, with failure to develop the capacity for tension-storage and for the postponement of gratifications. . . . Although their judgement and time concepts are poor, they usually have adequate intelligence and their reality testing in certain areas is quite effective (Group for the Advancement of Psychiatry, 1966, pp. 247–8).

Secondary and dysocial 'psychopathy'

The individual we have been discussing is sometimes referred to as the *primary*, *idiopathic*, or *classical* psychopath. These particular adjectives simply acknowledge the fact that many antisocial and aggressive acts are performed by individuals who are basically neurotic rather than psychopathic. Since the behavior of these individuals is assumed to be merely symptomatic of some emotional disturbance, they are sometimes called *secondary*, *symptomatic*, or *neurotic* psychopaths.

One of the difficulties with the use of terms like secondary and neurotic psychopathy is the implication that individuals so labelled are basically psychopaths. This is apt to be misleading, in my opinion, since the motivations behind their behavior, as well as their personality structure, life-history, response to treatment, and prognosis, are probably quite different from those of the psychopath. Moreover, unlike psychopaths, these individuals are able to experience guilt and remorse for their behavior and to form meaningful, affectional relationships with others. Since their antisocial behavior is apparently motivated by neurotic conflicts and tensions, it may be more appropriate to use terms that emphasize this neurotic element, e.g., *acting-out neurotic*, *neurotic delinquent*, etc. When dealing with children, the GAP suggests that the term *neurotic personality disorder* be used.

Many individuals exhibit aggressive, antisocial behavior, not because they are psychopathic or emotionally disturbed, but because they have grown up in a delinquent subculture or in an environment that fosters and rewards such behavior. Their behavior, while considered deviant by society's standards, is nevertheless consonant with that of their own group, gang, or subculture. Although they are sometimes called *dysocial psychopaths*, they are unlike the 'true' psychopath in that they are capable of strong loyalties, guilt, remorse, and warm relationships within the context of their own group. It therefore seems more appropriate to refer to them as *subcultural delinquents*. Where children are involved, the GAP prefers the term *socio-syntonic personality disorder*.

It is of interest that the clinical subdivision of antisocial behavior into psychopathic, neurotic and subcultural components is supported by several statistical studies of case history data. Jenkins and his associates (1964, 1966) have repeatedly isolated several clusters of personality traits (or syndromes) occurring in delinquent children and in guidance clinic referrals. The three most common clusters have been labeled the *unsocialized-aggressive syndrome* (assaultive tendencies, starting fights, cruelty, defiance of authority, malicious mischief, inadequate guilt feelings), the *over-anxious syndrome* (seclusiveness, shyness, apathy, worrying, sensitiveness, submissiveness), and the *socialized delinquency syndrome* (bad companions, gang activities, cooperative stealing, habitual truancy from school and home, out late at night).

Other studies have produced similar results. Thus, a series of factor analytic studies using behavior ratings (Quay, 1964b), case history data (Quay, 1964a), and responses to questionnaires (Peterson, Quay and Tiffany, 1961), has consistently yielded at least two main factors related to delinquency. The first factor, labeled *psychopathic delinquency*, reflects tough, amoral and rebellious qualities coupled with impulsivity, distrust of authority, and freedom from family ties. The second factor, labeled *neurotic delinquency*, also reflects impulsive and aggressive tendencies; however, in this case they are associated with tension, guilt, remorse, depression, and discouragement. A third factor has been identified in studies of personality questionnaires (Peterson, Quay and Tiffany, 1961). Labeled *subcultural delinquency*, the factor reflects the attitudes and values commonly believed to occur in delinquent groups; it is similar to Jenkins's socialized delinquency syndrome and to the dysocial 'psychopath' described above.

The results of several studies by Finney (e.g., 1966) provide further support for the distinction between psychopathic and neurotic forms of antisocial behavior. Using responses to a personality inventory, the MMPI, Finney isolated several factors, including one related to antisocial behavior and another related to anxiety distress and guilt. On the basis of his findings, Finney was able to distinguish between psychopathy (high in antisocial behavior, low in guilt), neurotic inhibition (low in antisocial behavior, high in guilt), and normalcy (low in antisocial behavior, low in guilt).

Although there is reasonably good agreement on the conceptual meaning of the term psychopathy (Albert, Brigante, and Chase, 1959: Gray and Hutchison, 1964), it is of course not always so easy to identify those individuals who warrant the label 'psychopathic'. In this respect, the concept shares a problem that is common to all diagnostic categories, viz., the problem of diagnostic reliability (Phillips, 1968; Zubin, 1967). Nevertheless, as has been pointed out elsewhere (Hare, 1970), the problem is not as great as some would have us believe – certainly it is not great enough to prevent worthwhile research from being carried out. Moreover, the use of reasonably explicit criteria, such as those outlined by Cleckley, would seem to provide a useful starting point for the development of a more objective, empirically-based conceptualization of psychopathy.

Before reviewing some of the recent research on autonomic activity and conditioning, there are several comments worth making. First, compared to other disorders (e.g., schizophrenia), very little research on psychopathy has been carried out.

This paucity of research is unfortunate but perhaps not too surprising. Most research is carried out in clinics and mental hospitals where the majority of patients are schizophrenic. Relatively few psychopaths are found in these institutions, and those that are there are likely to be considered nuisances rather than worthwhile subjects for research. Penal institutions provide the major source of psychopathic subjects, which leads to another problem – psychopathic criminals probably represent only a small proportion of the total population of psychopaths (Robins, 1966), viz., those whose behavior was unsuccessful (in a legal sense). Whether these individuals differ in important ways from those psychopaths whose behavior is legal or quasi-legal (though unethical and unscrupulous) is not known, although the possibility must be kept in mind when drawing conclusions from research that has used incarcerated psychopaths.

A second point is that there is as yet no well-developed, comprehensive theory of psychopathy. Instead, we have a large and diverse number of mini-theories and hypotheses, all of them incomplete or restricted to some selected aspect of psychopathy, and some of them untestable and without empirical foundation. Fortunately, this situation is beginning to change, largely as the result of the increasing use of procedures and conceptualizations derived from experimental psychology, including learning theory, motivation, and psychophysiology.

Finally, throughout the presentation to follow, I have avoided commenting upon the controversy over the most appropriate way of conceptualizing psychopathy. One viewpoint is that psychopathy is a relatively distinct clinical and behavioral entity – a specific combination or clustering of characteristics that, individually and in other combinations, may be found in other disorders as well as in normal persons. Many investigators, however, find it more appealing to conceptualize psychopathy in dimensional terms. According to this view, psychopaths as such do not exist, although some individuals may be considered more psychopathic than others if they occupy a more extreme position on some dimension that we choose to label 'psychopathy'. The difficulty here is that before we can really say that one person is more or less psychopathic than another, we need to know more about what the dimension consists of. This means that we have to determine not only the psychological and physiological characteristics that define the dimension, but also their relative importance (the weights assigned them). An individual's position on the dimension would then be determined by the number of relevant characteristics he exhibits, their severity, and the weights assigned them. It should be possible, of course, to use multivariate statistical techniques to obtain information of this sort, and to derive a score or set of scores indicative of an individual's degree and type of psychopathy. To a certain extent, of course, the clinician already makes use of this procedure, but instead of identifying and weighting relevant characteristics empirically, he does so subjectively and on the basis of his experience.

Perhaps the disagreement about whether psychopathy is best viewed as a typology or as a dimensional concept arises because both views are appropriate, representing, as it were, different sides of the same coin. It is also possible, as Zubin (1967) has put it, that 'The conflict between typology and dimensionality is a pseudoconflict dependent upon the state of knowledge of the field' (p. 398).

Autonomic correlates of psychopathy
Tonic activity

Several attempts have been made to obtain measures of tonic autonomic activity from Ss that could be considered to be in a 'resting' state or a state of relative quiescence. In general, this tonic activity is measured somewhere near the beginning of the experiment involved and after the S has had a chance to settle down. The results of most relevant studies are summarized in Table 1. Now, there are certain obvious difficulties involved in comparing the results of these studies. For example, several different procedures and criteria for the selection of Ss have been used. In some studies the comparisons are between psychopathic and nonpsychopathic inmates, while in others the comparisons are between psychopathic inmates and Ss who are not incarcerated, e.g., attendants, students, etc. In addition, studies differ in the extent to which stress is generated in the Ss participating. That is, 'resting' states represent the interaction between the characteristics of the *S* and the particular set of experimental conditions involved. It is difficult, therefore, to compare studies on the amount of stress involved, the motivational and psychological significance of the experiment to the *S*, etc.

In spite of these difficulties, the recent research literature has been reasonably consistent. As Table 1 indicates, most of the significant differences between groups, as well as most of the trends towards a difference, involved two aspects of electrodermal activity – palmar skin conductance (SC) and nonspecific

Table 1 Resting tonic level in psychopaths

Investigator	Subjects[1]	Variables[2]	Findings
Lindner (1942)	M, NPC	SR, HR, RR	No significant difference
Ruilmann & Gulo (1950)	M, NC	SR, HR, RR, BP	No significant difference
Lykken (1955)	P, M, NC	SR	Group P had lowest SR
Fox & Lippert (1963)	M, NPC	SC, NSP	Group M gave fewer NSP
Schachter & Latané (1964)	P, NPC	HR	No significant difference
Goldstein (1965)	M, NC	SC, HR, RR, BP, MAPs	No significant difference
Hare (1965b)	P, NPC, NC	SC	Group P had lowest SC
Lippert & Senter (1966)	M, NPC	SC, NSP	No significant difference though trend towards fewer NSP in Group M
Hare (1968)	P, M, NPC	SC, NSP, HR, P–T, RR	Groups P and M had lower SC than group NPC; tendency for Group P to give fewer NSP and smaller P–T
Schalling, Lidberg, Levander & Dahlin, (1968)	P, NPC	SC, NSP, NVC	Group P had fewer NSP and tendency toward lower SC
Blankstein (1969)	P, M, NC	SC, NSP, SP, HR, P–T	Group P had lowest SC and more (but smaller) NSP
Schmauk (1968)	P, M, NC	SC	No significant differences
Hare & Quinn (in press)	P, M, NPC	SC, NSP, HR, P–T, RR	Group P had lowest SC, P–T, and tendency toward fewer NSP

[1] P = psychopaths; M = mixed group; NPC = nonpsychopathic criminals or patients; NC = noninstitutionalized *S*s.

[2] SR = skin resistance; SC = skin conductance; NSP = nonspecific fluctuations in SC; SP = skin potential; HR = heart rate; RR = respiration rate; BP = blood pressure; P–T = peak-trough difference in heart rate; MAPs = muscle action potentials; NVC = non specific peripheral vasoconstriction; VC = peripheral vasoconstriction.

fluctuations in skin conductance (NSP), and the Ss in these studies usually included relatively well-defined groups of psychopaths (designated Group P). It should be noted, however, that three of the studies which found psychopaths to have an unusually low level of resting tonic skin conductance (Hare, 1965c, 1968; Hare and Quinn, in press) involved Ss from a single institution, the British Columbia Penitentiary. Although different Ss were used in each study, I earlier suggested (Hare, 1968) that until similar results have been provided by other investigators, the possibility must be considered that these results are specific to the population used. Since then several studies have provided supporting evidence (Blankstein, 1969; Schalling, Lidberg, Levander, and Dahlin, 1968), while another (Schmauk, 1968) found that psychopathic criminals and normal noncriminals did not differ in resting tonic skin conductance.

The situation with respect to the nonspecific fluctuations in skin conductance is somewhat clearer. Thus, the only relevant study which failed to find that psychopaths exhibit a relatively low level of nonspecific electrodermal activity was the one carried out by Blankstein (1969). He points out, however, that extremely small fluctuations were included in the analysis, and that the fluctuations given by the psychopathic Ss were much smaller than those given by the other Ss.

The only other aspect of tonic autonomic activity to differentiate between psychopaths and nonpsychopaths is mean peak–trough difference in heart rate (P–T). Several studies (Hare, 1968; Hare and Quinn, in press) indicate that tonic P–T difference is lower in psychopaths than in nonpsychopaths.

Some indication of the changes in tonic electrodermal activity and P–T differences that occur during the course of an experiment is given in Figures 1 and 2. The data in Figure 1 were obtained in a habituation study involving the presentation of sixteen 80db tones. It is evident that the differences between Groups P and NP generally increased throughout the experiment (from Period 1 to Period 2). Near the end of the experiment the Ss were required to solve a series of arithmetic problems. The cognitive activity involved in doing so (Period CA) produced a sharp increase in the SC and NSP activity of both groups, and in the P–T difference in the psychopaths. It is rather interesting that in the case of NSP activity and P–T differences in heart rate, cognitive activity washed out the differences between psychopaths and nonpsychopathic Ss.

The data in Figure 2 were obtained in a classical conditioning study involving tones as the conditioned stimuli (CS) and shock and slides of nude females as the unconditioned stimuli (UCS). Again, with the exception of SC, the tonic autonomic activity of

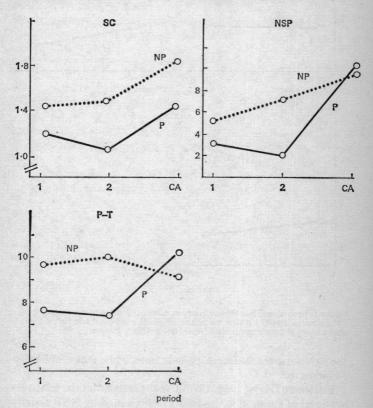

Figure 1 Tonic autonomic activity in psychopathic (P) and non-psychopathic (NP) inmates. Period 1 is near the beginning of the experiment and Period 2 is after a series of 16 80db tones. Period CA is during the solution of arithmetic problems (After Hare, 1968)

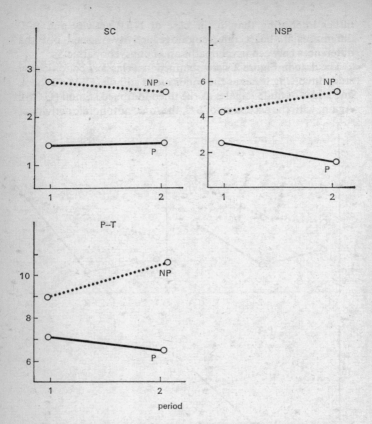

Figure 2 Tonic autonomic activity in psychopathic (P) and non-psychopathic (NP) inmates. Period 1 is near the beginning of the experiment and Period 2 is after a series of conditioning trials (After Hare & Quinn, in press)

the psychopathic Ss decreased over time, while that of the other Ss increased.

Elsewhere (Hare, 1968, 1970) I've suggested that the relatively low level of autonomic variability (represented by NSP activity and P–T differences in heart rate) are consistent with the hypothesis that psychopathy is characterized by a tendency towards chronic autonomic and cortical hypoarousal.

234 Psychopathy

Autonomic responsivity

The results of studies concerned with autonomic responsivity in psychopaths are summarized in Table 2. It is evident that several recent studies (Blankstein, 1969; Hare and Quinn, in press) support Lykken's (1955) earlier finding that psychopaths are electrodermally hyporesponsive to intense stimuli, including electric shock and loud tones. Although the evidence is not clear-cut, it appears that they may be normally responsive to other less noxious forms of stimulation.

There is some evidence that the cardiac response to novel auditory stimulation may be related to psychopathy. Figure 3 shows the mean deceleration to a series of fifteen identical 80db

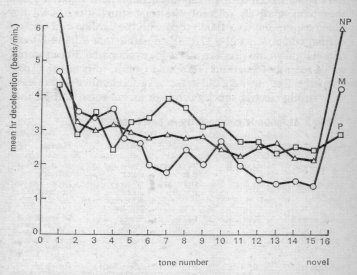

Figure 3 Mean cardiac deceleration to repetitive (Tones 1–15) and novel (Tone 16) stimulation P = psychopaths; M = mixed group; NP = non-psychopaths (after Hare, 1968)

tones and a sixteenth tone different in frequency and loudness. Note that the major difference between groups lay in the relatively small decelerative response given by the psychopaths to the two novel tones, viz., tones one and sixteen. Although the groups did not differ in electrodermal or digital vasomotor responsiveness to the sixteen tones, the heart rate data suggest that the cardiac component of the OR may be relatively small in psychopaths. I've indicated elsewhere (Hare, 1968) that the pattern of autonomic activity to repetitious stimulation exhibited by the psychopaths is similar to that observed in drowsy Ss (McDonald, Johnson and Hord, 1964).

Using more intense (100db) auditory stimulation, Blankstein (1969) found that nonpsychopaths gave a biphasic cardiac response (acceleration followed by deceleration) to the first (novel) tone in a series, while the psychopaths gave only a monophasic decelerative response. Since the psychopaths also gave small electrodermal responses, Blankstein suggested that they were relatively tolerant of strong stimulations, i.e., they failed to respond to a 100db tone with the cardiac and electrodermal components of a DR. It's possible that a more intense stimulation would produce a DR in psychopaths. For example, we've recently found out (Hare and Quinn, in press) that psychopaths, like other Ss, did in fact give accelerative responses to very strong electric shock (although as indicated earlier, they

Table 2 **Autonomic responsivity in psychopaths**

Investigator	Subjects[1]	Variables[2]	Situation	Findings
Lindner (1942)	M, NPC	EDR, HR, RR	Tones and shock	No significant difference
Ruilmann & Gulo (1950)	M, NC	EDR, HR, RR, BP	'Sensory stimuli' questions, arithmetic problems	Group M gave smaller EDRs
Lykken (1955)	P, M, NC	EDR	Tones and shock; lie detection	Groups P and M gave smaller EDRs to shock, tones signalling shock, and 'lying'
Gellhorn (1957)	M, NPC	BP	Injection of mecholyl	Group M showed smaller BP drop and quicker homeostatic recovery
Tong (1959)	M, NC	EDR	Heat, tones, tactile, frustration	Some group M more responsive some less
Schachter & Latane (1964)	P, NPC	HR	Injection of adrenalin	Group P more responsive
Goldstein (1965)	M, NC	EDR, HR, RR, BP, MAPs	White noise	No significant difference

Investigator	Subjects[1]	Variables[2]	Situation	Findings
Hare (1965c)	P, NPC, NC	EDR	Shock and threat of shock	No significant difference in responsitivity to shock; Group P least responsive to threat of shock
Hare (1965b)	P, NPC	EDR	Tones and shock	Group P less responsive to tones signalling shock
Hare (1968a)	P, M	EDR, HR, VC	80db tones	No significant difference in EDR; Group P showed smallest cardiac deceleration to novel tones, and slower habituation of cardiac and vasomotor responses
Schalling, Lidberg, Levander & Dahlin (1968)	P, NP	EDR, NSP, NVC	Tones	Group P gave fewer NSP
Schmauk (1968)	P, M, NC	EDR	Motor response	No significant differences in EDR; P gave smallest anticipatory EDRs when incorrect responses were associated with shock or social disapproval, but not with loss of money
Blankstein (1969)	P, M, NC	EDR, SPR, HR	100db tones	Group P gave smallest EDR and SPR; initial stimulus elicited biphasic cardiac response (accel-decel) in Groups M & NC, but only deceleration in Group P
Hare & Quinn (in press)	P, M, NPC	EDR, HR, VC, CVM	Tones, shock and slides of nude females	Group P gave smallest EDR to shock, slides and threat of shock; CVM response to shock was dilation in Group P and absent in Group NP

[1][2] Same as for Table 1, plus EDR = electrodermal response (GSR); SPR = skin potential response; CVM = cephalic vasomotor response.

also gave a small electrodermal response). We also found that psychopaths gave normal digital vasomotor responses to shock and slides of nude females, but that their cephalic vasomotor responses to shock were rather unusual. The latter are shown in Figure 4, along with responses to the slides of nude females. The

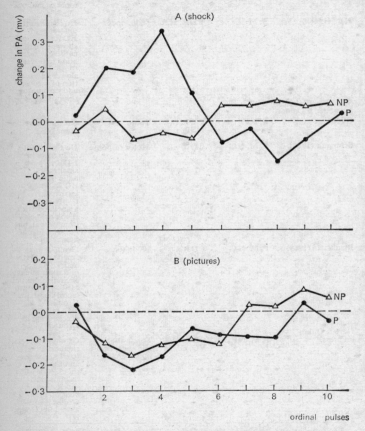

Figure 4 Mean cephalic vasomotor UCR to shock (A) and slides of nude females (B). Deviations above the baseline indicate dilation and those below constriction

data are plotted as deviations in pulse-amplitude (PA) from the prestimulus mean. The cephalic vasomotor response to the slides was a decrease in PA, i.e., vasoconstriction. This is, of course, contrary to what would be expected on the basis of Sokolov's (1963) conception of the orienting response (OR) – the OR is traditionally associated with cephalic vasodilation and the defensive response (DR) with cephalic vasoconstriction. However, several recent studies have found that cephalic vasoconstriction (taken as a reduction in PA) is the typical response to moderate and intense tones (Raskin, Kotses and Bever, 1969) and to slides of nude females and homicide victims (Hare, Wood, Britain and Shadman, 1970, 1971). The fact that *S*s in the Hare and Quinn study responded to the slides with cephalic vasoconstriction is therefore consistent with other research. On the other hand, the response of the psychopaths to the shock was cephalic vasodilation, while the nonpsychopaths were relatively unresponsive.

Conditioning and avoidance learning

Although psychopaths are traditionally considered to be unable to 'profit from experience', the available research literature (reviewed in Hare, 1970) indicates that any learning deficit may be largely confined to the classical conditioning of autonomic responses and the avoidance learning.

Lykken (1955), for example, using a combination of simple and delayed discrimination conditioning paradigms, found that the conditioned EDRs of psychopathic criminals were smaller and quicker to extinguish than were those of neurotic criminals and normal noncriminals. Similarly Hare (1965b), using a simple, delayed conditioning design, found that psychopathic criminals not only acquired conditioned EDRs slowly, but also that such responses, once acquired, were generalized less by psychopathic than by nonpsychopathic criminals.

In a slightly different context, there is some evidence (Hare, 1965c; Lippert and Senter, 1966; Schalling and Levander, 1967) that when explicitly informed that they will shortly receive a strong electric shock, psychopaths exhibit little electrodermal activity in the interval prior to the expected shock. For example, in one study (Hare, 1965c) *S*s were required to watch the consecutive numbers 1 to 12 (each 3 seconds in duration) appear in the window of a memory drum. After this first trial, each S was told that the series would be repeated several times and that each time the number 8 appeared he would receive an electric shock equal in intensity to one earlier determined to be the strongest he would tolerate. Skin conductance was monitored throughout the six trials given. During the first (nonshock) trial, all Ss showed a gradual decrease in skin conductance. The results for Trials 2 and 6 are shown in Figure 5. Compared with the nonpsychopathic criminals (NP) and non-criminal Ss (C), the psychopathic criminals (P) showed very little anticipatory electrodermal activity prior to the advent of shock. Presumably the anticipatory EDRs of the normal Ss reflect the reinstigation of earlier associations between warning cues and noxious events. With psychopaths, however, these earlier associations (or at least their emotional correlates) have either not been made or have failed to generalize to the experimental situation involved. Elsewhere (Hare, 1965a, 1965c) I've suggested that results such as these are consistent with the hypothesis that psychopaths are characterized by a relatively steep temporal gradient of fear arousal. That is, unless warning cues are in very close proximity to a noxious event, little anticipatory fear is elicited in the psychopath.

Conceptually, this relative inability to experience anticipatory fear is related to the other form of learning in which psychopaths seem to have difficulty, viz., avoidance learning. Learning to inhibit behavior likely to have unpleasant consequences may be viewed as a two-stage process involving the conditioning of fear to cues associated with punishment, and the subsequent reinforcement, by fear-reduction, of behavior that removes the individual from the fear-producing cues (Brown and Farber, 1968; Mowrer, 1947). The psychopath's apparent disregard for the future consequences of his behavior may therefore be seen as the failure of cues (visual, kinesthetic, symbolic, verbal, etc.) associated with punishment to elicit sufficient anticipatory fear for the instigation and subsequent reinforcement of avoidance responses. There is some empirical support for this position. Lykken (1955), using a complex 'mental maze', found that psychopaths learned a sequence of rewarded responses normally,

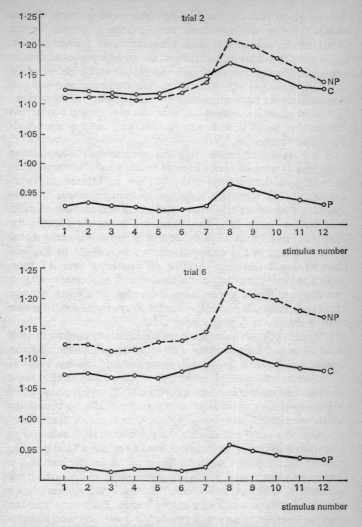

Figure 5 Log conductance level as a function of anticipated shock (administered at stimulus number S). P = psychopathic criminals; NP = non-psychopathic criminals; C = normal noncriminals (after Hare, 1965c)

but failed to learn to avoid responses punished with electric shock. Similar findings have been obtained by Schoenherr (1964), Schmauk (1968) and Schachter and Latane (1964). The latter investigators also found that an injection of adrenalin greatly enhanced the ability of the psychopathic Ss to avoid shocked responses. On the assumption that adrenalin-induced sympathetic activity augments the experience of fear, these results support the hypothesis that the psychopath's apparent inability to avoid punishment is related to inadequate anticipatory fear responses.

It is possible, of course, that the punishments used in these experiments are not really painful enough for the psychopath to make special attempts to avoid them (cf. Hare and Thorvaldson, 1970). Similarly, it is possible that the use of punishments that are more relevant to his value system would be more effective in controlling his behavior. Schmauk (1968), for example, found that while psychopaths made little attempt to avoid shock or social disapproval, they were quite willing and able to avoid responses leading to monetary loss. Further, avoidance of these latter responses was associated with a 'normal' amount of anticipatory electrodermal activity, activity that was absent when shock or social disapproval was involved.

In general, the conditioning studies of psychopathy have produced results that are not only conceptually consistent with those obtained from avoidance learning studies, but in addition make sense from a clinical point of view (e.g., Cleckley, 1964). It is important to note, however, that all of the conditioning studies cited used electric shock as the UCS and electrodermal activity as the response to be conditioned. Whether psychopaths would also condition poorly when other types of UCS (e.g., non-aversive ones) and other autonomic variables are involved was the subject of an experiment already referred to in another context (Hare and Quinn, in press). The study involved a delayed, differential conditioning paradigm in which three noticeably different conditioned stimuli (tones) were each presented sixteen times in random order. Each tone was ten seconds long; termination of two of the tones was accompanied by either a strong electric shock (CS^s) or a two-second slide of a nude female (CS^p). No UCS followed the third tone (CS). The

*S*s included eighteen psychopathic criminals (Group P), eighteen nonpsychopathic criminals (Group NP), and eighteen criminals about whom there was some doubt; the *S*s in this latter group probably represented a heterogeneous mixture of misclassified psychopaths and nonpsychopaths. The term mixed group (M) seems appropriate here. Dependent variables were electrodermal, cardiac, and both peripheral and cephalic vasomotor responses.

Electrodermal responses with a latency of from 4–11 seconds after CS onset were defined as anticipatory responses (AR). The mean amplitude of the electrodermal AR to each CS is plotted in Figure 6. It is evident that the main difference between groups

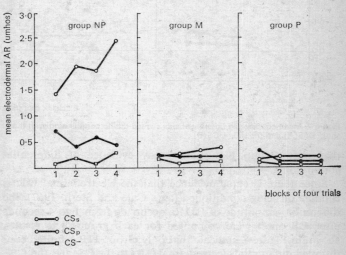

Figure 6 Mean electrodermal ARs elicited by each CS

lay in the size of the AR to the CS^s and, to a lesser extent, to the CS^p, with Group NP giving large, and the other groups small responses. In addition, Group NP was the only group to show clear-cut differentiation between CS^s and CS^-. Another way of presenting the data in Figure 6 is to plot them as differential ARs by subtracting the mean amplitude of the AR elicited by the CS^-, on a trial-by-trial basis, from the mean amplitude of the ARs elicited by the CS^s and by the CS^r. The resulting differential ARs are plotted in Figure 7, where it can be seen

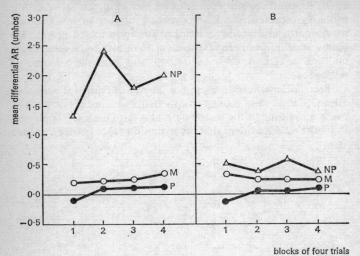

Figure 7 Mean conditioned differential aids elicited during conditioning with the shock 065(A) and the slide UCS(B)

that only Group NP showed any evidence of differential conditioning.

Since there is some evidence that the electrodermal OR is capable of being conditioned (e.g., Gale and Stern, 1967), the differential amplitude of EDRs occurring from 1 to 4 seconds after CS onset were computed for each group. The results, shown in Figure 8, indicate that only Group NP acquired conditioned differential electrodermal ORs to the CS^s and the CS^r.

Preliminary inspection of the data indicated that the cardiac response to the conditioned stimuli (generally deceleration) reached a maximum between 5 and 10 seconds after CS onset. The amplitude of the cardiac CR was therefore determined by computing the difference between the mean HR during this period and the mean HR during the 5 seconds immediately preceding CS onset. The differential cardiac CRs were averaged over blocks of four trials, and are plotted in Figure 9. It is

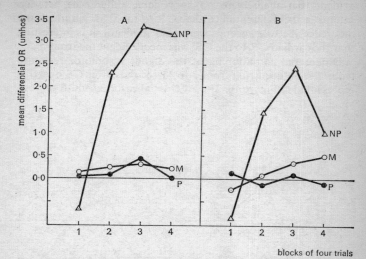

Figure 8 Mean differential electrodermal ORs elicited during conditioning with the shock UCS (A) and the slides UCS (B)

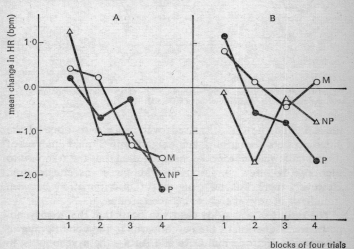

Figure 9 Mean differential cardiac CRs elicited during conditioning with the shock UCS (A) and the slides UCS (B). Deviations below the baseline indicate cardiac deceleration

evident that there were no appreciable differences between groups in the differential cardiac C R to the CSs. Although the differences between groups were not significant, it is interesting that the cardiac C R to the CS^P was most evident in Group P.

Differential conditioning of the digital vasomotor response (constriction occurring from 2 to 11 seconds after CS onset) is represented in Figure 10. The differential vasomotor C R to both

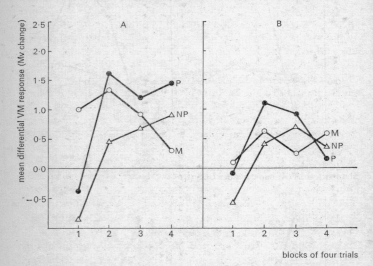

blocks of four trials

Figure 10 Mean differential digital vasomotor CRs elicited during conditioning with the shock UCS (A) and the slides UCS (B)

the CS^s and the CS^P increased over trials, with none of the differences between groups being significant. Similar analyses of the cephalic vasomotor responses revealed that the response to each of the three conditioned stimuli was vasoconstriction. However, there was no evidence of discrimination between stimuli, or of any differences between groups.

The results of this study clearly indicate that the nonpsychopaths were superior to the psychopaths in the conditioning of differential electrodermal O Rs and A Rs – the psychopaths, in fact, showed virtually no evidence of differential electrodermal conditioning, with the result that the differences between groups were rather dramatic, particularly where shock was involved as the UCS. Moreover, the responses given by the psychopaths were very small in an absolute sense. With shock as the UCS, the results are consistent with earlier research (Hare, 1965b; Lykken, 1955) and with the hypothesis that psychopaths do not acquire conditioned fear responses readily.

The situation with respect to the pictorial stimuli (nude females) is less clear. Although the psychopaths gave smaller differential electrodermal ORs and ARs to the CS^r, the differences between groups were not significant. The relatively small absolute responses given by the nonpsychopaths (compared with their responses to the CS^s) suggests that pictures of nude females were not a particularly effective UCS for electrodermal conditioning. Had more effective stimuli been used, it is quite possible that the differences between groups would have been more appreciable. An interesting point here is that even though clear-cut electrodermal conditioning did not occur with nude slides as the UCS, these same stimuli were very effective reinforcers for both psychopaths and non-psychopaths engaged in a simple operant conditioning task (Hare and Quinn, 1970). It is possible that the effectiveness of these slides in the conditioning paradigm used was reduced by virtue of the fact that they were used along with a somewhat more potent UCS, viz. shock.

The differences between groups in electrodermal conditioning did not extend to cardiac and vasomotor conditioning. The differential cardiac (decelerative) and digital vasomotor (constrictive) conditioning of the psychopaths was at least as good as that of the other Ss, and was similar to the results of other research with normal Ss (e.g., Gale and Stern, 1968; Obrist, 1968). Moreover, the failure of either psychopaths or non-psychopaths to show any evidence of differential cephalic vasomotor conditioning is consistent with a study by Brotsky (1969) in which normal Ss showed no evidence of cephalic vasomotor conditioning in spite of the fact that electrodermal conditioning took place.

It is clear from these results that simple generalizations about the psychopath's conditionability are not warranted unless restricted to electrodermal activity. However, beyond this, it is difficult to know what the implications are for a psychopath (or any S for that matter) who acquires cardiovascular conditioned responses readily but not electrodermal ones. Clearly, the psychopaths were able to make the connection between the CS and UCS on at least the cardiovascular level. Does this mean that they learned to anticipate, in an emotional sense, the advent of the unconditioned stimuli? Previous theory and research (*see* Hare, 1970) suggest that the psychopath's inability to avoid punishment is related to the *failure* to anticipate emotionally the consequences of his behavior, a suggestion based upon clinical observation and research involving electrodermal measures. The present electrodermal results are consistent with this suggestion, but the cardiovascular results are not. It is possible, of course, that electrodermal activity is a better (or simpler) indicant of emotional arousal in conditioning paradigms than is cardiovascular activity. Some indirect support for this possibility lies in the conceptual system relating psychopathy to electrodermal activity, fear arousal, and avoidance learning (see discussions by Hare, 1970; Schachter and Latane, 1964). It would be interesting here, both for psychopathy and for more general theories of behavior, to determine whether electrodermal conditionability is in fact a better predictor of avoidance learning (which is conceptually related to fear arousal) than is cardiovascular conditionability. Cardiovascular activity may be involved in fear arousal; however, it is also involved with the maintenance of bodily functioning and is characterized by complex interactions between the various components. Cardiac activity may also be related to attentiveness to environmental stimulation, and to the modulation of sensory input (Lacey, 1967). The point is that the behavioral and physiological functions of cardiovascular mechanisms and the implications of cardiovascular conditioning are complex and as yet poorly understood. With respect to conditioning, Obrist (1968) has suggested that the conditioned cardiac deceleration generally observed may represent one aspect of an inhibitory state initiated by the CS. This inhibitory state may serve either to attenuate the aversive qualities of the UCS (e.g., shock) or to facilitate the reception of a non-aversive UCS (e.g., nude pictures). Just why cardiac deceleration should have either inhibitory or facilitative functions, depending upon the situation, is unclear. Nevertheless, within the context of Obrist's suggestion, it is possible that the psychophysiological significance of the conditioned cardiac deceleration was not the same for the psychopaths as for the nonpsychopaths. Alternatively, it may be that the cardiovascular responses indicate that both groups of Ss were aware of and attentive to the stimuli and their contingencies, while the electrodermal responses reflect the fact that only the nonpsychopaths experienced anticipatory fear (in the case of shock).

References

ALBERT, R. S., BRIGANTE, T. R. and CHASE, M. (1959), 'The psychopathic personality: a content analysis of the concept', *J. gen. Psychol.*, vol. 60, pp. 17–28.

AMERICAN PSYCHIATRIC ASSOCIATION, (1952, 1968), *Diagnostic and Statistical Manual: Mental Disorders*, Washington, D.C.

BLANKSTEIN, K. R. (1969), 'Patterns of autonomic functioning in primary and secondary psychopaths', unpublished Master's thesis, University of Waterloo.

BROTSKY, S. J. (1969), 'Cephalic vasomotor responses as indices of the orienting reflex, and semantic conditioning and generalization. A failure to replicate Soviet research', *Psychonomic Sci.*, vol. 17, pp. 228–9.

BROWN, J. S. and FABER, I. E. (1968), 'Secondary motivational systems', in P. R. Farnsworth (ed.), *Ann. Rev. Psychol.*, vol. 19, Annual Review, Inc., pp. 99–134.

CLECKLEY, H. (1964), *The Mask of Sanity*, (4th edn), Mosby.

FINNEY, J. C. (1966), 'Relations and meaning of the new MMPI scales', *Psychol. Reports*, vol. 18, pp. 459–70.

FOX, R. and LIPPERT, W. (1963), 'Spontaneous GSR and anxiety level in sociopathic delinquents', *J. cons. Psychol*, vol. 27, p. 368.

GALE, E. N. and STERN, J. A. (1968), 'Classical conditioning of the peripheral vasomotor orienting response', *Psychophysiology*, vol. 4, pp. 342–8.

GELHORN, E. (1957), *Autonomic Imbalance and the Hypothalamus: Implications for Physiology, Medicine, Psychology, and Neuropsychiatry*, University of Minnesota Press.

GOLDSTEIN, I. B. (1965), 'The relationship of muscle tension and autonomic activity to psychiatric disorders', *Psychosomatic Medicine*, vol. 27, pp. 39–52.

GRAY, K. C. and HUTCHISON, H. C. (1964), 'The psychopathic personality: a survey of Canadian psychiatrists' opinions', *Canad. psychiat. Ass. J.*, vol. 9, pp. 452–61.

GROUP FOR THE ADVANCEMENT OF PSYCHIATRY (1966),
Psychopathological Disorders in Children: Theoretical Considerations and a Proposed Classification, Author, Report no. 62.

HARE, R. D. (1965a), 'A conflict and learning theory analysis of psychopathic behaviour', *J. Res. Crime and Delinquency*, vol. 2, pp. 12–19.

HARE, R. D. (1965b), 'Acquisition and generalization of a conditioned-fear response in psychopathic and non-psychopathic criminals', *J. Psychol.*, vol. 59, pp. 367–70.

HARE, R. D. (1965c), 'Temporal gradient of fear arousal in psychopaths', *J. ab. Psychol.*, vol. 70, pp. 442–5.

HARE, R. D. (1968), 'Psychopathy, autonomic functioning, and the orienting response', *J. Ab. Psych.*, Monograph Supplement, vol. 73, no. 3, Part 2, pp. 1–24.

HARE, R. D. (1970), *Psychopathy: Theory and Research*, Wiley.

HARE, R. D. and QUINN, M. J. (in press), 'Psychopathy and autonomic conditioning', *J. b. Psychol.*

HARE, R. D. and THORVALDSON, S. A. (1970), 'Psychopathy and response to electrical stimulation', *J. ab. Psychol.*, vol. 76, pp. 370–4.

HARE, R. D., WOOD, K., BRITAIN, S. and SHADMAN, J. (1970), 'Autonomic Responses to affective visual stimulation', *Psychophysiol.*, vol. 7, pp. 408–17.

HARE, R. D., WOOD, K., BRITAIN, S. and SHADMAN, J. (1971), 'Autonomic responses to affective visual stimulation: Sex differences', *J. Exper. Res. Person.*, vol. 5, pp. 14–22.

LACEY, J. I. (1967), 'Somatic response patterning and stress: Some revisions of activation theory', in M. H. Appley and R. Trumbull (eds.), *Psychological Stress: Issues in Research*, Appleton-Century-Crofts, pp. 14–44.

LINDNER, R. (1942), 'Experimental studies on constitutional psychopathic inferiority, Part 1. Systemic patterns', *J. crim. Psychol.*, vol. 3, pp. 252–76.

LIPPERT, W. W. and SENTER, R. J. (1966), 'Electrodermal responses in the sociopath', *Psychonomic Sci.*, vol. 4, pp. 25–6.

LYKKEN, D. T. (1955, 1956), 'A study of anxiety in the sociopathic personality', doctoral dissertation, University of Minnesota, University Microfilms No. 55–944, also in *J. ab. Psychol.*, vol. 55, pp. 6–10.

MCDONALD, D. C., JOHNSON, L. C. and HORD, D. J. (1964), 'Habituation of the orienting response in alert and drowsy subjects', *Psychophysiol.*, vol. 1, pp. 163–73.

MOWRER, O. H. (1947), 'On the dual nature of learning—a reinterpretation of "conditioning" and "problem-solving"', *Harvard Educ. Rev.*, vol. 17, pp. 102–48.

OBRIST, P. A. (1968), 'Heart rate and somatic motor coupling during classical aversive conditioning in humans', *J. exp. Psychol.*, vol. 77, pp. 189–93.

PETERSON, D. R., QUAY, H. C. and TIFFANY, T. L. (1961), 'Personality factors related to juvenile delinquency', *Child Devel.*, vol. 32, pp. 335–72.

PHILLIPS, L. (1968), 'A social view of psychopathology', in P. London and D. Rosenhan (eds.), *Foundations of ab. Psychol.*, Holt, Rinehart & Winston, pp. 427–59.

QUAY, H. C. (1964a), 'Dimensions of personality in delinquent boys as inferred from the factor analysis of case history data', *Child Devel.*, vol. 35, pp. 479–84.

QUAY, H. C. (1964b), 'Personality dimensions in delinquent males as inferred from the factor analysis of behaviour rating', *J. Res. Crime and Delinquency*, vol. 1, pp. 35–7.

RASKIN, D. C., KOTSES, H. and BEVER, J. (1969), 'Cephalic vasomotor and heart rate measures of orienting and defensive reflexes', *Psychophysiol*, vol. 6, pp. 149–59.

ROBINS, L. N. (1966), *Deviant Children Grown Up*, Williams and Wilkins.

RUILMANN, C. J. and GULO, M. J. (1950), 'Investigation of autonomic responses in psychopathic personalities', *S. med. J.*, vol. 43, pp. 953–6.

SCHACTER, S. and LATANE, B. (1964), 'Crime, cognition and the autonomic nervous system', in M. R. Jones, (ed.), *Nebraska Symposium on Motivation*, University of Nebraska Press, pp. 221–75.

SCHALLING, D. and LEVANDER, S. (1967), 'Spontaneous fluctuations in EDA during anticipation of pain in two delinquent groups differing in anxiety proneness', Report no. 30, Psychological Laboratory, University of Stockholm.

SCHALLING, D., LIDBERG, L., LEVANDER, S. and DAHLIN, Y. (1968), 'Relations between fluctuations in skin resistance and digital pulse volume and scores on the Gough DeScale', unpublished manuscript, University of Stockholm.

SCHMAUK, F. J. (1968), 'A study of the relationship between kinds of punishment, autonomic arousal, subjective anxiety and avoidance learning in the primary sociopath', unpublished Ph.D. dissertation, Temple University.

SCHOENHERR, J. C. (1964), 'Avoidance of noxious stimulation in psychopathic personality', doctoral dissertation, University of California, University Microfilms no. 64–8334.

TONG, J. E. (1959), 'Stress reactivity in relation to delinquent and psychopathic behaviour', *J. ment. Sc.*, vol. 105, pp. 935–56.

ZUBIN, J. (1967), 'Classification of the behaviour disorders', in P. R. Farnsworth (ed.), *Ann. Rev. Psychol.*, Annual Reviews, Inc., pp. 373–406.

Part Four
Psychosomatic Disorders

In recent years there has begun to emerge a central theme in the explanation of psychosomatic disorders. The theme rests upon the so-called *diathesis-stress* model. A disorder, according to this model, may arise when the proper combination of biological predisposition and external stress occurs. Without the predisposition, the environmental stress will be ineffective and, without the stress, the predisposed individual may escape the disorder.

The first paper by Dr Weiner and his colleagues has become a contemporary classic in the field of psychosomatic research. It is framed within the diathesis-stress model but is exceptional for the thoroughness with which the predisposition was assayed biologically before the disorder developed. Their findings leave open the question of the specificity of the stress that might be required before a disorder is triggered. Will any stress serve equally well? Grace and Graham, in an ingenious investigation, report data that suggest that specific kinds of psychological stress are pathogenic for particular kinds of psychosomatic disorder. Modern psychopathologists would probably feel that the question is still open; these two papers provide clear examples of the questions at issue.

12 H. Weiner, M. Thaler, M. F. Reiser and I. A. Mirsky

Etiology of Duodenal Ulcer

H. Weiner, M. Thaler, M. F. Reiser and I. A. Mirsky, 'Etiology of Duodenal Ulcer', *Psychosomatic Medicine*, vol. 19, No. 1, 1957, pp. 1–11.

The life history of a clinical syndrome and the various factors that contribute to the predisposition and precipitation of the syndrome in any particular person are usually inferred from data obtained after the clinical disorder has developed. Such inferences are frequently biased by the investigator's particular orientation. Thus, there are those who claim that the development of duodenal ulcer is determined solely by 'organic' factors, whereas others claim that 'psychic' factors are the sole determinants. Such polar attitudes are inevitable when the data being considered is *post hoc* in nature. The ideal approach for evaluating the determinants responsible for precipitating any clinical disorder is to study the subject who is going to develop the disorder before he does so. This *propter hoc* approach requires criteria that will permit the selection of individuals who are susceptible to the development of the particular syndrome.

Previous studies have established that the concentration of pepsinogen in the blood is dependent upon the rate of pepsinogen production by the stomach. In 87 per cent of patients with duodenal ulcer, the pepsinogen concentration is greater than the mean of values found in subjects without duodenal or other gastrointestinal disturbances. This observation is consistent with the general consensus that patients with duodenal ulcer tend to secrete more gastric juice, hydrochloric acid, and pepsin than do healthy subjects. The fact that the high concentration of pepsinogen in the sera of such patients was found to persist even after the duodenal lesion was healed, as does also the increased rate of gastric secretion, suggested that gastric hypersecretion is an essential but not the sole determinant in the development of the lesion.

The concentration of pepsinogen in the blood of 14 per cent of subjects without any gastrointestinal disturbance is greater than the mean of values found in patients with duodenal ulcer. Presumably, the stomachs of such 'healthy' subjects are hypersecreting pepsinogen. If gastric hypersecretion is an essential determinant in the development of duodenal ulcer, it may be postulated that the high pepsinogen secretors represent that segment of the population with a maximal secretory capacity that is most likely to develop duodenal ulcer when exposed to those circumstances responsible for precipitating the sequence of physiological events that result in the characteristic lesion. In accord with this hypothesis is the observation that apparently healthy subjects, without any previous history of gastrointestinal derangement, but with serum pepsinogen values in the range of those of patients with duodenal ulcer may go on to develop the lesion without any further significant increase in the concentration of pepsinogen in the blood.

The precise circumstances responsible for the precipitation of duodenal ulcer remain unknown. The consensus, however, is that psychic tension initiated by exposure to some environmental event is a prepotent factor. Although numerous studies have established that various manifestations of psychic tension can be related to a variety of gastrointestinal changes, no clue to the source of the tension became apparent until Alexander and his colleagues applied psychoanalytical principles to the study of patients with peptic ulcer. Such studies by Alexander and others led to the generalization that patients with duodenal ulcer have in common a conflict related to the persistence of strong infantile wishes to be loved and cared for, on the one hand, and the repudiation of these wishes by the adult ego or by external circumstances, on the other hand. This psychic conflict is postulated to be responsible for initiating a sequence of physiological changes that result in the development of the duodenal lesion. Yet, as Alexander and others have stressed, similar psychodynamic patterns can be demonstrated in subjects without any gastrointestinal disturbance or in subjects with some other derangement. Consequently, as Alexander indicated, psychic conflict, specific or otherwise, cannot be the sole determinant in the precipitation of duodenal ulcer.

It is generally acknowledged that the response to some environmental event is a major factor in initiating the process responsible for the precipitation of peptic ulcer. Yet, there is nothing specific about the social situation that so frequently precedes the precipitation of duodenal ulcer. The only inference that can be made is that the specific meaning of the environmental event to the particular individual determines whether or not the event is responded to as a noxious one.

From the preceding it would appear that there are three parameters which may contribute to the precipitation of duodenal ulcer: a physiological parameter, which determines the susceptibility of the duodenum to ulceration; a psychological parameter, which determines the relatively specific psychic conflict that induces psychic tension; and a social parameter, which determines the environmental event that will prove noxious to the particular individual. Accordingly, a duodenal ulcer should develop when an individual with a sustained rate of gastric hypersecretion and the aforementioned psychic conflict is exposed to an environmental situation that mobilizes conflict and induces psychic tension.

This report deals with part of a study designed to evaluate the role of the three parameters in the precipitation of duodenal ulcer. The degree of gastric secretion gauged by the concentration of pepsinogen in the serum comprised the physiological parameter; subjects with serum pepsinogen values beyond one standard deviation of the mean were regarded as hypersecretors, and subjects with pepsinogen values below one standard deviation of the mean were regarded as hyposecretors. The selection of subjects representative of those with the highest and lowest concentrations of pepsinogen in the blood permitted one group to serve as a control for the other. The style of interpersonal interactions that could be inferred from projective and other psychological techniques comprised the psychological parameter. The exposure to sixteen weeks of basic training comprised the environmental situation that might prove noxious to some and not to other subjects.

Method

A total of 2073 draftees between the ages of 17·5 years and 29·2 years were chosen at random while being processed at induction at an army camp. Before entering service all had resided in the northeastern United States. Ten ml. of blood was drawn from each man. The sample was identified by code number, refrigerated, and sent to one of us (I A M) for analysis. The concentration of pepsinogen in the serum was determined by a method described in an earlier paper. The Cornell Medical Index, the Saslow Screening Inventory, and a sociological rating scale[1] were administered to each man. Approximately 300 men were processed per week.

At the end of each week, the code numbers of twenty men were returned to the research group at the Induction Center without their levels of serum pepsinogen being revealed. These numbers identified men who were chosen for more detailed study because they were in the range of the highest and lowest values obtained in the group of men tested during the previous week. At the end of seven weeks, a total of 120 men had been selected for special study.

During the second week the twenty men who had been selected at the end of the first week were given a battery of psychological tests (Rorschach Test, Blacky Pictures, and Draw-A-Person Test). Each man was interviewed briefly by a psychiatrist and social worker, and each man was given a complete gastrointestinal roentgenological examination. The psychological tests were administered by a technician, and the test material was then sent to three of us (M.T., H.W., and M.R.) for evaluation.

After these studies were completed the men were sent to the basic training area. Subsequently, all but thirteen men were again given the psychological tests and roentgenological examinations some time between the eighth and sixteenth week of the basic training period.

The Rorschach results were submitted both to a formal scoring and to that devised by DeVos, which divides content into various categories and subcategories 'concerned with the symbolic expressions of affect'. Each drawing from the Draw-A-

1. Devised and evaluated by 1st Lt. Sidney Croog, W R A I R, Walter Reed Army Medical Center, Washington 12, D.C.

Person Test was classified as primitive, distorted, boyish, masculine, or adult. The Cornell Medical Index, Saslow and Blacky tests were scored as recommended by their originators. In addition, Card II of the Blacky Test was scored as to whether Blacky was seen as openly expressing anger or whether the expression of such affect was denied, rationalized, or ignored.

Results

Figure 1 illustrates the normal distribution of the values for the concentration of pepsinogen in the sera of the population of 2073 men who were screened. The hypersecretor group selected

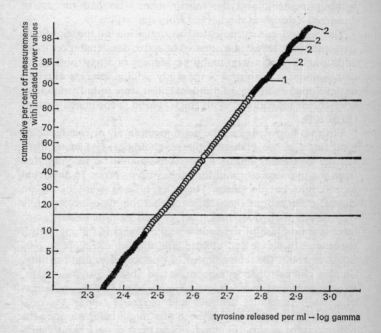

Figure 1 Distribution of blood serum pepsinogen concentrations: the frequency distribution of the logarithm of the concentration of the pepsinogen in the serum plotted on a probit scale. The subjects selected for special study were among those designated with closed circles. The numerals refer to individuals with duodenal ulcer

for special study consisted of sixty-three of the 300 men who comprised those with the upper 15 per cent of the serum pepsinogen values. The hyposecretor group selected for special study consisted of fifty-seven of the 179 men who comprised those with the lowest 9 per cent of the serum pepsinogen values.

The first roentgenological examination revealed evidences of a healed duodenal ulcer in three, and of an active ulcer in one of the sixty-three men with gastric hypersecretion. Of these four men with evidence of duodenal lesions at the outset, one became a disciplinary problem and was confined to the stockade, one went 'absent without leave', one went through his basic training without incident, and the fourth man, who had the active duodenal lesion, was discharged from the service.

The second roentgenological examination at the eighth to sixteenth week revealed evidences of active duodenal ulcer in an additional five men who had no evidences of a gastrointestinal derangement at the outset of the study. All the subjects who had or developed evidences of duodenal ulcer were found among the sixty-three individuals with high blood pepsinogen values (Figure 1).

With no knowledge of the pepsinogen levels or roentgenological findings, we evaluated the psychological test material to test the hypothesis that the hypersecretor could be differentiated from the hyposecretor and that men with or prone to duodenal ulcer could be identified. These hypotheses were based on clinical observations that suggested that the hypersecretor, like the patient with duodenal ulcer, would exhibit evidences of intense infantile oral dependent wishes, marked 'immaturity', tendencies to please and placate, and difficulties revolving particularly about the management of oral impulses and hostility. Similar clinical observations suggested that the hyposecretor, like the patient with pernicious anaemia, would exhibit evidences of pseudo-masculine defenses and paranoid trends. Accordingly, in order to categorize those who might belong among the hypersecretor group, the psychological test material was examined specifically for the presence of strong direct references to the acts of feeding, of being fed, and of incorporation. Indirect or inferred oral symbolism such as talking, smoking, kissing, blowing, etc., and responses referable to heat and cold (e.g., snow, people warming themselves, flowers growing in the snow) were also sought. It was anticipated that the hypersecretors would reveal diffuse anxiety in their answers, that many records might be characterized by depressive associations, and that the drawings would be those of boys, or primitive and gross, or asexual.

To categorize those who might belong to the hyposecretor group, special attention was paid to indications of problems referable to activity and passivity, submissiveness and assertiveness, femininity and masculinity, as evidenced by responses suggesting conflict over sexual identification, passive sexual longing, and anal symbolism. It was postulated that the test material of the hyposecretors, in contrast to the hypersecretors, would show little or no oral, depressive, or anxiety content and a paucity of indications of a need to please and placate.

Using the above criteria, one psychologist and two psychiatrists independently rated the test records to determine whether the subject belonged to the hypersecretor or hyposecretor group. On the basis of a majority opinion, 61 per cent of the 120 men – 71 per cent of the hypersecretors and 51 per cent of the hyposecretors – were correctly designated on the basis of the postulated traits.

It had been anticipated that the psychological test material and social histories would permit the prediction of the way in which each individual would react to the social situation represented by the period of basic training. This anticipation, however, proved incorrect since no technique could be devised *post hoc* to permit the selection of individuals who would react to the situation as if it were a noxious one. Consequently, based on previous experience with test patterns from patients with duodenal ulcer and on inferences derived from psychoanalytical and other clinical observations of such patients, an attempt was made to predict which individual would develop a duodenal ulcer during the sixteen weeks of basic training. It was postulated that the subject most likely to develop an ulcer during the period of basic training would show all the characteristics of the hypersecretor but with a much greater intensity than the individual who was not likely to develop the lesion. Accordingly, the psychological test material of the inductees was evaluated *before* the biochemical and roentgenological data became available.

Ten men were selected as those most likely to develop an ulcer because their test material not only suggested that they belong to the group of hypersecretors but also showed evidences of intense needs to maintain relationships with others. Their anxieties centered around a fear of expressing hostility lest there be a loss of supplies for their needs; they went out of their way to rationalize, deny, and displace such feelings. The need to please and placate authority figures as potential sources of affection was particularly striking. The predictions were accurate in seven out of the ten. Of the three who did not have or did not develop an ulcer, two were hypersecretors.

Post hoc studies revealed that all of the nine men who had or developed a duodenal ulcer during the period of basic training had been classified correctly as belonging to the group with high serum pepsinogen values on the basis of the psychological criteria given above. Other than the intensity of their attempt to maintain relationships, no criterion was found to distinguish the hypersecretor who developed an ulcer from the hypersecretor who did not.

The attempt to differentiate the hypersecretors from the hyposecretors on the basis of clinical impressions of the available psychological test material indicated that the criteria used for such differentiation were inadequate. To develop a more accurate diagnostic tool, a variety of criteria from the test material of the hypersecretors and hyposecretors were analysed statistically. Only those criteria that were significant at less than the 5 per cent level of confidence were used for a final classification. By means of a cluster of twenty such criteria it was possible to distinguish the two groups to the extent that 85 per cent of the 120 men could be assigned accurately to their group at a 0·001 level of confidence. Thus, of the 120 men, only six hypersecretors and twelve hyposecretors could not be correctly classified on the basis of the cluster of psychological test criteria.

The twenty criteria that permitted the relatively correct differentiation of the hypersecretor from the hyposecretor are listed in Table 1. No single criterion permitted the separation of the two groups with an accuracy exceeding 64·2 per cent, but all were significant at the 5 per cent level of confidence or better. The combinations of items, however, permitted the more accurate designation.

The overall impression of the psychological makeup of hypersecretors gained from the use of these scoring criteria was one of marked dependency in their relationships to others, of compliance, and of passiveness. Thus the affect of a greater number was childishly toned (criteria 1 and 2); they gave more texture responses (criterion 3), suggesting a greater awareness of, or need for tactile contact with others. A greater incidence of responses symbolizing oral needs (criterion 4) and dependency on authority figures (criterion 2) were given by the hypersecretors. This group also displayed a greater incidence of immature body images on human drawings (criterion 5).

The majority of the hypersecretors gave responses symbolizing the expression, explicit or implicit, of anxiety (criterion 6), the source of which appeared to be hostile impulses (criterion 7) that they felt must not be revealed or directly expressed (criteria 8, 9, and 10). This was inferred from the resulting formal evidences of depression that were evident in the Rorschach scores (criteria 11 and 12). The hypersecretors had relatively few complaints about bodily symptoms, be they of discomfort, physical illness (criterion 13), or of the anxiety reaction (criterion 13), or of the anxiety reaction (criterion 14). It is noteworthy, however, that the Rorschach associations of some individuals indicated both the presence of anxiety (criterion 6) in freely associated material, and a tendency not to complain of its physical concomitant and not to be aware of and/or acknowledge its presence on direct questioning (criteria 13 and 14). Thus, of the twenty-seven individuals with high serum pepsinogen levels who gave anxiety associations (criterion 6), twelve denied that they felt anxious on the Saslow questionnaire. Yet anxiety associations (criterion 6) were given by fourteen hyposecretors, eleven of whom admitted their anxiety openly (criterion 14).

Although the above features, so common to many of the hypersecretors, were also present in twelve of the hyposecretors, the incidence of such features was insignificant among the latter (criteria 1, 2, 4, and 5). The greater 'immaturity' of the hyper-

Table 1 Criteria distinguishing subjects with high and low concentration of pepsinogen in the blood

Criterion	Responses: Cut-off score	Serum pepsinogen concentration		Number correctly classified	% of total corr. classified	X^2	P Level
		High	Low				
1. Rorschach: Color-form	Present Absent	31 32	17 40	71	59·2	4·684	< ·05
2. Rorschach: Childish and authority-dependency	Present Absent	37 26	21 36	73	60·8	5·741	< ·02
3. Rorschach: texture	Present Absent	33 30	18 39	72	60·0	5·299	< ·05
4. Rorschach: oral symbolism	31% or more 30% or less	35 28	19 38	73	60·8	5·971	< ·02
5. Draw-A-Person: boyish drawings	Present Absent	24 39	8 49	73	60·8	7·67	< ·01
6. Rorschach: openly symbolized hostility	3 or more 2 or less	27 36	14 43	70	58·3	5·010	< ·05
7. Rorschach: per cent hostile responses	24% or less 25% or more	50 13	30 27	77	64·2	9·624	< ·01
8. Blacky test: anger on Card II	Absent Present	32 31	18 39	71	59·2	4·546	< ·05
9. Blacky test: denial of aggression, card IIIb	Present Absent	29 34	16 41	70	48·3	4·119	< ·05

Criterion	Category			No.	%	χ²	p
10. Saslow test: anger expressed (N = 110)	No	36	22	66	60·0	4·296	< ·05
	Yes	22	30				
11. Rorschach: per cent small details	8% or more	36	20	73	60·8	5·849	< ·02
	7% or less	27	37				
12. Rorschach: poorly perceived responses	20% or less	31	32	74	61·7	7·755	< ·01
	21% or more	14	43				
13. Cornell Medical Index: Number of items	15 or less	46	16	75	62·5	9·153	< ·01
	16 or more	26	29				
14. Saslow Text: anxiety expressed (N = 109)	No	30	28	67	61·5	6·64	= ·01
	Yes	14	37				
15. Rorschach: hostile-sado-masochistic content	Absent	52	11	72	60·0	4·853	< ·05
	Present	37	20				
16. Rorschach: feminine identification	Absent	52	11	72	60·0	4·853	< ·05
	Present	37	20				
17. Rorschach: anxious face details	Absent	62	1	70	58·3	5·010	< ·05
	Present	49	8				
18. Rorschach: hybrid combinations	1 or less	62	1	72	60·0	7·335	< ·01
	2 or more	47	10				
19. Rorschach: per cent unpleasant content	39% or less	33	30	72	60·0	5·299	< ·05
	40% or more	18	39				
20. Rorschach: per cent neutral content	35% or more	33	30	72	60·0	5·299	< ·05
	34% or less	18	39				
Total classification (20 criteria)	10 or more	57	45	102	85·0	. . . .	< ·001

Table 2 Check list of 'disturbed' records

Sign	Responses: Cut-off score	Serum pepsinogen concentration		Number correctly classified	% of total (120) corr. classified	X^2	P Level
		High	Low				
1. Formal Rorschach. N-33							
(a) P%	12% or less	8	7	20	60·0		N. S.
	13% or more	6	12				
(b) F minus % and i% combined	49% or more	9	9	19	57·0		N. S.
	48% or less	5	10				
(c) W%	20% or less	9	8	20	60·0		N. S.
	21% or more	5	11				
(d) Feminine on card 3	Absent	14	12	21	63·0	4·417	< ·05
	Present	0	7				
(e) Elaboration	Absent	14	10	23	69·0	6·76	< ·01
	Present	0	9				
2. DeVos scoring:							
(f) Ahyb	1 or less	13	13	19	57·0		N.S.
	2 or more	1	6				
(g) AA and Aa combined	2 or more	13	6	26	78·0	9·874	< ·01
	1 or less	1	13				
(h) Oral	2 or more	10	6	23	69·0	4·515	< ·05
	1 or less	4	13				

secretors, when compared with the hyposecretors, is also revealed in the fact that they consistently showed two of the three categories which best reveal juvenile traits (criteria 1, 2, and 5) when these criteria were combined to evaluate this feature.

Another distinction between the two groups was that the hyposecretors showed high hostility scores (criterion 7) in which sadomasochistic associations figured prominently (criterion 15), or they openly expressed their anger (criteria 8 and 10).

To test the consistency with which the hypersecretor group appeared to avoid or evade the evidences of the expression of hostility, responses to criteria 7, 8, 9, 10, and 15 were combined. Using a simple majority tally as a cut-off score, the direct expression of hostility was found to be rarer among the hypersecretors than among the hyposecretors (P < 0·001).

Bodily preoccupation (criterion 13) and more complaints about bodily symptoms generally characterized individuals in the group with low serum pepsinogen concentrations. The hyposecretors gave a mean of nineteen complaints, whereas the hypersecretors gave a mean of twelve complaints. Furthermore, using Brodman's criterion of thirty or more complaints as an indicator of potentially inadequate military performance, there were four hypersecretors and fifteen hyposecretors who gave thirty or more of these answers; the difference is statistically significant (P < 0·01).

Twenty of the fifty-seven hyposecretors drew very masculine and adult figures on the Draw-A-Person Test, but twenty of these had an apparent difficulty in sexual identity, revealed by

Table 3 **Overall clinical judgment of Rorschach record**

DeVos index number of responses	Hypersecretors		Hyposecretors	
	Not disturbed (49)	Disturbed (14)	Not disturbed (38)	Disturbed (19)
0	32	4	22	5
1	12	1	9	3
2 and more	5	9	7	11
	$X^2 = 8·75$		$X^2 = 7·399$	
	$p < ·01$		$p < ·01$	

their identifying the figures on the third Rorschach card as women or by giving only female human content on the entire test.

That a small number of hyposecretors handle their anxiety by focusing on profile details on the Rorschach test is indicated by criterion 17. Other subjects gave two or more autistic and hybrid combinations of humans and animals (criterion 18).

In the overall group of 120 soldiers, there were thirty-three (fourteen hypersecretors and nineteen hyposecretors) whose test records on inspection indicated sufficient psychological difficulties to rate the protocols as 'disturbed'. The contrast between 'disturbed' hyper- and hyposecretors was consistent with the inference drawn above for the entire group. In fact, the 'disturbed' records of hypersecretors revealed that their anxieties were the product of variants of primitive oral impulses in dependent relationships. The hyposecretors, in contrast, evidenced marked somatic preoccupation, predominantly projective defenses, and an elaborate form of thought disorder.

Discussion

In the present study, the criterion chosen as an index of the susceptibility to the development of duodenal ulcer was the concentration of pepsinogen in the serum. This criterion was selected because long-term studies still in progress have indicated that duodenal ulcer develops only in those with high serum pepsinogen concentrations.

The data reported herein reveal a remarkable correlation between the concentration of pepsinogen in the serum and specific personality characteristics of a group of young men inducted into the army. The group of subjects with high serum pepsinogen concentrations show intense needs that are principally 'oral' in nature and which are exhibited in terms of wishing to be fed, to lean on others, and to seek close bodily contact with others. Satisfaction of these needs for external support and external sources for satiation is attempted by many means. When such attempts fail, the resultant frustration arouses anger that cannot be expressed lest there ensue a loss of supply for their needs. Consequently these subjects usually do not make complaints or express any feelings of anger.

In contrast to the above, the subjects with low concentrations of pepsinogen in the serum exhibit fewer problems about and less dependency on external sources of supply and support. They are more narcissistic and exhibit more problems relative to internal, bodily discomfort, and react to the sources of the discomfort with intense hostility which they express relatively freely. They show evidences of a disturbance in language style by elaboration and pretentiousness. Some of the subjects show a hostile feminine identification which they defend themselves against by a masculine overcompensation. Projective defenses against anxiety are common.

In accord with the hypothesis stated at the outset, the men who had or developed a duodenal lesion were among those with high concentrations of pepsinogen in the circulation; that is, among the hypersecretors. Further, the personality characteristics of those who did develop a duodenal ulcer are essentially the same as most of the subjects comprising the hypersecretor group. Although the predictions were accurate in seven of nine subjects who had or developed duodenal ulcer, it proved impossible in the present study to use the available data to determine why only some of the hypersecretors reacted as they did to the social situation or developed the duodenal lesion. In another study in which psychoanalytically oriented anamnestic interviews were conducted, however, it has been possible to predict the character of the social situation that would prove noxious to the specific individual, and subsequently to observe that when such exposure occurred, a duodenal ulcer ensued. These observations, as well as the mechanism whereby exposure to a social event that is noxious to the individual induces the development of a duodenal lesion, will be described in another communication.

The present study does not provide an explanation for the high correlation between the serum pepsinogen concentration and the relatively specific personality characteristics. Studies on siblings and twins reveal that the secretory capacity of the gastric mucosa as gauged by the serum pepsinogen concentrations is genetically determined. Even at birth, the concentration of serum pepsinogen is distributed normally with some newborn infants having values that are beyond the mean of patients with duodenal ulcer. Consequently, it is improbable that the psychological characteristics described above are responsible for the physiological state of the stomach. Although the psychological development of the infant is largely dependent upon his human environment, the secretory capacity of the stomach with which the child is born may play a significant role in his relationship with that environment. Studies on the manner in which the quantitative aspects of a physiological system influences the child-mother unit and thereby the child's psychological development are in progress and should provide data that may clarify the mechanisms involved.

Although it is possible to postulate that the inherited secretory capacity of the stomach plays a role in determining not only the psychological development of the infant but also his physiological predisposition, it does not account for the marked individual differences that characterize the manner in which the needs described above are handled. Study of these individual differences suggest that the vagaries of each person's life experiences determine the manner in which impulses and wishes are mastered, whereas the hypersecretor's persistent wishes for support and succor from the external environment are determined by early childhood factors. The manner in which he handles these wishes is determined by all his life experiences, that is, by the factors that determine his integrative capacity.

Summary

1. Serum pepsinogen was determined for each of 2073 army inductees. Sixty-three with values in the upper 15 per cent and fifty-seven with values in the lower 9 per cent of the blood pepsinogen distribution were selected for special study. Each of these was given the Rorschach, Blacky, Draw-A-Person, Cornell Medical Index, and Saslow tests, and a complete upper gastrointestinal roentgenological examination before being sent to basic training.

2. One hundred and seven subjects were reexamined between the eighth and sixteenth week of basic training. The first roentgenological examination revealed healed duodenal ulcers in three subjects and an active ulcer in one. The second roentgenological examination revealed active duodenal ulcers in five additional

men. All nine subjects with peptic ulcer were in the upper 15 per cent of the blood pepsinogen distribution, eight of them being in the upper 5 per cent. Thus, 15 per cent of men in the top 5 per cent developed peptic ulcer.

3. Independent evaluation of the psychological data revealed that subjects with peptic ulcer displayed evidence of major unresolved and persistent conflicts about dependency and oral gratification, the characteristics of which are described.

4. Classification of the selected test population into two groups on the basis of criteria derived from the psychological tests was found to correlate (85 per cent) with the two groups (hyper- and hypo-pepsinogen secretors) derived from the physiological tests.

5. The study indicates that neither a high rate of gastric secretion nor a specific psychodynamic constellation is independently responsible for development of peptic ulcer.

Together, however, these two parameters constitute the essential determinants in the precipitation of peptic ulcer on exposure to social situations noxious to the specific individual.

References

ALEXANDER, F. (1934), 'The influence of psychologic factors upon gastrointestinal disturbances: General principles, objectives and preliminary results', *Psychoanalyt. Q.*, vol. 3, p. 501.

ALEXANDER, F. (1950), *Psychosomatic Medicine*, Norton.

BECK, S. J. (1947), *Rorschach's Test*, Grune and Stratton.

BLUM, G. S. (1951), 'Revised scoring system for research use of the Blacky pictures', (male form-1951), University of Michigan.

BRODMAN, K., ERDMANN, A. J. JR., LORGE, I., DEUTSCHBERGER, J., and WOLFF, H. G. (1954), 'The Cornell Medical Index-Health Questionnaire VII: The prediction of psychosomatic and psychiatric disabilities in army training', *Amer. J. Psychiat.*, vol. 111, p. 37.

DEVOS, G. (1952), 'A quantitative approach to affective symbolism in Rorschach responses', *J. Proj. Tech.*, vol. 16, p. 133.

GILDEA, E. G. (1949) 'Special features of the personality which are common to certain psychosomatic disorders', *Psychosom. Medicine*, vol. 11, p. 273.

GARMA, A (1953), 'Internalized mother as harmful food in peptic ulcer patients', *Int. J. Psychoanal.*, vol. 34, p. 102.

HUNT, J. N. and KAY, A. W. (1954), 'The nature of gastric hypersecretion of acid in patients with duodenal ulcer', *Brit. Med. J.* vol. 2, p. 1444.

IVY, A. C., GROSSMAN, M. I. and BACHRACH, W. H. (1950), *Peptic Ulcer*, Blakiston.

JONES, F. A. (1956), 'The problem of peptic ulcer', *Ann. Int. Medicine*, vol. 44, p. 63.

KAPP, F. T., ROSENBAUM, M. and ROMANO, J. (1947), 'Psychological factors in men with peptic ulcer', *Amer. J. Psychiat.*, vol. 103, p. 700.

LEVIN, E., KIRSNER, J. B. and PALMER, W. L. (1948), 'Twelve-hour nocturnal gastric secretion in uncomplicated duodenal ulcer patients: Before and after healing', *Proc. Soc. exper. biol. Medicine*, vol. 69, p. 153.

MINSKI, L. and DESAI, M. M. (1955), 'Aspects of personality in peptic ulcer patients', *Brit. J. Med. Psychol.*, vol. 28, p. 113.

MIRSKY, I. A., FUTTERMAN, P., KAPLAN, S. and BROH-KAHN, R. H. (1952), 'Blood plasma pepsinogen: I. The source, properties, and assay of the proteolytic activity of plasma at acid reactions', *J. lab. and clin. Medicine*, vol. 40, p. 17.

MIRSKY, I. A., FUTTERMAN, P. and KAPLAN, S. (1952), 'Blood plasma pepsinogen; II. The activity of the plasma from "normal" subjects, patients with duodenal ulcer, and patients with pernicious anemia', *J. lab. and clin., Medicine*, vol. 40, p. 188.

MIRSKY I. A. (1953), 'Psychoanalysis and the biological sciences', in Alexander and Ross, *Twenty Years of Psychoanalysis*, Norton and Co.

RUESCH, J. (1948), 'The infantile personality', *Psychosom. Medicine*, vol. 10, p. 134.

RUESCH, J., CHRISTIANSEN, C., DEWEES, S., HARRIS, R. E., JACOBSON, A. and LOEB, M. B. (1948), *Duodenal Ulcer, a Sociopsychological Study of Naval Enlisted Personnel and Civilians*, University of California Press.

SASLOW, G., COUNTS, R. M. and DUBOIS, P. H. (1951), 'Evaluation of a new psychiatric screening test', *Psychosom. Medicine*, vol. 13, p. 242.

STREITFELD, H. S. (1954), 'Specificity of peptic ulcer to intense oral conflicts', *Psychosom. Medicine*, vol. 16, p. 315.

THALER, M. B., WEINER, H. and REISER, M. F. (1955), 'An exploration of the doctor-patient relationship through projective techniques', presented at 111th annual meeting, American Psychiatric Association, Atlantic City, N. J.

ZANE, M. (1947), 'Psychosomatic considerations in peptic ulcer', *Psychosom. Medicine*, vol. 2, p. 372.

13 W. J. Grace and D. T. Graham

Relationship of Specific Attitudes and Emotions to
Certain Bodily Diseases

W. J. Grace and D. T. Graham, 'Relationship of Specific Attitudes and
Emotions to Certain Bodily Diseases', *Psychosomatic Medicine*, vol. 14,
1952, pp. 243–51.

There is now evidence that many symptoms and diseases occur
in settings of difficult life situations. In spite of this, however,
the reason why some individuals suffer from one disease or
symptom and others from another continues to arouse considerable discussion.

Previous attempts to find something in common among persons with any given disease, other than the disease itself, fall into
several loosely defined and not mutually exclusive categories. In
the first place, there have been attempts to demonstrate a particular kind of personality pattern in all patients with the same
disease. Migrainous individuals, for example, have been described as having 'feelings of insecurity with tension, manifested
as inflexibility, conscientiousness, meticulousness, perfection-
ism, and resentment'. A modification of this has consisted of the
identification of a single personality trait or characteristic, defined in terms of overt behavior in association with a particular
disease, as for instance, 'obsessive-compulsive behavior' and
'subnormal assertiveness' with arterial hypertension or 'non-
participation' with rhinitis. A prominent psychoanalytic point
of view, which could in some instances be combined with the
preceding, is that the common denominator in individuals with
the same disease is a 'nuclear conflict' or 'dynamic configuration' unique to the disease in question, the significant factors
being largely unconscious. An older formulation is the notion
of 'organ inferiority', the assumption that certain individuals
have particular organs predisposed to disturbance, so that in
some persons any kind of life stress will result in gastric dysfunction, for example.

A somewhat different approach to the problem has revolved

around an investigation of what has happened to the patient previously, especially in childhood, with relatively little attention paid to the aspects of the present situation which are important to his disease. An example of this is the search for toilet-training conflicts in the histories of patients with constipation and diarrhoea.

Finally, there have been efforts to correlate the occurrence of particular symptoms with particular situations, as, for instance, asthmatic attacks with withdrawal of a mother's love. These have usually not been rigidly restricted to an objective description of the situation, however, since some qualification in terms of the patient's perception of it is ordinarily introduced. Perhaps the closest approach to the views expressed in the present paper is Groen's statement that the onset of ulcerative colitis occurred at times of 'acute love-loss and painful humiliation'.

These formulations contain considerable truth and have contributed significantly to our understanding and knowledge of human behavior, but they have been unsatisfactory in some respects. There are, for example, some persons with migraine who do not show the personality features described to an outstanding degree, just as there are individuals who show these features and do not have migraine. Also, many patients manifest a great variety of symptoms during their lives, often with fairly rapid changes; this phenomenon is difficult to reconcile with the notion of fixed personality patterns belonging to different diseases. The same objection can be raised against the idea of 'organ inferiority'. (In addition, an organ such as the colon cannot be considered 'weak' if it is working all the time.) We have seen one patient who had at different times angina pectoris, eczema, vasospastic retinopathy, diarrhoea, vomiting, and backache; and there are many persons who show at least two diseases, such as vasomotor rhinitis and ulcerative colitis, or peptic ulcer and migraine. It seems, in fact, that the majority of patients if followed for an extended period will show more than one symptom, although of course one may predominate over the others.

The concept of the single, significant personality trait has not been much explored. It is an attractive notion, since a single individual may have many traits. It does appear, however, that traits will be found in many persons free of the corresponding diseases and that some with a disease may not have the trait in question. The correlations of 'obsessive-compulsive behavior' and 'subnormal assertiveness' with arterial hypertension, for example, although significant statistically, were far from perfect. Obvious difficulties arise also in connection with the definition of traits and in their measurement. Similar considerations apply to the 'specific dynamic configuration' theory, and it has been explicitly stated that there are persons who have the configuration without having the disease in question. In both of these approaches there is a relative lack of emphasis on correlating definite events in the individual's life with exacerbations of symptoms.

Attempts to find common factors in early life experiences of individuals with the same disease have not met with uniform success. For instance, difficulty in early toilet training seemed to play no part in ulcerative colitis. There may well be such factors, however, which have been missed because the relevant variables have not been isolated.

Finally, there is not necessarily any striking external similarity among the situations which provoke exacerbations of any one disease in the same patient or in different patients; nor is the same situation always associated with attacks. The greater the extent to which the patient's way of looking at the situation is introduced into this formulation, the more closely it approaches the thesis of the present paper. No one, however, has given clear-cut statements of the patients' attitudes.

In the course of attempting to resolve these difficulties it became apparent that there was associated with each symptom a definite attitude which was peculiar to it, and without which it did not occur. In order to explore this approach further, a systematic method of questioning patients was employed.

Method

One hundred and twenty-eight patients, who had one or more of the twelve symptoms or diseases studied, were followed in treatment in the outpatient department. Interviews with the patients by one or the other of the authors were the only method of obtaining the information used in this paper. Interviews usually lasted about one hour, and took place as often as twice a week and as infrequently as once in three months. Most of the patients made a total of ten or more visits to the clinic.

In the interviews, emphasis was first placed on defining the situations temporally associated with attacks of the patient's symptoms. After such a situation had been identified, the next step was to obtain from him a description of his *attitude, by which is meant a clear and unambiguous statement of what he felt was happening to him, and what he wanted to do about it, at the time of the occurrence of the symptom.* This last point is of major importance, as it was found that often an individual felt in one way about the precipitating event during an interview, but in another way at the time symptoms were developing. Conventional names of 'emotions', etc., were not accepted without further definition.

It was noted, in the first place, that many of the patients with the same symptom-complex spontaneously referred to their life-situations and their own reactions in the same way. Those who did not were asked to describe the situation in the terms outlined above. Patients who were still unable to grasp the task were given a set of possibilities from among which they were told to select those most applicable to themselves.

No attempt was made to utilize dream or associative material in collecting the data used in this study. All of the conclusions are based entirely on direct statements by the patients.

Surprisingly little difficulty was encountered with most patients in obtaining unequivocal answers to the questions asked. Obstacles arose chiefly with reticent or bland individuals in trying to discover exactly what the stressful situation was. Without this information the method described of eliciting the patient's attitude cannot be employed. There was an occasional patient who, although willing to say that he was 'upset' by some event, refused to go any further without strong urging.

Results

All patients with the same symptom-complex described their attitudes toward the situation which precipitated it in essentially the same way.

The following attitudes and physiological disturbances were found to be associated:

1. Urticaria (thirty-one patients) occurred when an individual saw himself as being mistreated. This mistreatment might take the form of something said to him or something done to him. He was preoccupied entirely with what was happening to him, and was not thinking of retaliation or of any solution of his problem. Typical statements were: 'They did a lot of things to me and I couldn't do anything about it.' 'I was taking a beating.' 'My mother was hammering on me.' 'The boss cracked a whip on me.' 'My fiancée knocked me down and walked all over me but what could I do?'

2. Eczema (twenty-seven patients) occurred when an individual felt that he was being interfered with or prevented from doing something, and could think of no way to deal with the frustration. His preoccupation was with the interference and the persons or things thwarting him, rather than with the goals or aims which concerned migraine patients. Typical statements were: 'I want to make my mother understand, but I can't.' 'I couldn't do what I wanted but there wasn't anything I could do about it.' 'It upset me because it interfered with what I wanted to do.' 'I felt terribly frustrated.'

In addition, however, minor attacks of urticaria or exacerbations of eczema occurred when the individual felt that he was being looked at and had no response to make – the feeling commonly called 'embarrassment'. An additional feature in many instances of eczema was the aggression directed toward the self, expressed in the statement, 'I take it out on myself.'

3. Cold and moist hands (ten patients) occurred when an individual felt that he should undertake some kind of activity, even though he might not know precisely what to do. Typical statements were: 'I wanted to hit him.' 'I just had to be doing something.' 'Something ought to be done.' 'I wanted to do something.' In Raynaud's disease (four patients) the coldness of the hands is carried to the extreme. The action contemplated by those with Raynaud's disease was characteristically a hostile one. Typical statements were 'I wanted to hit him.' 'I wanted to put a knife through him.' 'I wanted to strangle him.'

W. J. Grace and D. T. Graham 277

4. Vasomotor rhinitis (twelve patients) occurred when an individual was facing a situation with the wish that he didn't have to do anything about it, or that it would go away, or that somebody else would take over the responsibility. The essential feature was the desire to have nothing to do with the situation at all, to deal with it by excluding it. Typical statements were: 'I wanted them to go away.' 'I didn't want to have anything to do with it.' 'I wanted to blot it all out, I wanted to build a wall between me and him.' 'I wanted to hole up for the winter.' 'I wanted to go to bed and pull the sheets over my head.'

5. Asthma (seven patients) occurred in association with attitudes exactly like those associated with vasomotor rhinitis. Presumably in asthma the feelings are more intense, but since no measure of strength of attitude was employed, this cannot be categorically stated. It is consistent with this formulation that attacks of asthma are almost invariably accompanied by vasomotor rhinitis, although the reverse is not true. In short, the two seem to be essentially the same disease, the difference between them being one of severity. Typical statements were: 'I wanted them to go away.' 'I didn't want to have anything to do with it.' 'I just couldn't face it.'

6. Diarrhoea (twenty-seven patients) occurred when an individual wanted to be done with a situation or to have it over with, or to get rid of something or somebody. One man who developed severe diarrhoea after he had purchased a defective automobile said: 'If I could only get rid of it!' 'I want to dispose of it.' Typical statements of others were: 'If the war was only over with.' 'I wanted to get done with it.' 'I wanted to get it finished with.'

7. Constipation (seventeen patients) occurred when an individual was grimly determined to carry on even though faced with a problem he could not solve. Typical statements were: 'I have to keep on with this, but I know I'm not going to like it.' 'It's a lousy job but it's the best I can do.' 'This marriage is never going to be any better but I won't quit.' 'I have to keep on with this but I don't like it.' 'I'll stick with it even though nothing good will come of it.'

8. Nausea and vomiting (eleven patients) occurred when an individual was thinking of something which he wished had never

happened. He was preoccupied with the mistake he had made, rather than with what he should have done instead. Usually he felt responsible for what had happened. Typical statements: 'I wish it hadn't happened.' 'I was sorry I did it.' 'I wish things were the way they were before.' 'I made a mistake.' 'I shouldn't have listened to him.'

9. Duodenal ulcer (nine patients) occurred when an individual was seeking revenge. He wished to injure the person or thing that had injured him. Typical statements were: 'I wanted to get even.' 'I wanted to get back at him.' 'I wanted revenge.' 'He hurt me so I wanted to hurt him.' 'I did it for spite.'

10. Migraine headache (fourteen patients) occurred when an individual had been making an intense effort to carry out a definite planned program, or to achieve some definite objective. The headache occurred when the effort had ceased, no matter whether the activity had been associated with success or failure. The essential features were striving and subsequent relaxation. Typical statements were: 'I had to get it done.' 'I had to meet a deadline.' 'I had a million things to do before lunch.' 'I was trying to get all these things accomplished.'

11. Arterial hypertension (seven patients) occurred when an individual felt that he must be constantly prepared to meet all possible threats. Typical statements were: 'I had to be ready for anything.' 'It was up to me to take care of all the worries.' 'Nobody is ever going to beat me, I'm ready for everything.'

12. Low back pain (eleven patients) occurred when an individual wanted to carry out some action involving movement of the entire body. The activity which such patients were most commonly thinking about was walking or running away. One sixteen-year-old girl spent most of her waking hours contemplating various schemes for running away from home. Typical statements were: 'I just wanted to walk out of the house.' 'I wanted to run away.' 'I wanted to get out of there.' 'I felt like taking a flying leap off that island.'

Comment

It is interesting to inquire whether a generalization concerning these observed relations can be found. It appears that in many cases the attitude can be considered as a description of the function of the physiological process with which it is associated. This is an extension of the formulation previously made particularly by Cannon and Wolff.

1. Vasodilation is the reaction of the skin to trauma. Whealing occurs when vasodilatation is intense. The patient with urticaria feels that he is receiving a blow, and that there is nothing he can do about it.

2. Cold skin is the result of cutaneous vasoconstriction. Its occurrence in the individual who is contemplating some kind of action probably represents the functioning of a mechanism to raise body temperature by reducing heat loss. That an elevated body temperature is desirable for the active organism is suggested by the fact that the elevation occurs to the same extent with a standard amount of exercise whether heat loss is experimentally facilitated or interfered with.

3 and 4. The reaction of the respiratory mucous membrane to a noxious agent is to exclude it by swelling of the membrane with consequent narrowing of the passageway, and to dilute it and wash it out by hypersecretion. When these changes are limited to the nose, the reaction is called vasomotor rhinitis; when they are sufficiently intense to include the bronchi, so that wheezing occurs, the name 'asthma' is applied.

5. Defecation is a way of ridding the body of substances which have been taken in but are no longer useful. Diarrhoea, or frequent defecation, occurs in the setting of an intense desire to get something over with or to dispose of something.

6. Constipation is a phenomenon of holding on without change. This corresponds to the patients' attitudes of trying to continue with things as they are, without hope of immediate improvement, or definite desire to do anything different.

7. Vomiting is a way of undoing something which has been done. It thus corresponds to the patient's wishes to restore things to their original situation, as if nothing had ever happened.

8. Duodenal ulcer is probably the end-result of protracted gastric hyperfunction. It has been suggested that such hyperfunction is part of the preparation for eating. Directing aggres-

sion into the particular channel of eating seems to make sense biologically, for the only way an injured animal can use the animal which injured him as a source of materials for tissue repair is to devour him. An individual with duodenal ulcer desires revenge – that is, he wishes to hurt the person who hurt him.

9. The backache which accompanies the desire of the individual to walk out of his situation is probably consequent to the tension of the lumbar muscles. The latter fix the spinal column in preparation for locomotion. It has been shown that thinking about lifting a weight is associated with increased electrical activity in the appropriate muscles. It has also been demonstrated that sustained contraction of skeletal muscles can be painful.

The biological function of the bodily changes underlying others of the symptoms is obscure. The value of elevation of the diastolic blood pressure is not clear at present, although it seems probable that there are circumstances under which it is a useful response. The vasodilatation of frustration, seen in eczema, may possibly represent a method of heat loss by an organism which has abandoned its readiness for action. The occurrence in the head of vasoconstriction followed by vasodilation, which underlies migraine, has no useful function which is obvious at present.

Discussion

The present approach differs from those discussed in its emphasis on the nature of the patient's reaction to the situations which precipitate attacks of his illness. The reaction of an adult human being consists of an *attitude*, which can be expressed verbally, and accompanying *bodily changes*. By 'attitude' is meant the way in which he perceives his own position in the situation, and the action, if any, which he wishes to take to deal with it. The bodily changes, if sufficiently intense and prolonged, give rise to experiences which have names and are called 'symptoms', such as palpitations or diarrhoea. If the phenomena recur or persist, and especially if they lead to structural changes, they are said to represent a 'disease'. Most of the common diseases can be viewed as the outcome of physiological adjustments which, although perfectly appropriate in some circumstances, may eventually entail discomfort, disability and danger to the organism.

It will be noted that, although the above definition of attitude has two aspects, in many of the specific attitudes discussed – for example that accompanying diarrhoea – there is no mention of the first component. The reason for this is that no consistencies were discovered in the statements of patients in question about what they felt was happening to them, although they all wished to deal with the traumatic situation in the same way. It is possible that further investigation in certain of the syndromes will reveal common denominators in the first component of the attitude as well as the second, and to this extent the attitude statements given may be incomplete. It may be, for instance, that persons with duodenal ulcer always regard the situations responsible for their symptoms as injuries of a particular kind.

The results of this study suggest that each attitude is associated with its own unique set of bodily changes. The possibility of the existence of such a relationship has been suggested by Bull. Nothing is implied in this connection about a cause-and-effect relation between 'mental' and 'physical' events, and, indeed, it seems unprofitable to look at the matter in this light.

This conclusion is in opposition to the widely-held view that there is no predictable relation between the 'emotion' felt and the physiological changes which accompany it. There seem to have been at least three reasons for the adoption of this position. The first was the attempt to work with an inadequate vocabulary, so that the range of possible attitudes was not sufficiently explored. Second, questioning was not conducted in such a way that precise attitudes were ascertained, the experimenter or therapist remaining content with the 'name' of the emotion supplied by the subject or patient, or suggested by his own appraisal of the situation. This introduces the difficulty that not all individuals attach the same meanings to the common words denoting feeling-states. Third, only a very few of the large number of possible physiological variables were measured, for example cardiovascular changes and the galvanic skin responses.

These considerations suggest the advisability of defining the word emotion,[1] so that it means *an attitude and the associated*

1. There is considerable dissatisfaction with present definitions of emotion

bodily changes. This implies that there are a very large number of possible emotions, probably many more than are conventionally considered, since there are a large number of possible attitudes toward situations. It also implies that there is no such thing as 'non-emotional' behavior, since it is presumably impossible to do anything or think about anything without adopting some attitude. In ordinary speech, however, emotions are not recognized until they reach a certain intensity.

Looked at in this way, it becomes apparent that most emotions have no specific or appropriate name. There are, however, suitable words in the English language to describe some of them, with at least some degree of exactness. According to Webster's Collegiate Dictionary (1939), for instance, *resentment* is a 'feeling of indignant displeasure because of something regarded as a wrong, insult, etc.' This is a good description of the attitude of patients who have urticaria. *Hostility* is 'antagonism, especially as manifested in action'. Wishes to take hostile action are associated with Raynaud's disease. *Regret* is 'a wishing that something had not happened' (Funk and Wagnalls College Standard Dictionary, 1933). This is the attitude associated with vomiting.

Anxiety is a term which is widely used in psychiatry, but one for which there is no generally accepted precise definition. If one considered those individuals who have the symptoms ordinarily considered those of 'anxiety', it is fairly evident that their attitude consists of two major components. The first is *apprehension*, the feeling that something bad is about to happen, and the second is an urge to action of some kind, a feeling that something must be done (even though there is no clear idea of what to do) which may be named *tension*. The names are not important, but it is important that there are such feelings, and that they can be clearly expressed by patients. The complete anxiety syndrome, then, consists of a feeling that something bad will happen, together with an urge to do something. The physiological correlates of these attitudes, however, have not been clarified. It is suggested that the term 'anxiety' be reserved for

---

especially with respect to the distinction between 'emotional' and 'non-emotional' behavior. See, for example, the series of papers on emotion in *Psychological Review* during 1948 and 1949.

the coexistence of these two attitudes with their accompanying physiological changes.

It may be well to emphasize again that the correlation of attitudes with bodily changes given above is based entirely on the patient's statements about their feelings, and not on inter-pretations of dream or fantasy material with inferences concern-ing the content of the unconscious. In other words, a clear-cut statement of any attitude was accepted at its face value. It is, in fact, surprising how aware patients are of their attitudes toward particular circumstances, and how readily they can verbalize them. The reasons, on the other hand, which determine the way a situation is viewed are very likely to be unconscious.

It is commonly held that patients' declarations about their feelings are of little significance. Some individuals, for example, may say of a situation which is repeatedly associated with attacks of their symptoms, 'It doesn't bother me.' It is, however, highly significant that if a patient admitted to an awareness of any emotional disturbance at all, and could be made to describe his attitude toward the precipitating event in the terms outlined above, he always did so in the same way as all the other patients with the same syndrome. The importance of such statements is supported by the correlations between them and the observed physiological changes. If what the patients said was really com-pletely 'unreliable', no consistent relation between verbaliza-tions and bodily changes would be possible.

It sometimes happened that a patient expressed about some situation one of the attitudes listed, without developing the cor-responding symptoms. This is presumably because the feeling was not sufficiently intense or long-lasting, so that only tran-sitory and minor physiological changes occurred. Such findings are therefore not evidence against the thesis of this paper. What is crucial, however, is that no attack of any of the symptoms mentioned occurred in the absence of the appropriate attitude. It is probable that all human beings develop at one time or another the attitudes and associated somatic changes described. The person who gets symptoms severe enough to make him a patient simply feels a particular way very intensely and for a long time.

Most persons show some consistency in the attitudes they

have. A single individual, in other words, 'selects' from the wide range of possible attitudes one or a few which he develops often and intensely, to the relative exclusion of others. Since different attitudes lead to different kinds of overt behavior, one would predict some correlation between personality traits and diseases. This individual consistency in attitude seems also to be of importance in keeping disease processes active. Asthmatics, for instance, often state that they wish not to have to think about or deal with their asthma, and persons with diarrhoea say that they wish to be rid of their symptoms.

It is important to know what it is in the life history of a patient which predisposed him to adopt the response (attitude and bodily change) which eventually culminated in disease. Are there common factors in the lives of persons with asthma, for instance, which have made them especially prone to wish to shut unpleasant things away from them? It seems probable that there are certain experiences, particularly exposure to attitudes and behavior of parents, which result in the development of predictable attitudes in any individual exposed to them, and that all patients with the same disease have had lives with these experiences in common. Their reactions to their present situations are, of course, in large part determined by their previous learning. There is, however, reason to think that certain situations encountered for the first time in adult life may have intrinsically a high potentiality for evoking particular attitudes and bodily changes, just as they would in a child.

It is probably also true that some persons have been exposed to environments producing more than one kind of traumatic situation, repeated often enough to be significant. These individuals are presumably those who react as adults with many different symptoms, the nature of which is determined by the situation.

With a few of the common syndromes it has been possible to identify experiences of early life which seem highly relevant to adult attitudes and diseases, and which are found in the background of many of the patients with the syndrome. One girl whose chief complaint was backache, for instance, had a mother who constantly threatened to pack her bags and walk out of the home. Another woman, who developed severe vomiting as a reaction to her life situation, had been thoroughly indoctrinated with the idea of the impossibility of atonement for sin, so that having once done something which she felt was wrong she was completely preoccupied with wishing it hadn't happened.

This is a first report, and greater objectivity in the evaluation of attitudes is desirable in order to obviate the criticism that patients' statements are so loose as to be open to any number of interpretations, or that suggestion by the therapist may have played a part. The method of questioning was designed to avoid these difficulties, but, in addition, a questionnaire has been made up to be presented to patients after the event responsible for an attack of their symptoms has been clearly defined. It consists of about fifty questions representing a variety of possible attitudes toward life situations, the patient answering 'yes' to those he thinks best represent his attitudes at the time the symptoms developed. For example, questions pertinent to diarrhoea are, 'Did you feel that you wanted to get rid of someone or something?', and 'Did you feel that there was something you wanted to get over with or done with?'

Summary and conclusions

1. One hundred and twenty-eight patients, who had one or more of the following symptoms or diseases as responses to life situations, were studied: urticaria, eczema, cold hands, vasomotor rhinitis and asthma, diarrhoea, constipation, nausea and vomiting, duodenal ulcer, migraine, arterial hypertension, low back pain.

2. It was found that each of these conditions was associated with a particular, completely conscious, attitude toward the precipitating situation. There were, in other words, physiological changes specific to each attitude.

3. These changes are biologically appropriate to the attitudes they accompany.

4. It is proposed that 'emotion' be defined to mean 'an attitude with its associated physiological changes'.

References

ALEXANDER, F. G. (1950), *Psychosomatic Medicine, Its Principles and Applications*, W. W. Norton and Co.

ALMY, T. P., KERN, F. and ABBOT, F. (1950), 'Constipation and diarrhoea,' *A. Res. nerv. and ment. Dis., Proc.*, vol. 29, p. 724.

BROBECK, J. R. (1949), 'Regulation of energy exchange', in J. F. Fulton, *A Textbook of Physiology*, (16th edn), W. B. Saunders Co.

BULL, N. (1945), 'Toward a clarification of the concept of emotion', *Psychosom. Medicine*, vol. 7, p. 210.

CANNON, W. B. (1929), *Bodily Changes in Pain, Hunger, Fear and Rage*, Appleton–Century–Crofts.

DUNBAR, F. (1947), *Emotions and Bodily Changes* (edn 3), Columbia University Press.

GRACE, W. J., WOLF, S. and WOLFF, H. G. (1951), *The Human Colon*, Paul B. Hoeber, Inc.

GRAHAM, D. T. (1950), 'The pathogenesis of hives', *A. Res. nerv. and ment. Dis., Proc.*, p. 987.

GRESSEL, G. C., SHOBE, F. O., SASLOW, G., DUBOIS, P. H. and SHREODER, H. A. (1949), 'Personality factors in arterial hypertension', *J.A.M.A.*, vol. 140, p. 265.

GROEN, J. (1947), 'Psychogenesis and psychotherapy of ulcerative colitis', *Psychosom. Medicine*, vol. 9, p. 151.

HALLIDAY, J. L. (1948), *Psychological Medicine*, W. W. Norton and Co.

HOLMES, T. H., GOODELL, H., WOLF, S. and WOLFF, H. G. (1950), *The Nose*, Charles C. Thomas.

JACOBSON, E. (1932), 'Electrophysiology of mental activities', *Amer. J. Psychol.*, vol. 44, p. 677.

Life Stress and Bodily Disease: Proceedings of the Association for Research in Nervous and Mental Disease, December 2, and 3, (1949, 1950), Williams and Wilkins, Co.

MAHONEY, V. P., BOCKUS, H. L., INGRAM, M., HUNDLEY, J. W. and YASKIN, J. C. (1950), 'Studies on ulcerative colitis', *Gastroenterology*, vol. 13, p. 547.

MUNN, N. L. (1946), *The Fundamentals of Human Adjustment*, Houghton Mifflin

NIELSEN, M. (1948), 'Die Regulation der Körpertemperatur bei Muskelarbeit', *Skandinav. Arch. f. Physiol.*, vol. 79, p. 193.

SIMONS, D. J., DAY, E., GOODELL, H. and WOLFF, H. G. (1943), 'Experimental studies on headache; muscles of the scalp and neck as sources of pain', *A. Res. nerve. ment. Dis., Proc.*, vol. 23, p. 228.

STEINDLER, A. (1935), *Mechanics of Normal and Pathological Locomotion*, Charles C. Thomas.

WOLF, S. and WOLFF, H. G. (1947), *Human Gastric Function* (edn 2), Oxford University Press.

WOLFF, H. G. (1947), 'Protective reaction patterns and disease', *Ann. Int. Medicine*, vol. 27, p. 944.

WOLFF, H. G. (1948), *Headache and Other Head Pain*, Oxford University Press.

Part Five
Psychoneurotic Disorders

Although some psychopathologists have concentrated upon the issue of constitutional factors in susceptibility to psychoneurosis, the major effort has been directed at the processes whereby the environment generates neurotic behaviour in individuals. Behaviourists and psychoanalysts have both regarded anxiety as the core experience, and susceptibility to anxiety as the chief difference between neurotic and non-neurotic individuals.

Wolpe presents a behavioural account of the role of anxiety in neurosis, an account that has been of particular significance in the thinking of the behaviour therapists. However, the ranks of the supporters of a learning-theory approach to neurosis are far from united. Wolpe's position has been subject to criticism from other behaviourists who argue that it has weaknesses both as an account of neurosis and as an exercise in the application of behavioural principles. Breger and McGaugh have been at the forefront of this criticism and their paper should be read as a counterbalance to Wolpe's own views.

14 J. Wolpe

The Etiology of Human Neuroses

Excerpted from J. Wolpe, *Psychotherapy by Reciprocal Inhibition*, Stanford University Press, 1958, pp. 83–95.

The causal relations of pervasive ('free-floating') anxiety

Under certain circumstances it is not only to well-defined stimulus configurations that anxiety responses are conditioned, but also to more or less omnipresent properties of the environment, of which extreme examples would be light, light and shade contrasts, amorphous noise, spatiality, and the passage of time. Since each of these enters into most, if not all, possible experience, it is to be expected that if any of them becomes connected to anxiety responses the patient will be persistently, and apparently causelessly, anxious. He will be suffering from what is erroneously called 'free-floating' anxiety, and for which a more suitable label would be *pervasive* anxiety.

It must be unequivocally stated, in case it is not quite self-evident, that there is no sharp dividing line between specific anxiety-evoking stimuli and stimuli to pervasive anxiety. The pervasiveness of the latter is a function of the pervasiveness of the stimulus element conditioned; and there are degrees of pervasiveness ranging from the absolute omnipresence of time itself through very common elements like room walls to rarely encountered configurations like hunchbacks.

What reason is there for believing that pervasive anxiety has definable stimulus sources?

Questioning of patients with pervasive anxiety usually reveals that definable aspects of the environment are especially related to this anxiety. For example, one patient reported increased anxiety in the presence of any very large object; another an uncomfortable intrusiveness of all sharp contrasts in his visual field – even the printed words on a page, and particularly contrasts in the periphery of the field. A third felt overwhelmed by physical space. Frequently, patients with pervasive anxiety observe that noise causes a rise in the level of their anxiety. In some cases the noise need not be loud, and in some even music is disturbing.

Although pervasive anxiety is usually felt less when the patient lies down and closes his eyes, it does not disappear. To some extent this may be explained on the basis of perseveration due to prolonged reverberation of the effects of the stimulus in the nervous system. But this does not account for the fact that usually *some* anxiety is already felt at the moment of waking. An obvious explanation is that anxiety evocable by stimuli that enter into the very structure of experience is likely to be produced by the first contents of the awakening subject's imagination. Anxiety increases when the outside world makes its impact; and it is consonant with this that, very commonly, the level of pervasive anxiety gradually rises as the day goes on.

This diurnal rise in level is less likely to occur when the general level of pervasive anxiety is low; for then there is a greater likelihood of the arousal, during a normal day's experience, of other emotions which may be physiologically antagonistic to anxiety, so that the anxiety will be inhibited and its habit strength each time slightly diminished. On the other hand, invariably (in my experience) the patient with pervasive anxiety also has unadaptive anxiety reactions to specific stimuli, and if he should encounter and react to any one of the latter during that day, the level of pervasive anxiety will promptly rise. In the normal course of events it is to be expected that level of pervasive anxiety will fluctuate because of 'chance' occurrences which strengthen or weaken its habit strength.

Sometimes, when a patient is fortunate enough not to meet with any specific disturbing stimuli over an extended period, his pervasive anxiety may practically cease, but subsequent response to a relevant specific anxiety-revoking stimulus will condition it lastingly again. This reconditioning was beautifully demonstrated in one of my patients, who, in addition to pervasive anxiety, had a number of severe phobias on the general theme of illness. The pervasive anxiety responded extremely well to La Verne's carbon dioxide-oxygen inhalation therapy. The patient stopped coming for treatment until several months later when the pervasive anxiety was reinduced after he had witnessed an epileptic fit in the street. The pervasive anxiety was again speedily removed by carbon dioxide–oxygen and the patient again stopped treatment after a few more interviews. The essence of this sequence was repeated about ten times before the patient finally allowed desensitization to the phobic stimuli to be completed.

The question naturally arises: What factors determine whether or not pervasive anxiety will be part of a patient's neurosis? At the moment two possible factors may be suggested on the basis of clinical impressions. One seems to be the intensity of anxiety evocation at the time of the induction of the neurosis. It is hypothesized that the more intense the anxiety the more stimulus aspects are likely to acquire *some* measure of anxiety conditioning. Indirect support for this hypothesis comes from the observation that, on the whole, it is the patient who reacts more severely to specific stimuli who is also likely to suffer from pervasive anxiety.

The second possible factor is a lack of clearly defined environmental stimuli at the time of neurosis induction. For example, one patient's pervasive anxiety began after a night in a hotel during which he had attempted intercourse with a woman to whom he felt both sexual attraction and strong revulsion. He had felt a powerful and strange, predominantly nonsexual excitation, and ejaculation had occurred very prematurely without pleasure. The light had been switched off, and *only the dark outlines of objects could be seen*. After this, so great was his feeling of revulsion to the woman that he spent the remainder of the night on the carpet. This experience left him, as he subsequently found, with an anxiety toward a wide range of sexual objects, along with much pervasive anxiety, characterized by a special intrusiveness of all heavy dark objects.

The causal process in hysteria

Hysterical reactions are clearly distinguishable from the rather diffuse discharges of the autonomic nervous system that characterize anxiety reactions. In most instances hysterical reactions do not find expression in the autonomic nervous system at all, but in the sensory system, the motor system, or groups of functional units involved in the production of imagery or of consciousness in general. Thus, they may take the form of anaesthesias, paraesthesias, hyperaesthesias, or disturbances of vision or hearing; of paralyses, pareses, tics, tremors, disturbances of balance, contractures or fits; of amnesias, fugues, or 'multiple personality' phenomena. Occasionally, hysterical reactions do appear to involve functions within the domain of the autonomic nervous system – in the form of vomiting (or nausea) or enuresis, but it is noteworthy that each of the two functions involved is to some extent within voluntary control.

Anxiety frequently accompanies hysterical reactions and then they occur side by side as two distinct forms of *primary* neurotic response. This state of affairs must be sharply distinguished from that in which sensory or motor phenomena are secondary effects of the normal components of anxiety, and as such do not qualify as hysterical. For example, a headache due to tension of the temporal muscles, backache due to tension of the longitudinal spinal muscles, or paresthesia due to hyperventilation are not to be regarded as hysterical.

It is necessary also to differentiate hysterical from obsessional reactions. Hysterical reactions are at a relatively low level of organization, affecting well-defined sensory areas and specific motor units, and causing changes in the general character of consciousness or the exclusion from consciousness of 'blocks' of experience limited in terms of a time span or some other broad category. The details of the reactions tend to be fixed and unchanging. Obsessional reactions consist by contrast of highly organized movements or of elaborate and complex thinking, in either of which there is a great variety in the individual instances of expression of a specific constant theme.

Like other neurotic reactions, hysterical reactions are acquired by learning. It is intriguing to note that Freud's very early observations on hysterical subjects could easily have led him to this conclusion had he not been sidetracked by a spurious deduction from observations on therapeutic effects. In a paper published in 1893, speaking of the relation of the symptoms of hysteria to the patients' reactions at the time of the precipitating stress, he states:

The connection is often so clear that it is quite evident how the exciting event has happened to produce just this and no other manifestation; the phenomenon is determined in a perfectly clear manner by the cause; to take the most ordinary example, a painful effect, which was originally excited while eating, but was suppressed, produces nausea and vomiting, and this continues for months, as hysterical vomiting. A child who is very ill at last falls asleep, and its mother tries her utmost to keep quiet and not to wake it; but just in consequence of this resolution (hysterical counterwill) she makes a clucking noise with her tongue. On another occasion when she wishes to keep absolutely quiet this happens again, and so a tic in the form of tongue-clicking develops which for a number of years accompanies every excitement. . . . A highly intelligent man assists while his brother's ankylosed hip is straightened under an anaesthetic. At the instant when the joint gives way with a crack, he feels a violent pain in his own hip joint which lasts almost a year. . . [pp. 25–6].

The attack then arises spontaneously as memories commonly do; but they may also be provoked, just as any memory may be aroused according to the laws of association. Provocation of an attack occurs either by stimulation of a hysterogenic zone or by a new experience resembling the pathogenic experience. We hope to be able to show that no essential difference exists between the two conditions, apparently so distinct; and in both cases a hyperaesthetic memory has been stirred [p. 40].

Apart from the reference to the possibility of attacks arising 'spontaneously' (which Freud later explicitly repudiated) we have here an account of the formation by learning of stimulus-response connections. That Freud did not *see* this was mainly because, having observed patients cured when they recalled and narrated the story of the precipitating experience, he concluded that the symptoms were due to the imprisonment of emotionally disturbing memories. He states '. . . we are of opinion that the psychical trauma, or the memory of it, acts as a kind of foreign body constituting an effective agent in the present, even long after it has penetrated. . . .' There can be little doubt that this statement would not have been made, and the mind-structure theory that is psychoanalytic theory would not have been born, if Freud could have known that memories do not exist in the form of thoughts or images in some kind of repository within us, but depend on the establishment, through the learning pro-

J. Wolpe 295

cess, of specific neural interconnections that give a *potentiality* of evocation of particular thoughts and images when and only when certain stimulus conditions, external or internal, are present.

When a clear history of the onset of hysterical symptoms is obtained, it is usually found, as illustrated in Freud's cases quoted above, that the hysterical reaction displays a repetition of features that were present in response to the initiating disturbing experience. The stimulus to the reaction varies. Sometimes it is a fairly specific sensory stimulation. For example, a thirty-three-year-old woman had as a hysterical reaction an intolerable sensation of 'gooseflesh' in her calves in response to any rectal sensation such as a desire to defecate, ever since, three years previously, a surgeon had unceremoniously performed a rectal examination upon her, while, drowsy from premedication with morphia, she was awaiting the administration of an anaesthetic for an abdominal operation.

In other cases it appears that the hysterical reaction is aroused by ubiquitous stimuli, being then the hysterical equivalent of pervasive ('free-floating') anxiety. An example of this is wryneck that is present throughout the working day and relaxes the moment the patient falls asleep. In yet others anxiety appears to *mediate* the hysterical reaction. The hysteria of one of my patients had both a pervasive component and an anxiety-mediated component. This was a fifty-eight-year-old woman who eighteen months earlier had encountered a deadly snake in a copse. She had been terrified and momentarily paralyzed; her ears were filled with the sound of waves and she had been unable to speak for two hours. The sound of waves had never left her, and any considerable anxiety such as might arise from tension in her home would intensify this sound and then lead to vertigo, loss of balance, and a feeling of great weakness in all her limbs, so that she sometimes fell.

The central feature of hysterical reactions is the conditioning, in situations of stress, of neurotic reactions other than anxiety, although anxiety is often also conditioned as well. It is necessary to ask what determines this. There are two possible answers. One is that these reactions are conditioned when they happen to be evoked in addition to anxiety. The other is that although such reactions may be evoked by stress in all subjects, they become the neurotic responses conditioned only in those in whom some special factor is present that gives preference to nonanxiety conditioning. Since, in fact, the immediate response to neurotigenic stimulation always seems to implicate all response systems, the latter possibility is the more likely to be relevant. And there is evidence that it is people with distinct personality features who usually develop hysterical reactions.

Jung (1923) long ago observed that hysterics tend to exhibit extravert character traits while other neurotic subjects tend to be introverted. In this partition of personalities he was followed by other writers who, while differing in many ways, agreed, as Eysenck (1947, p. 58) concluded from a survey, in the following particulars: (a) the introvert has a more subjective, the extravert a more objective outlook; (b) the introvert shows a higher degree of cerebral activity, the extravert a higher degree of behavioral activity; (c) the introvert shows a tendency to self-control (inhibition), the extravert a tendency to lack of such control. Eysenck (1955b), has pointed out on the basis of experiments performed by Franks (1956) and himself (1955a) that extraverted subjects besides learning more poorly also generate reactive inhibition more readily than introverts do. He postulates (1955b, p. 35) that subjects in whom reactive inhibition is generated quickly and dissipated slowly 'are predisposed thereby to develop extraverted patterns of behaviour and to develop hysterico-psychopathic disorders in cases of neurotic breakdown'. Clearly what his facts actually demonstrate is that the hysterical type of breakdown is particularly likely in subjects in whom reactive inhibition has the feature stated. The *causal* rôle of reactive inhibition is not shown, nor is a possible mechanism suggested.

A possibility is this: that in addition to their easily generated and persistent reactive inhibition (and perhaps in some indirect way bound up with it) extraverted people have one or both of the following characteristics: (a) when exposed to anxiety-arousing stimuli they respond with relatively low degrees of anxiety so that other responses are unusually prominent; (b) when anxiety and other responses are simultaneously evoked in them, contiguous stimuli become conditioned to the other

responses rather than to the anxiety – by contrast with introverts.

This hypothesis lends itself readily to direct experimentation.
In the meantime a survey from my records of the twenty-two
patients with hysterical symptoms has yielded some suggestive
evidence. Nine of them (41 per cent) had initial Willoughby
scores below thirty. This is in striking contrast to 273 non-
hysterical neurotic patients, in only fifty (18 per cent) of whom
were the initial scores below this level. The Kolmogorov-
Smirnov test shows the difference to be significant at the ·05
level. It is interesting to note that insofar as this supports our
hypothesis it accords with the time-worn conception of the
hysterical patient with little or no anxiety – *la belle indifférence*.
It is relevant to the same point that the hysterical patients with
low Willoughby scores all benefited by procedures that varied
greatly but did not obviously affect anxious sensitivity. By contrast, in the thirteen patients whose hysterical reactions were
accompanied by much anxiety there was a direct correlation
between diminution of anxious sensitivity and decreased
strength of hysterical reactions except in two cases where this
consisted purely of amnesia, which was unaffected. (In one of
these the events of the forgotten period were later retrieved
under hypnosis, in the other they remained forgotten. It seemed
to make no difference either way to the patient's recovery.)

Summarizing the above facts, it may be said that hysterical
reactions may either accompany anxiety or occur on their own.
In the former case their treatment is the treatment of anxiety,
in the latter it is different in a way that will be discussed in the
chapter on treatment. It is supposed that anxiety is a feature
when hysteria occurs in subjects relatively far from the extraverted extreme of Eysenck's introversion-extraversion dimension, just because the hypothetical preferential conditioning of
responses other than anxiety to neurotigenic stimuli is less
marked in these people. This supposition needs to be tested.

Meanwhile it may be noted that there is experimental evidence of a competitive relationship in certain contexts between
autonomic and motor responses. Mowrer and Viek (1948),
using two groups of rats, placed each animal after a period of
starvation on the electrifiable floor of a rectangular cage and

offered him food on a stick for ten seconds. Whether the animal ate or not, shock was applied ten seconds later. In the case of one group of ten rats, jumping into the air resulted in the experimenter switching off the shock (shock-controllable group). Each animal in this group had an experimental 'twin' to which the shock was applied for the same length of time as it had taken its counterpart to jump into the air (shock-uncontrollable group). One trial a day was given to each animal. The animals in each group whose eating responses during the ten seconds were inhibited (by conditioned anxiety responses resulting from the shocks) were charted each day, and it was found that in the shock-controllable group the number of eating inhibitions was never high and declined to zero, whereas in the shock-uncontrollable group the number rose to a high level and remained there. Apparently, the constant evocation of jumping in the former group resulted in a gradual development of conditioned inhibition of anxiety. By contrast with this, in the typical Cornell technique for producing experimental neuroses (p. 43) a very localized musculo-skeletal conditioned response comes to be increasingly dominated by autonomic anxiety responses. This whole matter has been discussed in more detail elsewhere (Wolpe, 1953).

Obsessional behavior

Sometimes, besides the autonomic discharges characteristic of anxiety, ideational, motor, and sensory responses are prominent in a neurosis. If simple and invariate in character, they are labeled *hysterical* (see p. 293). The term *obsessional* is applied to behavior that is more complex and variable in detail, consisting of well-defined and often elaborate thought sequences or relatively intricate acts which, though they may differ in outward form from one occasion to the next, lead or tend to lead to the same kind of result. The term is applicable even to those cases characterized by an obstinate impulse to behavior that rarely or never becomes manifest. Examples of obsessions predominantly of thought are a woman's insistent idea that she might throw her child from the balcony of her apartment, or a man's need to have one of a restricted class of 'pleasant' thoughts in his mind before he can make any well-defined movement such as entering a doorway or sitting down. Exhibitionism and compulsive handwashing are characteristic examples of predominantly motor obsessional behavior.

Sometimes the word *compulsive* has been preferred to obsessional for those cases in which motor activity predominates. However, as most cases display both elements, there is little practical value in the distinction. Furthermore, the term compulsive is open to the objection that *all* behavior is compulsive in a sense, for causal determinism implies that the response that occurs is always the only one that could have occurred in the circumstances. The feature of any example of obsessional behavior is not its inevitability but its *intrusiveness*. Its elicitation or the impulse toward it is an encumbrance and an embarrassment to the patient.

If hysterical and obsessional reactions involve similar elements, we may expect that borderline cases will be found. An example of this is a forty-seven-year-old male nurse employed in an industrial first-aid room who for seventeen years had an uncontrollable impulse to mimic any rhythmic movements performed before him, e.g., waving of arms or dancing, and to obey any command no matter from whom. In this was combined the basic simplicity of hysteria and the situationally determined variability of obsessional behavior.

It may be stated almost as dogma that the strength and frequency of evocation of obsessional behavior is directly related to the amount of anxiety being evoked in the patient. Pollitt (1957) in a study of 150 obsessional cases noted that obsessional symptoms became more severe and prominent 'when anxiety and tension increased for whatever causes'. However, it is not always that the source of the anxiety is irrelevant. Sometimes the obsessional behavior is evident only when anxiety arises from specific, usually neurotic sources. For example, an exhibitionist experienced impulses to expose himself when he felt inadequate and inferior among his friends but not when he was anxious about the results of a law examination.

Anxiety-elevating obsessions

Two types of obsessional behavior are clearly distinguishable in clinical practice. One type appears to be part and parcel of the immediate response to anxiety-evoking stimulation and has secondary effects entirely in the direction of increasing anxiety. When a motor mechanic of forty-five had neurotic anxiety exceeding a certain fairly low level, he would have a terrifying though always controllable impulse to strike people. From the first moment of awareness of the impulse he would feel increased anxiety, and if at the time he was with an associate or even among strangers – for example, in a bus – he would thrust his hands firmly into his pockets 'to keep them out of trouble'. In the history of such patients one finds that behavior similar to that constituting the obsession was present during an earlier situation in which conditioning of anxiety took place. In 1942 this motor mechanic, on military service, had been sentenced to thirty days' imprisonment in circumstances which he had with some justice felt to be grossly unfair. Then, as he had resisted the military police rather violently in protest, he was taken to a psychiatrist who said there was nothing wrong with him and that the sentence should be carried out. At this his feeling of helpless rage had further increased and he was taken out by force. Then for the first time he had had 'this queer feeling' in his abdomen and had struck a military policeman who tried to compel him to work. Horror at the implications of this act intensified his disturbed state. The obsession to strike people made its first appearance in 1953, eleven years later. He had been imprisoned overnight (for the first time since 1942) because, arriving home one night to find his house crowded with his wife's relatives, he had shouted and been violent until his wife had called the police. After emerging from jail, burning with a sense of injustice much like that experienced during his imprisonment in the army, he had felt the impulse to strike a stranger who was giving him a lift in an automobile, and then again, much more strongly, a few days later toward his wife at their first meeting since his night in jail. This time he had gone into a state of panic, and since then, for a period of five months, the obsession had recurred very frequently and in an increasing range of conditions, e.g., at work he would often have a fear-laden desire to hit fellow workmen with any tool he happened to be holding. (There was subsequently a secondary conditioning of anxiety to the *sight* of tools, including knives and forks.)

Anxiety-reducing obsessions

The second type of obsessional behavior occurs as a *reaction* to anxiety, and its performance *diminishes* anxiety to some extent, for at least a short time. It occurs in many forms – tidying, hand-washing, eating, buying – activities which are of course 'normal' when prompted by usual motivations and not by anxiety; rituals like touching poles, perversions like exhibitionism, and various thinking activities. In some of these cases secondary heightening of anxiety occurs as a response to some aspect of the obsessional behavior. For example, in a case of obsessional eating, the anxiety was at first reduced by the eating, and then its level would rise in response to the idea of getting fat.

Obsessional behavior of this kind owes its existence to the previous conditioning of anxiety-relieving responses. This has been strikingly demonstrated in a recent experiment by Fonberg (1956). This writer conditioned each of several dogs to perform a definite movement in response to several auditory and visual stimuli using food reinforcement. When these instrumental conditioned responses had been firmly established, she proceeded to elaborate defensive instrumental conditioned responses, employing stimuli and responses distinct from those of the alimentary training. The noxious stimulus used was either an electric shock to the right foreleg or a strong air puff to the ear. As a result of this conditioning, upon presentation of the conditioned stimulus an animal would be able to avert the noxious stimulus – for example, by lifting a particular foreleg. The dogs were then made neurotic by conditioning an excitatory alimentary response to a strong tone of fifty cycles and an inhibitory response to a very weak tone of the same frequency, and then bringing the two differentiated tones nearer and nearer to each other from session to session either by progressive strengthening of the inhibitory tone or by both strengthening the inhibitory and weakening the excitatory. In all animals, as soon as neurotic behavior appeared it was accompanied by the previously elaborated defensive motor reaction. Besides this deliberately conditioned reaction, 'shaking off' movements were observed in those dogs in whom the noxious stimulation had originally been air puffed into the ear. The more intense the general disturbance the more intense and frequent were the defensive movements. The alimentary conditioned reflexes disappeared completely. With the disappearance of general disturbed symptoms, the defensive movements subsided, reappearing with any new outburst of behavioral disturbance.

It appears clear from these observations that in elaborating the conditioned defensive reaction to the auditory stimulus, anxiety-response-produced stimuli were also conditioned to evoke the defensive reaction, and this reaction was consequently evocable *whenever* the animal had anxiety responses, no matter what the origin of these may have been.

Similarly, in the history of patients displaying this kind of obsessional behavior, it is found that at an earlier period, some important real threat was consistently removed by a single well-defined type of behavior, and this behavior later appears as a response to *any* similar anxiety. The behavior must owe its strength to its association with exceptionally strong reinforcement-favoring conditions – either very massive or very numerous anxiety-drive reductions or both. Its development is also, no doubt, greatly favored when from the outset no other significant anxiety-relieving activity has occurred to compete with it. Its maintenance depends upon the reduction of anxiety it is able to effect at each performance.

One patient was the youngest daughter of a man who despised females and would not forgive his wife for failing to bear him a son. She was very clever at school, and found that intellectual achievement, and that alone, could for brief periods abate her father's blatant hostility and therefore her own anxiety. Consequently, 'thinking things out' became her automatic response to *any* anxiety. Since there are many objective fears for which careful thought is useful, there were no serious consequences for years. But when a series of experiences in early adult life led to a severe anxiety state in her, she automatically resorted to her characteristic 'problem-solving' behavior. Because the anxiety responses now arose from such sources as imaginary social disapproval, and could not be removed by the solution of a well-defined problem, she began to set herself complex problems in which she usually had to decide whether given behavior was morally 'good' or 'bad'. Partial and brief alleviation of anxiety followed both the formulation of a 'suitable' problem and the solution thereof, while prolonged failure to solve a problem increased anxiety sometimes to terror. Although the anxiety soon returned in full force, its temporary decrements at the most appropriate times for reinforcement maintained the problem-finding and problem-solving obsessions, and could well have continued to do so indefinitely.

In other cases obsessional behavior is less episodically determined because everyday circumstances contain aspects of the special situation in which the obsessional mode of behavior alone brought relief from severe anxiety. A history of more than undetected thefts of money by a seventeen-year-old university student began at the age of five when his mother joined the army and left him in the care of an elder sister who beat him severely or tied him to a tree for a few hours if he was slightly dirty or did anything 'wrong'. He feared and hated her and retaliated by stealing money from her. He was never caught and the possession of the stolen gains gave him a feeling of 'munificence and security'. The kleptomania continued all through the early home life and school life and was clearly connected with the chronic presence of punishment-empowered authority in the shape of parents or teachers.

It is not surprising, if obsessional behavior is so consistently followed by reduction of anxiety drive, that it is apt to become conditioned to other stimuli too, especially any that happen to be present on repeated occasions. Thus, after therapy had rendered the young woman with the problem-solving obsession mentioned above practically free from neurotic anxieties, mild problem-solving activity was still occasionally aroused by a trifling question, such as 'Is it cloudy enough to rain?' The conditioned stimulus was apparently the mere awareness of doubt. Similarly an exhibitionist whose exhibiting had almost entirely disappeared with the overcoming of his anxious sensitivities, still had some measure of the impulse when he saw a girl dressed in a school ('gym') uniform, because he had in the past exhibited to schoolgirls particularly frequently and with special relish. Of course, in this instance sex-drive reduction may have played as important a role in the reinforcement as anxiety-drive reduction.

Amnesia and 'Repression'

The amnesias that are usually encountered in the course of neurotic states can be conveniently divided into two classes, according to the emotional importance of the incidents forgotten. Patients who are in a chronic state of emotional disturbance frequently fail to register many trifling events that go on around them. For example, a patient may go into a room and conduct a brief conversation with his wife and an hour later have no recollection whatever that he went into that room at all. Here we seem to have a simple case of deficient registration of impressions (retrograde amnesia). Apparently, the patient's attention is so much taken up by his unpleasant anxious feelings that very little is left to be devoted to what goes on around him.

The forgetting of the contents of highly emotionally charged experiences has been given foremost importance by Freud and his followers as the cause of neurosis. It seems, however, that forgetting of this character is rather unusual, and when it does occur it appears to be merely one more of the conditionable occurrences in the neurotigenic situation. It does not appear that the repression as such plays any part in the maintenance of neurosis. It is quite possible for the patient to recover emotionally although the forgotten incidents remain entirely forgotten. The following case illustrates this.

A thirty-seven-year-old miner was seen in a state of intense anxiety. He had had a very marked tremor and total amnesia for the previous four days. He gave a story that his wife, on whom he was greatly dependent, had cunningly got him to agree to 'temporary divorce' six months before and was now going to marry a friend of his. No attempt was made at this juncture to recall the lost memories. The patient was made to realize how ineffectual his previous attitudes had been and how he had been deceived. As a result, he angrily 'had it out' with his wife (and a few others, incidentally); anxiety rapidly decreased, and he soon felt strongly motivated to organize his whole life differently. At his fifth interview (ten days after treatment began) he said that he felt 'a hundred per cent' – and looked it – and he was full of plans for the future. Yet he had still recalled nothing whatever of the forgotten four days.

Since the possible effects of restoring the memories at this stage were obviously a matter of great interest, the patient was then deeply hypnotized and told to recount the story of the four days. He narrated in detail how he had traveled 300 miles to his rival, meaning to strangle him; how he had been fobbed off, and how, on returning and at last hearing from his wife's own lips that she was in love with the rival, he had staggered out of the house, had made his way to his sister's house, and there collapsed. He told all this quietly, with little emotion, except where he described meeting his rival. Then he moved his hands as if about to throttle someone. He was given the posthypnotic suggestion that he would remember the whole story on waking. When he woke, he told it again briefly, expressing slight amusement at it and surprise at having remembered. There were no important consequences. A few months later he married another woman and was apparently very well adjusted generally. After four years there was no evidence of relapse.

References

EYSENCK, H. J. (1947), *Dimensions of Personality*, Routledge & Kegan Paul.

EYSENCK, H. J. (1955a), 'A dynamic theory of anxiety and hysteria', *J. ment. Sci.*, vol. 101, pp. 28–51.

EYSENCK, H. J. (1955b), 'Cortical inhibition, figural after-effect and the theory of personality', *J. ab. and soc. Psychol.*, vol. 51, pp. 94–106.

FONBERG, E. (1956), 'On the manifestation of conditioned defensive reactions in stress', *Bull. Soc. Sci. Letters., Lodz, Class III*, Vol. 7, No. 1.

FRANKS, C. M. (1956), 'Conditioning and personality: A study of normal and neurotic subjects,' *J. ab. soc. Psychol.*, vol. 52, pp. 143–50.

FREUD, S. (1893), 'On the physical mechanisms of hysterical phenomena', in *Collected Works of Sigmund Freud, Vol. 1*, Hogarth Press, 1949.

JUNG, C. G. (1923), *Psychological Types*, Harcourt Brace. & World.

MOWRER, O. H. and VIEK, P. (1948), 'Experimental analogue of fear from a sense of helplessness', *J. ab. soc. Psychol.*, vol. 43, pp. 193–200.

POLLITT, J. (1957), 'Natural history of obsessional states: A study of 150 cases', *Brit. Med. J.*, vol. 1, pp. 194–8.

WOLPE, J. (1953), 'Learning theory and "abnormal fixations"', *Psychol. Rev.*, vol. 60, pp. 111–16.

15 Louis Breger and James L. McGaugh

Critique and Reformulation of 'Learning-Theory'
Approaches to Psychotherapy and Neurosis

Louis Breger and James L. McGaugh, 'Critique and Reformulation of
"Learning-Theory" Approaches to Psychotherapy and Neurosis',
Psychological Bulletin, vol. 63, 1965, No. 5, 338-58.

'Learning-theory' interpretations of neuroses and the behavioral treatment techniques based on these interpretations are
critically reviewed. The particular learning principles advocated
by the behavior-therapy group are found to be outmoded and
unable to account for evidence from laboratory studies of learning. Particularly open to criticism are: (*a*) the emphasis on the
peripheral response, (*b*) the assumption that concepts taken
from Pavlovian and operant conditioning can be used as explanatory principles, and (*c*) the use of the concept of reinforcement.
The inadequate conception of learning phenomena in terms of
conditioned responses and reinforcement is paralleled by an
equally inadequate conception of neurosis in terms of discrete
symptoms. Next, the claims put forth for the effectiveness of
behavioral techniques is independently examined. The lack of
control over sampling, observer biases, and the lack of control
over the variety of activities that constitute behavioral therapy
all argue strongly against accepting the claims of success at face
value. Finally, a reformulation is offered in which the learning
process is viewed as the acquisition and storage of information,
emphasizing the role of central processes.

A careful look at the heterogeneous problems that are brought
to psychotherapy points up the urgent need for new and varied
theories and techniques. While some new methods have been
developed in recent years, the field is still characterized by
'schools' – groups who adhere to a particular set of ideas and
techniques to the exclusion of others. Thus, there are dogmatic
psychoanalysts, Adlerians, Rogerians, and, most recently, dogmatic behaviorists.

It is unfortunate that the techniques used by the behavior-therapy group (Bandura, 1961; Eysenck, 1960; Grossberg, 1964; Wolpe, 1958) have so quickly become encapsulated in a dogmatic 'school', but this seems to be the case. Before examining the theory and practice of behavior therapy, let us first distinguish three different positions, all of which are associated with the behaviorism or 'learning-theory' label. These are: (a) Dollard and Miller (1950) as represented in their book, (b) the Wolpe-Eysenck position as represented in Wolpe's work (1958; Wolpe, Salter and Reyna, 1964) and in the volume edited by Eysenck (1960), and (c) the Skinnerian position as seen in Krasner (1961) and the work that appears in the *Journal of the Experimental Analysis of Behavior*.

Dollard and Miller present an attempt to translate psychoanalytic concepts into the terminology of Hullian learning theory. While many recent behavior therapists reject Dollard and Miller because of their identification with psychoanalysis and their failure to provide techniques distinct from psychoanalytic therapy, the Dollard-Miller explanation of neurotic symptoms in terms of conditioning and secondary anxiety drive is utilized extensively by Wolpe and his followers. Wolpe's position seems to be a combination of early Hullian learning theory and various active therapy techniques. He relies heavily on the idea of reciprocal inhibition, which is best exemplified by the technique of counter-conditioning. In line with this Hullian background, Wolpe, Eysenck, and others in this group use explanations based on Pavlovian conditioning. They define neurosis as 'persistent unadaptive habits that have been conditioned (that is, learned)' (Wolpe *et al.*, 1964, p. 9), and their explanation of neurosis stresses the persistence of 'maladaptive habits' which are anxiety reducing.

The Skinnerian group (*see* Bachrach in Wolpe *et al.*, 1964) have no special theory of neurosis; in fact, following Skinner, they tend to disavow the necessity of theory. Their approach rests heavily on *techniques* of operant conditioning, on the use of 'reinforcement' to control and shape behavior, and on the related notion that 'symptoms', like all other 'behaviors', are maintained by their effects.

Our discussion will be directed to the Wolpe-Eysenck group

and the Skinnerians, keeping in mind that some of the points we will raise are not equally applicable to both. Insofar as the Skinnerians disavow a theory of neurosis, for example, they are not open to criticism in this area.

It is our opinion that the current arguments supporting a learning-theory approach to psychotherapy and neurosis are deficient on a number of grounds. First, we question whether the broad claims they make rest on a foundation of accurate and complete description of the basic data of neurosis and psychotherapy. The process of selecting among the data for those examples fitting the theory and techniques while ignoring a large amount of relevant data seriously undermines the strength and generality of the position. Second, claims for the efficacy of methods should be based on adequately controlled and accurately described evidence. And, finally, when overall claims for the superiority of behavioral therapies are based on alleged similarity to laboratory experiments and alleged derivation from 'well-established laws of learning', the relevance of the laboratory experimental findings for psychotherapy data should be justified and the laws of learning should be shown to be both relevant and valid.

In what follows we will consider these issues in detail, beginning with the frequently voiced claim that behavior therapy rests on a solid 'scientific' base. Next, we will examine the nature and adequacy of the learning-theory principles which they advocate. We will point out how their learning theory is unable to account for the evidence from laboratory studies of learning. That is to say, the laws or principles of conditioning and reinforcement which form the basis of their learning theory are insufficient explanations for the findings from laboratory experiments, let alone the complex learning phenomena that are encountered in psychotherapy. Then we will discuss how the inadequate conception of learning phenomena in terms of conditioned responses is paralleled by an equally inadequate conception of neurosis in terms of discrete symptoms. Within learning theory, conceptions of habit and response have been shown to be inadequate and are giving way to conceptions emphasizing 'strategies', 'plans', 'programs', 'schemata', or other complex central mediators. A central point of this paper is that conceptions of habit and response are also inadequate to account for neuroses and the learning that goes on in psychotherapy and must here too be replaced with conceptions analogous to strategies. Next we will turn our attention to an evaluation of the claims of success put forth by the proponents of behavior therapy. Regardless of the adequacy of their theory, the claims that the methods work are deserving of careful scrutiny. Here we shall raise a number of questions centering around the issue of adequate controls. Finally, we shall attempt a reformulation in terms of more recent developments within learning, emphasizing the role of central processes.

Science issue

Claims of scientific respectability are made with great frequency by the behavior therapists. Terms such as laboratory based, experimental, behavioral, systematic, and control are continually used to support their position. The validity of a theory or method must rest on empirical evidence, however. Thus, their use of scientific sounding terminology does not make their approach scientific, but rather seems to obscure an examination of the evidence on which their claims are based.

Let us examine some of this evidence. Bandura (1961) provides the following account of a typical behavior-therapy method (Wolpe's counterconditioning):

On the basis of historical information, interview data, and psychological test responses, the therapist constructs an anxiety hierarchy, a ranked list of stimuli to which the patient reacts with anxiety. In the case of desensitization based on relaxation, the patient is hypnotized, and is given relaxation suggestions. He is then asked to imagine a scene representing the weakest item on the anxiety hierarchy and, if the relaxation is unimpaired, this is followed by having the patient imagine the next item on the list, and so on. Thus, the anxiety cues are gradually increased from session to session until the last phobic stimulus can be presented without impairing the relaxed state. Through this procedure, relaxation responses eventually come to be attached to the anxiety evoking stimuli [p. 144].

Without going into great detail, it should be clear from this example that the use of the terms stimulus and response are only remotely allegorical to the traditional use of these terms in psychology. The 'imagination of a scene' is hardly an objectively defined stimulus, nor is something as general as 'relaxation' a specifiable or clearly observable response. What the example shows is that counterconditioning is no more objective, no more controlled, and no more scientific than classical psychoanalysis, hypnotherapy, or treatment with tranquilizers. The claim to scientific respectability rests on the misleading use of terms such as stimulus, response, and conditioning, which have become associated with some of the methods of science because of their place in experimental psychology. But this implied association rests on the use of the same *words* and not on the use of the same *methods*.

We should stress that our quarrel is not with the techniques themselves but with the attempt to tie these techniques to principles and concepts from the field of learning. The techniques go back at least as far as Bagby (1928), indicating their independence from 'modern learning theory'. Although techniques such as these have received little attention in recent years (except from the behavior therapists) they are certainly worth further consideration as potentially useful techniques.[1]

The use of the term conditioning brings us to a second point, that the claims to scientific respectability rest heavily on the attempts of these writers to associate their work with the prestigious field of learning. They speak of something called modern learning theory, implying that psychologists in the area of learning have generally agreed upon a large number of basic principles and laws which can be taken as the foundation for a 'scientific' approach to psychotherapy. For example, Eysenck (1960) states:

Behavior therapy . . . began with the thorough experimental study of the laws of learning and conditioning in normal people and in animals; these well-established principles were then applied to neurotic disorders. . . . It may be objected that learning theorists are not always in agreement with each other and that it is difficult to

1. Another early application of behavioral techniques has recently been brought to our attention: Stevenson Smith's use of the Guthrie approach to learning in his work at the children's clinic at the University of Washington. Guthrie's interpretation of reinforcement avoids the pitfalls we discuss shortly, and contemporary behaviorists might learn something from a review of his work (see Guthrie, 1935).

apply principles about which there is still so much argument. This is only very partially true; those points about which argument rages are usually of academic interest rather than of practical importance. . . . The 10% which is in dispute should not blind us to the 90% which is not – disagreements and disputes naturally attract more attention, agreements on facts and principles are actually much more common. Greater familiarity with the large and rapidly growing literature will quickly substantiate this statement [pp. 14–15].

As we shall show in the next section, this assertion is untenable. 'Greater familiarity with the large and rapidly growing literature' shows that the very core of 'modern learning theory', as Eysenck describes it, has been seriously questioned or abandoned in favor of alternative conceptualizations. For example, the notion that the discrete response provides an adequate unit of analysis, or that reinforcement can be widely used as an explanation of both learning and performance, or that mediational processes can be ignored are being or have been rejected. Eysenck's picture of the field as one with 90 per cent agreement about basic principles is quite simply untrue. The references that Eysenck himself give for this statement (Hilgard, 1956; Osgood, 1953) do not support the claim. Hilgard presented many theories, not one 'modern learning theory', some of which (Gestalt, Tolman, Lewin) might just as easily be said to be in 90 per cent disagreement with behavioristic conditioning approaches. In the same vein, Osgood's text was one of the first to give heavy emphasis to the role of mediation, in an attempt to compensate for the inadequacies of a simple conditioning or one-stage S-R approach. Eysenck seems largely unaware of the very problems within the field of learning which necessitated the introduction of mediational concepts, even by S-R theorists such as Osgood.

These inadequacies center, in part, around the problem of generalization. The problem of generalizing from the level of conditioning to the level of complex human behavior has been recognized for a long time (Lewin, 1951; Tolman, 1933). It is a problem that is crucial in simple laboratory phenomena such as maze learning where it has resulted in the introduction of a variety of mediational concepts, and it is certainly a problem when complex human behavior is being dealt with. For example,

Dollard and Miller (1950) began their book with an attempt to explain neurosis with simple conditioning principles. A careful reading of the book reveals, however, that as the behavior to be explained became more and more complex, their explanations relied more and more on mediational concepts, including language. The necessity for these mediators arises from the inadequacy of a simple *peripheral* S-R model to account for the generality of learning, the equivalence of responses, and the adaptive application of behavior in novel situations. We shall return to these points shortly; here we just wish to emphasize that the field of learning is not 'one big happy family' whose problems have been solved by the widespread acceptance of a simple conditioning model. The claim to scientific respectability by reference back to established laws of learning is, thus, illusory.

Learning and learning theories

We have already noted the differences between the Wolpe-Eysenck and the Skinnerian approaches; let us now examine the similarities. Three things stand out: the focus on the overt response, the reliance on a conditioning model, and the notion of reinforcement. First, there is the belief that the response, consisting of some discrete aspect of overt behavior, is the most meaningful unit of human behavior. While this should ideally refer to a specific contraction of muscles or secretion of glands, with the possible exception of Guthrie (1935), traditional S-R theorists have tended to define response in terms of an effect on the environment rather than as a specific movement of the organism. The problems raised by the use of the response as a basic unit, both in traditional learning phenomena and in the areas of neuroses and psychotherapy, will be discussed in the section entitled What is Learned? A second common assumption is that the concepts taken from conditioning, either as described by Pavlov or the operant conditioning of Skinner, can be used as explanatory principles. The assumption in question here is that conditioning phenomena are the simplest kinds of learning and that all other behavior can be explained in terms of these 'simple' principles. We shall deal with the problems that arise from this source in a second section. The third assumption is that rewards play an essential role in all learning phenomena. We shall consider the problems that stem from this assumption in a third section.

What is learned?

Since its inception in the early twentieth century, behaviorism has taken overt stimuli and responses as its core units of analysis. Learning, as the behaviorist views it, is defined as the tendency to make a *particular response* in the presence of a *particular stimulus*; what is learned is a discrete response. Almost from its inception, however, this view has been plagued by a number of problems.

First, findings from studies of perception, particularly the fact of perceptual constancy, provide embarrassment for a peripheral S-R theory. Perceptual constancy findings show, for example, that the stimulus is much more than peripheral receptor stimulation. For example, once we have learned a song in a particular key (i.e., particular stimulus elements), we can readily recognize it or sing it in other keys. We are amazingly accurate in recognizing objects and events as being 'the same' or equivalent, even though the particular stimulation they provide varies considerably on different occasions (Gibson, 1950). Although the bases of perceptual constancies (size, shapes, brightness, etc.) are not yet well understood, the facts of perceptual constancy – invariance in percept with variation in perceptual stimulation – are not in question. The related phenomenon of transposition has received considerable attention in animal experimentation. Animals, infrahuman as well as human, respond to relations among stimuli (Köhler, 1929). For a number of years, transposition was not considered to pose a serious problem for a peripheral S-R theory since it was thought that it could be adequately handled by principles of conditioning and stimulus generalization (Spence, 1937). This view has not been supported by later experiments, however (Lawrence and DeRivera, 1954; Riley, 1958). It now appears more likely that stimulus generalization is but a special case of the more general complex phenomenon of stimulus equivalence. The absolute theory of transposition was important and instructive because it revealed in clear relief the nature and limitations of a peripheral S-R approach to behavior. The effective stimulus is clearly more 'central' than receptor excitation. The chapters on learning in the recent Koch series make it clear that workers in this area have seen the need for coming to terms with the facts of perception (Guttman, 1963; Lawrence, 1963; Leeper, 1963; Postman, 1963).

Second, the facts of response equivalence or response transfer posed the same kind of problem for a peripheral S-R view. A learned response does not consist merely of a stereotyped pattern of muscular contraction or glandular secretion. Even within the S-R tradition (e.g., Hull, Skinner) there has been a tendency to define responses in terms of environmental achievements. Anyone who has trained animals has recognized that animals can achieve the same general response, that is, make the same environmental change, in a variety of different ways once the response is learned. 'What is learned', then, is not a mechanical sequence of responses but rather, *what needs to be done in order to achieve some final event*. This notion is not new; Tolman stressed it as early as 1932 when he wrote of 'purposive behavior', and it has been strongly supported by a variety of experimental findings (e.g., Beach, Hebb, Morgan and Nissen, 1960; Ritchie, Aeschliman and Peirce, 1950). As this work shows, animals somehow seem to be able to bypass the execution of specific responses in reaching an environmental achievement. They can learn to go to particular places in the environment in spite of the fact that to do so requires them to make different responses from trial to trial. The learning of relatively specific responses to specific stimuli appears to be a special case which might be called stereotyped learning (canalization) rather than a basic prototype on the basis of which all other learning may be explained.

It should be noted further that even the stereotyped learning that forms the basic model of S-R conditioning does not hold up under close scrutiny. First, once a subject has learned a stereotyped movement or response, he is still capable of achieving a goal in other ways when the situation requires it. Thus, while we have all learned to write our names with a particular hand in a relatively stereotyped fashion, we can switch to the other hand, or even write our name with a pencil gripped in our teeth if we have to, in spite of the fact that we may not have made this specific response in this way before. Second, even a response that is grossly defined as constant, stable, or stereotyped does not appear as such a stereotyped pattern of muscular contractions when it is closely observed.[2] These findings in the area of response transfer indicate that a response seems to be highly variable and equipotential. This notion is, of course, quite old in the history of psychology, and it has been stressed repeatedly by numerous investigators including Lashley (*see* Beach *et al.*, 1960), Osgood (1953), Tolman (1932), and Woodworth (1958).

The facts of both response transfer and stimulus equivalence seem much more adequately handled if we assume that what is learned is a *strategy* (alternatively called cognitive maps, programs, plans, schemata, hypotheses, e.g., Krechevsky, 1932) for obtaining environmental achievements. When we take this view, habits, in the traditional behaviorist sense, become a later stage of response learning rather than a basic explanation (building block) for later, more complex learning.

Perhaps this whole problem can be clarified if we look at a specific example such as language learning. As Chomsky (1959) has demonstrated in his excellent critique of Skinner's *Verbal Behavior* (1957), the basic facts of language learning and usage simply cannot be handled within an S-R approach. It seems clear that an adequate view of language must account for the fact that humans, at a rather early age, internalize a complex set of rules (grammar) which enable them to both recognize and generate meaningful sentences involving patterns of words that they may never have used before. Thus, in language learning, what is learned are not only sets of responses (words and sentences) but, in addition, some form of internal strategies or plans (grammar). We learn a grammar which enables us to generate a variety of English sentences. We do not merely learn specific English sentence habits. How this grammar or set of strategies is acquired, retained, and used in language comprehension and generation is a matter for serious research effort; but it is clear that attempts to understand language learning on the basis of analogies from barpressing experiments are doomed before they start. To anticipate, we will argue shortly that if we are to make an attempt to understand the phenomena of neurosis, using

2. G. Hoyle, personal communication, 1963.

analogies from the area of learning, it will be much more appropriate to take these analogies from the area of psycholinguistics and language learning rather than, as has typically been done, from studies of classical and operant conditioning. That is, the focus will have to be on response transfer, equipotentiality, and the learning of plans and strategies rather than on sterotyped response learning or habituation.

Use of a conditioning model

As we indicated earlier, when writers in the behaviorist tradition say 'learning theory', they probably mean a conditioning theory; most of the interpretations of clinical phenomena are reinterpretations in terms of the principles of conditioning. Thus, a phobic symptom is viewed as a conditioned response, maintained by the reinforcement of a secondary fear drive or by a Skinnerian as a single operant maintained by reinforcement. Two types of conditioning are involved in these explanations by reduction. The first is Pavlovian or classical conditioning, frequently used in conjunction with later Hullian concepts such as secondary drive; the second is operant conditioning of the kind proposed by Skinner. The use of both of these models to explain more complex phenomena such as transposition, response transfer, problem solving, language learning, or neurosis and psychotherapy poses a number of difficulties.

The basic assumption that underlies the use of either kind of conditioning as an explanation for more complex phenomena is that basic laws of behavior have been established in the highly controlled laboratory situation and may thus be applied to behavior of a more complex variety. When we look at the way conditioning principles are applied in the explanation of more complex phenomena, we see that only a rather flimsy analogy bridges the gap between such laboratory defined terms as stimulus, response, and reinforcement and their referents in the case of complex behavior. Thus, while a stimulus may be defined as an electric shock or a light of a certain intensity in a classical conditioning experiment, Bandura (1961) speaks of the 'imagination of a scene'; or, while a response may consist of salivation or a barpress in a conditioning experiment, behavior therapists speak of anxiety as a response. As Chomsky (1959) puts it, with regard to this same problem in the area of language:

He (Skinner in *Verbal Behavior*) utilizes the experimental results as evidence for the scientific character of his system of behavior, and analogic guesses (formulated in terms of a metaphoric extension of the technical vocabulary of the laboratory) as evidence for its scope. This creates the illusion of a rigorous scientific theory with a very broad scope, although in fact the terms used in the description of real-life and of laboratory behavior may be mere homonyms, with at most a vague similarity of meaning [p. 30].

A second and related problem stems from the fact that the behavior-therapy workers accept the findings of conditioning experiments as basic principles or laws of learning. Unfortunately, there is now good reason to believe that classical conditioning is no more simple or basic than other forms of learning. Rather, it seems to be a form of learning that is in itself in need of explanation in terms of more general principles. For example, a popular but naïve view of conditioning is that of stimulus substitution – the view that conditioning consists merely of the substitution of a conditioned stimulus for an unconditioned stimulus. Close examination of conditioning experiments reveals that this is not the case, however, for the conditioned response is typically *unlike* the unconditioned response (Zener, 1937). Apparently, in conditioning, a new response is learned. Most of the major learning theorists have taken this fact into account in abandoning the notion of conditioning as mere stimulus substitution.

More than this, the most important theoretical developments using essentially Pavlovian conditioning principles have not even stressed overt behavior (Osgood, 1953). Hull and the neo-Hullians, for example, have relied quite heavily on Tolman's (1932) distinction between learning and performance, performance being what is observed while learning (conditioning) but is one essential ingredient contributing to any instance of observed performance. The most important, and perhaps the most sophisticated, developments in Hullian and neo-Hullian theory concern the attempts to explain complicated goal-directed behavior in terms of the conditioning of fractional responses. Unobserved, fractional responses (already we see the drift away from the overt behavior criteria of response) are assumed to serve a mediating role in behavior. Once a fractional response is conditioned in a particular situation, it is assumed to occur to the stimuli in that situation when those stimuli recur. The stimulus consequences of the fractional response referred to as the rg are assumed to serve as guides to behavior either by serving as a cue or by activating responses or by serving to reinforce other responses by secondary reinforcement. The latter-day proponents of a conditioning point of view (Bugelski, 1956; Osgood, 1953) have come to rely more and more heavily on concepts like the fractional response to bridge the gap between stimulus and overt behavior and to account for the facts of response transfer, environmental achievements, and equipotentiality. What this indicates is that a simple conditioning paradigm which rests solely on observable stimuli and responses has proved inadequate even to the task of encompassing simple conditioning and maze-learning phenomena, and the workers within this tradition have come to rely more and more heavily on mediational (central, cognitive, etc.) concepts, although they still attempt to clothe these concepts in traditional conditioning garb. To add to the problem, a number of recent papers (Deutsch, 1956; Gonzales and Diamond, 1960) have indicated that the r_g interpretations of complex behavior are neither simple nor adequate.

When we look again at the way conditioning principles have been applied to clinical phenomena, we see an amazing unawareness of these problems that have been so salient to experimental and animal psychologists working with conditioning.

While the above discussion has been oriented primarily to classical conditioning, the general argument would apply equally well to those attempts to make the principles of learning derived from operant conditioning the basis of an explanation of neurosis and psychotherapy (as in Krasner, 1961). The Skinnerians have been particularly oblivious to the wide variety of problems that are entailed when one attempts to apply concepts and findings from laboratory learning experiments to other, and particularly more complex, phenomena. While we will deal more directly with their point of view shortly, a few comments might be in order now concerning their use of the operant-conditioning paradigm as a basis for the handling of more complex data.

When Skinnerians speak of laws of learning, they have reference to the curves representing rate of responding of rats pressing bars (Skinner, 1938), and pigeons pecking (Forster and Skinner, 1957) which are, in fact, a function of certain highly controlled contingencies such as the schedule of reinforcement, the amount of deprivation, the experimental situation itself (there is very little else to do in a Skinner box), and the species of animals involved. These experiments are of some interest, both as exercises in animal training under highly restricted conditions, and for what light they may shed on the more general question of partial reinforcement. It is dubious that these findings constitute laws of learning that can be applied across species (see Breland and Breland, 1961) or even to situations that differ in any significant way from the Skinner box.

Use of reinforcement

Advocates of the application of learning theory to clinical phenomena have relied heavily on the 'law of effect' as perhaps their foremost established principle of learning. We shall attempt to point out that a good deal of evidence from experimental animal studies argues strongly that, at the most, the law of effect is a weak law of performance.

Essentially, the controversy can be reduced to the question of whether or not reward is necessary for learning. The initial source of evidence indicating that it was not came from the findings of latent learning studies (Blodgett, 1929; Tolman and Honzik, 1930) in which it was found, for example, that rats who were allowed to explore a maze without reward made fewer errors when learning the maze than controls who had no opportunity for exploration. Thus, these early latent learning studies, as well as a variety of more recent ones (Thistlethwaite, 1951) indicate that learning can take place without reward but may not be revealed until a reward situation makes it appropriate to do so (or to put it another way, the reward elicits the performance but plays little role during learning). Other sources which point to learning without reward come from studies of perceptual learning (Hebb, 1949), imitation (Herbert and Harsh, 1944), language learning (Chomsky, 1959), and imprinting (Moltz, 1960).

Defenders of the point of view that reinforcement is necessary for learning have attempted to handle results such as these in a variety of ways. One has been by appealing to the concept of secondary reinforcement (e.g., a maze has secondary reinforcing properties which account for the learning during exploration). When this sort of thing is done, even with respect to experiments where attempts were made to minimize secondary reinforcements (Thistlethwaite, 1951), it seems clear that this particular notion of reinforcement has become incapable of disproof. Another way of handling these potentially embarrassing results has been by the invention of a new set of drives (curiosity drive, exploratory drive, etc.) but this too has a *post hoc* flavor to it, and one wonders what kind of explanation is achieved by postulating an 'exploratory drive' to account for the fact that animals and humans engage in exploration. In fact, the assumption that exploration reduces an exploratory drive makes it difficult to explain why a rat's tendency to enter an alley of a maze *decreases* after he has explored the alley (Watson, 1961). Finally, there are those (particularly the Skinnerians) who tend to define reinforcement so broadly that neither the findings from latent learning nor any other source can prove embarrassing, since whenever learning has taken place this 'proves' that there has been reinforcement. To better understand this problem, however, we had best look for a moment at the general problem of defining reinforcement in a meaningful way.

Obviously, if the view that reinforcement is necessary for learning is to have any meaning, what constitutes a reinforcement must be defined independently from the learning situation itself. There has been a great deal of difficulty in getting around a circular definition of the law of effect, and it might be worthwhile to examine some of the attempts that have been made in the past.

One of the best known was the attempt to relate the reinforcing properties of stimuli to their drive-reducing characteristics (Hull, 1951). The drive-reduction model has had to be abandoned, however, because of evidence from a variety of areas including latent learning, sensory preconditioning (Brogden, 1939), and novelty and curiosity (Berlyne, 1960). Other evidence such as that of Olds and Milner (1954) on the effect of direct brain stimulation have strengthened the conviction that the drive-reduction interpretation of reinforcement is inadequate; and, in fact, original adherents of this view have begun to abandon it (e.g., Miller, 1959).

The other most frequent solution to the circularity problem has been by way of the 'empirical law of effect', an approach typified by Skinner's definition of reinforcement as any stimulus that can be demonstrated to produce a change in response strength. Skinner argues that this is not circular since some stimuli are found to produce changes and others are not, and they can subsequently be classified on that basis. This seems to be a reasonable position if it is adhered to; that is, if care is taken to define reinforcement in terms of class membership *independently* of the observations that show that learning has taken place. When we examine the actual use of the term reinforcement by Skinner (*see* especially *Verbal Behavior*, 1957) and by other Skinnerians (Lundin, 1961), we find that care is only taken in this regard within the context of animal experiments, but that when the jumps are made to other phenomena, such as language and psychotherapy, care is usually *not* taken to define reinforcement independently from learning as indicated by response strength. This leads to a state of affairs where any observed change in behavior is said to occur *because of* reinforcement, when, in fact, the change in behavior is itself the only indicator of what the reinforcement has been. Chomsky (1959) reviews the use of the concept of reinforcement by Skinner with regard to language and reaches the following conclusion:

From this sample, it can be seen that the notion of reinforcement has totally lost whatever objective meaning it may ever have had. Running through these examples, we see that a person can be reinforced though he emits no response at all, and the reinforcing 'stimulus' need not impinge on the reinforced person or need not even exist (it is sufficient that it be imagined or hoped for). When we read that a person plays what music he likes (165), says what he likes (165), thinks what he likes (438–9), reads what books he likes (163), etc., *because* he finds it reinforcing to do so, or that we write books or inform others of facts *because* we are reinforced by what we hope will be the ultimate behavior of reader or listener, we can only conclude that the term 'reinforcement' has a purely ritual function. The phrase 'X is reinforced by Y (stimulus, state of affairs, event, etc.)' is being used as a cover term for 'X wants Y', 'X likes Y', 'X wishes that Y were the case', etc. Invoking the term 'reinforcement' has no explanatory force, and any idea that this paraphrase introduces any new clarity or objectivity into the description of wishing, liking, etc., is a serious delusion [pp. 37–8].

This problem is exemplified in the area of psychotherapy by the attempts to use the studies of verbal conditioning (Krasner, 1958) as analogues to psychotherapy. First we should note that if these studies are taken at face value (i.e., if subjects are conditioned to increase the emission of certain responses because of reinforcement, without their awareness of this fact) it appears that a simple conditioning model is inadequate since subjects are presumably responding in terms of a class of responses (e.g., plural nouns, etc.) rather than in terms of a specific response (e.g., bar press), such classes implying response transfer and mediation. Second, and more to the point, a number of recent investigators (Erikson, 1962) have begun to question whether verbal conditioning does occur without the subject's awareness. If it does not, the whole phenomenon begins to look like nothing more than a rather inefficient way to get subjects to figure out what the experimenter wants them to do (telling them directly to emit plural nouns would probably be much more efficient) after which they can decide whether they want to do it or not. In any case, there seems to be enough question about what goes on in verbal conditioning itself to indicate that it cannot be utilized as a more basic explanation for complex phenomena such as psychotherapy. Psychotherapists of many persuasions would agree that rewards of some kind are important in work with patients. Thus, the view that the psychotherapist is a 'reinforcement machine' is trivial. The difficult problems are in specifying just what therapist activities are rewarding, in what ways, to what sorts of patients, and with what effects.

The above discussion should make clear that the use of the concept of reinforcement is only of explanatory usefulness when it is specified in some delimited fashion. As an empirical law of performance almost everyone in and out of psychology would accept it, including Lewin, Freud, Tolman, and others outside the traditional S-R movement. But this amounts to

Louis Breger and James L. McGaugh   323

saying nothing more than that some events, when presented, tend to increase the probability of responses that they have followed. The hard job, but the only one that will lead to any meaningful use of the concept of reinforcement, is specifying what the various events called reinforcers have in common. Some have argued that since this is such a difficult task, we should restrict ourselves to listing and cataloging so-called reinforcers. But this is nearly impossible, in a general way, because reinforcers differ from individual to individual, from species to species, from situation to situation, and from time to time (the saying 'one man's meat is another man's poison' is trite but true). Meaningful analysis must stem from a comprehensive study of the particular learning phenomena in question, whether it is language learning, the development of perceptual and perceptual-motor skills (Fitts, 1964; Hebb, 1949), the acquisition of particular species behavior patterns during critical periods of development (Scott, 1962), the learning of a neurosis, or the learning that takes place during psychotherapy. Experience with all of these phenomena has revealed that different kinds of events seem to be involved and that these can only be understood in the context of the phenomena in question. Lumping all these events together under the single term reinforcement serves to muddle rather than to clarify understanding.

The staunch reinforcement adherent might respond that all these complicated arguments may be true but we can ignore them, since all we are really interested in is predicting what the organism will do, and we can do this when we know the organism's reinforcement history. The answer to this is that the experimental literature does not support such a claim; rather, it shows that, in many instances, performance *cannot* be predicted on the basis of a knowledge of the history of reinforcement.

Latent learning studies indicate this quite clearly. Perhaps of more interest are the findings of discrimination-reversal learning studies (Goodwin and Lawrence, 1955; Mackintosh, 1963). Here we find that subjects that have been trained on a series of discrimination reversals learn to select the correct stimulus with very few errors even though they may have been rewarded *much more frequently and more recently for responding to another stimulus*. Similarly, in the double drive discrimination studies

(Thistlethwaite, 1951) animals chose alleys leading to food when they were hungry and water when they were thirsty, even though they have been rewarded equally frequently on the alleys on previous trials. In other words, 'what is learned' was not equivalent with 'reinforcement history'. The law of effect is not disproved by these studies; it is merely shown to be irrelevant.

To summarize: The 'law of effect', or reinforcement, conceived as a *law of learning*, occupies a very dubious status. Like the principles of conditioning, it appears to be an unlikely candidate as an explanatory principle of learning. As a strong law of learning it has already been rejected by many of the theorists who previously relied on it. As an empirical 'law of *performance*' it is noncontroversial, but usually so generally stated as to be of little explanatory value.

Conception of neurosis

In this section we will explicate the conception of neurosis that forms the basis of the behavior-therapy approach (particularly of the Wolpe-Eysenck group) and attempt to demonstrate its inadequacies both in terms of learning theory and as a way of accounting for the observed facts of neurosis. Our argument in the first instance will be that the conception of neurosis in terms of symptoms and anxiety parallels the general conception of learning in terms of overt responses, conditioning, and secondary drives, and suffers from the same inadequacies that we have outlined in the preceding section. With regard to the facts of neurosis, we will argue that the behavior-therapy position is inadequate at a descriptive level as well as being conceptually incorrect. It should be pointed out again that we are discussing the explanation or theory of neurosis here and not the techniques used by the behavior therapists. The strict Skinnerian may excuse himself at this point if he adheres to a 'no-theory' position and is only concerned with the effects of environmental manipulation. Furthermore, certain techniques themselves may be useful and have some of the effects attributed to them regardless of the theory.

In its essence, the conception of neurosis put forth by the behavior therapists is that neuroses are conditioned responses or habits (including conditioned anxiety) and *nothing else*, though it should be noted that they do not adhere to this argument when they describe the success of their methods. Wolpe, for example, while ostensibly treating overt symptoms, describes his patients as becoming more productive, having improved adjustment and pleasure in sex, improved interpersonal relationships, and so forth. The argument that removal of a troublesome symptom somehow 'generalizes' to all of these other areas begs the question. Their conception is typically put forth as an alternative to a psychodynamic viewpoint, which they characterize as resting on a distinction between symptoms and underlying causes (unconscious conflicts, impulses, defenses, etc.). They stress the point that inferences about underlying factors of this sort are unnecessary and misleading and that a more parsimonious explanation treats symptoms (which are typically equated with behavior or that which can be objectively observed) as the neurosis *per se*. They argue that by equating neurosis with symptoms, and symptoms, in turn, with habits (conditioned responses), they are able to bring 'modern learning theory' with its 'well-established laws' to bear on the understanding and treatment of neurosis.

As we have labored to show in the preceding section, the well-established laws of learning to which they refer have considerable difficulty within the area of simple animal behavior. More specifically, it seems clear that a wide variety of behaviors (from maze learning to more complex forms) cannot be adequately dealt with when the overt response and conditioned habit are the units of analysis. Furthermore, their learning position leads the behavior therapists into postulating an isomorphic relationship between antecedent learning and present behavior in which observed differences are accounted for in terms of principles of generalization. This is a key issue, and we shall explore it a little further at this time.

Much of the behaviorist conception of neurosis rests on a rejection of the distinction between symptoms and underlying causes (Eysenck, 1960) as typified by Yates' (1958) argument against 'symptom substitution'. By focusing attention on overt symptoms and banishing all underlying causes, however, the behavior therapists are faced with the same problem that has long confronted behaviorism; namely, the difficulty of explaining how *generality* of behavior results from specific learning experiences. The problem of *generality* (i.e., as exemplified by the facts of transposition and response transfer) has, in fact, brought about the downfall of peripheral S-R learning, of the conditioned habit as a basic unit, and tangentially, is leading to the dethroning of the law of effect. With regard to neurosis, this view has led the behavior therapists into the position where they must posit a specific learning experience for each symptom of a neurosis. They have partly avoided this problem by focusing their attention on those neuroses that can be described in terms of specific symptoms (bed-wetting, if this is a neurosis, tics, specific phobias, etc.) and have tended to ignore those conditions which do not fit their model, such as neurotic depressions, general unhappiness, obsessional disorders, and the kinds of persistent interpersonal entanglements that characterize so many neurotics. This leaves them free to explain the specific symptom in terms of a specific learning experience, as, for example, when a fear of going outdoors is explained in terms of some previous experience in which the stimulus (outdoors) has been associated with (conditioned to) something unpleasant or painful and has now, through generalization, spread to any response of going outdoors. As our previous analysis should make clear, however, even a simple conceptualization such as this, in terms of stimuli, responses, and conditioning is extremely cumbersome and begs the important questions. Within an S-R framework, in which generalization occurs along the dimension of physical stimulus similarity, it is difficult, if not impossible, to show how a previous experience such as being frightened in the country as a child could generalize to the 'stimulus' outdoors without a great deal of *mediation* in which the concept of 'outdoors' carried most of the burden of generalization. As we have pointed out, most workers in the field of learning recognize this and rely heavily on mediational concepts in their explanations of complex behavior. Dollard and Miller (1950), for example, return again and again to mediational explanations once they move beyond the 'combat neuroses' which lend themselves more readily to a simple isomorphic explanation.

A second important facet of the behaviorist conception of

neurosis is the use of the concept of anxiety as a secondary drive. Here, Wolpe and Eysenck and some others seem to follow the explanatory model laid down by Dollard and Miller. Anxiety is viewed as the main motivating force for symptoms and, in general, occupies a central place in their thinking. Briefly, it is worth pointing out that the concept of drive reduction, the distinction between primary drives and secondary drives, as well as the early thinking about the uniquely persistent qualities of fear-motivated behavior have had serious difficulty within learning theory (Watson, 1961; Solomon, 1964). The use of these concepts to explain clinical phenomena thus rests on an exceedingly shaky foundation.

Let us turn our attention now to the phenomena of neuroses. We shall try to point out that underlying the dispute over symptoms versus underlying causes is a real difference in definition that arises at the descriptive level, which, in a sense, antedates disagreements at the level of theory and explanation.

To keep the presentation simple, we will adopt the terms psychodynamic to refer to all those theorists and therapists, following Freud, whose view of neurosis and its treatment deals with motives (conscious and unconscious), conflict, etc. This covers a wide variety of workers, in addition to the more or less traditional followers of Freud, including Sullivan and his adherents (Fromm-Reichman, 1950), other neo-Freudians, and that broad group of psychiatrists and clinical psychologists who have been strongly influenced by the Freudian and neo-Freudian viewpoints even though they may not claim allegiance to any of the formal schools.

The point we wish to make here is that disagreement between the behaviorist and psychodynamic viewpoints seems to rest on a very real difference at the purely descriptive or observational level. The behaviorist looks at a neurotic and sees specific symptoms and anxiety. The psychodynamicist looks at the same individual and sees a complex intra- and interpersonal mode of functioning which may or may not contain certain observable fears[3] or certain behavioral symptoms such as compulsive motor

3. The term anxiety is frequently used as a theoretical inference, i.e., a patient deals with personal material in an overly intellectual fashion, and this is described as a defense mechanism – intellectualization – whose purpose is to ward off anxiety.

acts. When the psycho-dynamicist describes a neurosis, his referent is a cohering component of the individual's functioning, including his characteristic ways of interacting with other people (e.g., sweet and self-effacing on the surface but hostile in covert ways), his characteristic modes of thinking and perceiving (e.g., the hysteric who never 'remembers' anything unpleasant, the obsessive whose memories are overelaborated and circumstantial, etc.), characteristic modes of fantasy and dreaming, a variety of secondary gain features, and the like. Specific or isolatable symptoms may sometimes be a part of such an integrated neurotic pattern, but, even viewed descriptively, they in no sense constitute the neurosis *per se*.

So far, we have considered the behavior therapists' position at face value. In actuality, a good case can be made that they *behave* in a way which is quite inconsistent with their own position. A specific example, taken from one of Wolpe's own case descriptions, will illustrate this point, and, at the same time, show what the psychodynamicist sees when he looks at a neurotic. Wolpe (1960) presents the following case:

Case 5 – An attractive woman of 28 came for treatment because she was in acute distress as a result of her lovers' casual treatment of her. Every one of very numerous love affairs had followed a similar pattern – first she would attract the man, then she would offer herself on a platter. He would soon treat her with contempt and after a time leave her. In general she lacked assurance, was very dependent, and was practically never free from feelings of tension and anxiety.

What is described here is a complex pattern of interpersonal relationships, psychological strategies and misunderstandings (such as the way she became involved with men, the way she communicated her availability to them, her dependency, etc.), expectations that she had (presumably that men would not react with contempt to her generosity, that being dependent might lead to being taken care of, etc.), and thoughts and feelings about herself (lack of assurance, acute distress, etc.). Many of the statements about her (e.g., the description of the course of her love affairs) are abbreviations for very complex and involved processes involving two people interacting over a period of time. It is this, the psychodynamicist would argue, that *is* the neurosis. The tension and anxiety may be a part of it in this particular case (though there might be other cases in which there is no complaint of anxiety but, rather, its reverse – seeming inability to 'feel' anything) – but it is secondary and can be understood only in relation to the other aspects of the patient's functioning. Wolpe's case histories are classic testaments to the fact that he cannot, and does not, apply the symptom approach when working with actual data. As a further example, consider the argument against a symptom-substitution point of view (Yates, 1958) in which it is implied that anything other than symptoms is some sort of metaphysical inference. While it may be true that theories such as psychoanalysis deal with a number of inferential and higher-order constructs in their attempts to integrate the complex mass of data that constitutes a neurosis, it is also true that much more than symptoms exist at the level of observation. Secondary-gain features of a neurosis, in which it is apparent that a variety of goals may be served by a set of interchangeable symptoms, are the rule in most neurotic individuals. We are not defending the view (attributed to psychoanalysis by Yates) that if one symptom is removed another pops up to take its place; rather, we are arguing that the empirical phenomena of neurosis does not fit the symptom or response theory, but is much more compatible with a theory built around central mediators. Whether unconscious conflicts and defense mechanisms are adequate ways of conceptualizing the problem is an entirely separate question. What is clear is that a view stressing central mediators in which specific responses are seen as equipotential means of reaching certain goals is necessary to encompass the data of neurosis just as it has proven necessary to encompass the phenomena of animal learning.

To sum up, it would seem that the behaviorists have reached a position where an inadequate conceptual framework forces them to adopt an inadequate and superficial view of the very data that they are concerned with. They are then forced to slip many of the key facts in the back door, so to speak, for example, when all sorts of fantasy, imaginary, and thought processes are blithely called responses. This process is, of course, parallel to what has gone on within S-R learning theory where all sorts of central and mediational processes have been cumbersomely handled with S-R terminology (e.g., Deutsch, 1956). Thus, we have a situation where the behavior therapists argue strongly against a dynamic interpretation of neurosis at some points and at other points behave as if they had adopted such a point of view. This inconsistency should be kept in mind in reading the next section in which we evaluate the claims of success put forth by the behaviorist group. Insofar as there is disagreement as to what constitutes the descriptive facts of neurosis, it makes little sense to compare the effectiveness of different methods. However, since the behaviorist group adopts very broad (or psychodynamic, if you will) criteria for improvement, and since their *techniques* may have some effectiveness, in spite of theoretical and conceptual inadequacies, it is crucial that we look carefully at the empirical results that they lay claim to.

Claims of success

While much of the writing of the behavior therapists consists of arguments and appeals to principles of science and learning, the claims that are made for the success of the methods seem open to empirical analysis. No doubt a great deal of the appeal of behavior therapy lies right here. Here seem to be methods whose application can be clearly described (unlike such messy psychodynamic methods as 'handling countertransference' or 'interpreting resistance'), whose course is relatively short, and which seem to achieve a large number of practical results in the form of removal of symptoms. Wolpe (1960), for example, presents the following data: of 122 cases treated with behavioral techniques, 44 per cent were 'apparently cured', 46 per cent were 'much improved', 7 per cent were 'slightly or moderately improved', and 3 per cent were 'unimproved'. Combining categories, he claims 90 per cent 'apparently cured or much improved', and 10 per cent 'improvement moderate, slight or nil'. (Criteria of improvement consists of 'symptomatic improvement, increased productiveness, improved adjustment and pleasure in sex, improved interpersonal relationships and ability to handle ordinary psychological conflicts and reasonable reality stresses'.)

He compares this with data from the Berlin Psychoanalytic Institute (Knight, 1941) which shows 62–40·5 per cent in the first category and 38–59·5 per cent in the second. Wolpe concludes, as have others (Bandura, 1961; Eysenck, 1960; Lazarus, 1963), that this demonstrates the superiority of the behavior therapy methods. The fact that the psychoanalytic method showed as much as 62 per cent improvement is explained as being due to whatever accidental 'reciprocal inhibition' occurred during the therapy. (There is, however, no analysis or description of how this might have happened.) The behavioral methods achieve superior results presumably because of the more explicit application of these techniques.

It is fair to say that if these results can be substantiated they present a very strong argument in favor of behavioral *techniques* – even granting the theoretical and empirical inconsistencies we have discussed. However, we must ask if these claims are any better substantiated than those made by the practitioners of other methods of psychotherapy. Insofar as claims such as Wolpe's are based on uncontrolled case histories, they may reflect the enthusiasm of the practitioner as much as the effect of the method. History shows that new methods of therapy (ECS, tranquilizing drugs, as well as various schools of psychotherapy) have been oversold by their original proponents. Thus, a careful look at what lies behind the claims of the behavior-therapy group is in order.

The following does not purport to be a comprehensive review of the behavior-therapy literature. Rather, it is based on a survey of all the studies reported in the two reviews that have appeared (Bandura, 1961; Grossberg, 1964). The most striking thing about this large body of studies is that they are almost all case studies. A careful reading of the original sources reveals that only one study (Lang and Lazovik, 1963) is a controlled experiment, and here the subjects were not neurotics but normal college students. Thus, most of the claims (including those of Wolpe which have been widely quoted) must be regarded as no better substantiated than those of any other enthusiastic school of psychotherapy whose practitioners claim that their patients get better. Behavior therapy has appeared to differ on this score because of its identification with experimental psychology and with 'well-established laws of learning'. We have already dealt with this issue, so let us now turn to some problems in evaluating psychotherapy as a technique.

The problems here are essentially those of control, and they may be broken down into three areas: (a) sampling biases, (b) observer bias, and (c) problems of experimental control. While research in psychotherapy presents particular difficulties in controlling 'experimental input', more sophisticated workers (Frank, 1959) have attempted to deal with at least the sampling and observer problems. It thus comes as somewhat of a surprise that the behavior-therapy workers, despite their identification with experimental psychology, base their claims on evidence which is almost totally lacking in any form of control. Let us examine these issues in greater detail.

Sampling biases

Obviously a claim such as Wolpe's of 90 per cent success has meaning only when we know the population from which the sample of patients was drawn and the way in which they were selected. Ideally, a comparison of treatment techniques would involve the random assignment of patient from a common population pool to alternative treatments. Since, in practice, this is rarely feasible, it is essential for anyone making comparisons of different treatment methods to, at the very least, examine the comparability of the populations *and* of the methods used in selecting from these populations. Neither Wolpe's data nor that of Lazarus (1963) contains this evidence. Wolpe reports, for example, that:

Both series (seventy patients reported on in 1952 and fifty-two patients reported on in 1954 on which the 90 per cent figure is based) include only patients whose treatment has ceased after they have been afforded a reasonable opportunity for the application of the available methods; i.e., they have had as a minimum both a course of instruction on the changing of behavior in the life situation and a proper initiation of a course of relaxation-desensitization. This minimum takes up to about fifteen interviews, including anamestic interviews and *no patient who has had fifteen or more interviews has been omitted from the series* [emphasis added].

We may conclude from this that some patients (how many we do not know) having up to fourteen interviews have been excluded from the sample – a procedure highly favorable to the success of the method but which violates the simplest canons of sampling. Wolpe's final sample of 122 consists of those patients most likely to show improvement, since both they and he were satisfied enough with the first fourteen (or less) interviews to warrant proceeding further. Those patients least likely to improve are those most likely to drop out early (fourteen sessions or less) and not be included in the computation of success rate. The fact that a large number of poor-prognosis patients would very likely be eliminated during these early sessions is supported by a variety of research findings (Strickland and Crowne, 1963), which show that most dropping-out of untreatable or unsuccessful cases occurs during the first ten sessions. This serious sampling bias would be expected to spuriously inflate the per cent showing improvement.

When we add this to whatever unknown factors operate to delimit the original population (presumably there is some self-selection of patients who seek out this form of treatment), it becomes apparent that little confidence can be given to the reports of success.

Observer bias

Psychologists have long been aware that human beings are fallible observers, particularly when they have predispositions or vested interests to protect. In controlled studies, we try to protect judges from their own biases by not acquainting them with the hypotheses, or with the nature of the groups they are judging, or by using blind and double-blind designs. This problem is particularly acute with regard to psychotherapy because both therapist and patient have investments of time, involvement, competence, and reputation to protect. For these reasons, workers in the area have become extremely skeptical of claims put forth for any method which rests on the uncontrolled observation of the person administering the treatment. At a minimum we expect some sort of external evidence. Beyond this minimum we hope for an independent judge who can compare differentially treated groups without knowing which is which.

In addition, there is the problem of the patient's freedom to report effects which may be seriously curtailed when all his reports go directly to the person who has treated him. It seems reasonable to assume that some patients are prevented from expressing dissatisfaction with treatment when they must report directly to the therapist, either because they do not want to hurt his feelings, or are afraid, or are just saying what they think is being demanded of them, or are being polite, or for some other reason. Again, it would be highly appropriate to provide the patients with the opportunity of reporting results in a situation as free from such pressure as possible.

Examination of the twenty-six studies reviewed by Bandura reveals a surprising lack of concern with these problems. Of the twenty-six studies sampled, only twelve report evaluation of results by persons other than the treating therapist; four of these use ratings of the hospital staff (who may be acquainted with the treatment), four use mothers or parents reporting on their children to the treating therapist, one is a wife reporting on her husband to the therapist, and three use a second observer. Obviously, whatever factors enter in to cause observer and reporter biases are allowed full rein in most of these cases. While we cannot conclude from this that the reported results are *due to* observer and reporter biases (as is clearly indicated with the sampling biases), it is impossible to rule them out. Furthermore, a great deal of evidence from many areas of psychology leads us to be very skeptical of claims in which biases of this sort go uncontrolled.

Experimental control

While control of sampling and observer effects are basic to a wide variety of research activities, including field and clinical research, more exacting control over experimental conditions has long been the *sine qua non* of the laboratory methods of experimental psychology. The power of the experimental method stems, in part, from keeping careful control over all but a few conditions, which are experimentally varied, with the subsequent effects of these variations being observed. Since psychotherapy is not a controlled experiment, it is probably unfair to expect this type of control. However, there are more and less accurate descriptions of what goes on during any form of therapy, and we can demand as accurate a description as possible in lieu of experimental control. Thus, while we are led to believe that methods, such as counterconditioning, extinction of maladaptive responses, methods of reward, and the like, are applied in a manner analogous to their laboratory counterparts – examination of what is *actually done* reveals that the application of the learning techniques is embedded in a wide variety of activities (including many of the traditional therapy and interview techniques) which make any attribution of effect to the specific learning techniques impossible. Let us consider a few examples. From Wolpe (1960):

Case 4 – The patient had sixty-five therapeutic interviews, unevenly distributed over twenty-seven months. The greater part of the time was devoted to discussions of how to gain control of her interpersonal relationships and stand up for herself. She had considerable difficulty with this at first, even though it had early become emotionally important to her to please the therapist. But she gradually mastered the assertive behavior required of her, overcame her anxieties and became exceedingly self-reliant in all interpersonal dealings, including those with her mother-in-law.

From Lazarus and Rachman (1957) on systematic desensitization:

Case 1 – The patient was instructed in the use of assertive responses and deep (non-hypnotic) relaxation. The first anxiety hierarchy dealt with was that of dull weather. Starting from 'a bright sunny day' it was possible for the subject to visualize 'damp overcast weather' without anxiety after twenty-one desensitization sessions, and ten days after the completion of this hierarchy, she was able to report that, 'the weather is much better, it doesn't even bother me to look at the weather when I wake up in the morning' (previously depressing). . . . During the course of therapy, part of the reason for the development of the anxiety state in this patient was unearthed. When she was seventeen years old she had become involved in a love affair with a married man twelve years her senior. This affair had been conducted in an extremely discreet manner for four years, during which time she had suffered from recurrent guilt feelings and shame – so much so, that on one occasion she had attempted suicide by throwing herself into a river. It was her custom to meet her lover after work *in the late afternoon*. The dull weather can be accounted for, as this affair took place in London.

From Rachman (1959):

Interview number 12. The patient having received a jolt in her love relationship, this session was restricted to a sort of nondirective, cathartic discussion. No desensitizing was undertaken because of A.G.'s depressed mood and obvious desire to 'just talk'.

These excerpts have been presented because they seem representative of the practices of the behavioral therapists. As can be seen, the number and variety of activities that go on during these treatment sessions is great, including, in these few examples, discussions, explanations of techniques and principles, explanations of the unadaptiveness of anxiety and symptoms, hypnosis of various sorts, relaxation practice and training with and without hypnosis, 'nondirective cathartic discussions', 'obtaining an understanding of the patient's personality and background', and the 'unearthing' of a seventeen-year-old memory of an illicit affair. The case reports are brief and presented anecdotically so that it is really impossible to know what else went on in addition to those things described. What should be abundantly clear from these examples is that there is no attempt to restrict what goes on to learning techniques. Since it seems clear that a great variety of things do go on, any attribution of behavior change to specific learning techniques is entirely unwarranted.

In summary, there are several important issues that must be differentiated. First, a review of both learning theory and of the empirical results of behavior therapy demonstrates that they can claim no special scientific status for their work on either ground. Second, there are important differences of opinion concerning the type of patient likely to be affected by behavior therapy. Grossberg (1964), for example, states that: 'Behavior therapies have been most successful when applied to neurotic disorders with specific behavioral manifestations [p. 81].' He goes on to point out that the results with alcoholism and sexual disorders have been disappointing and that the best results are achieved with phobias and enuresis. He later states that 'desensitization only alleviates those phobias that are being treated, but other coexisting phobias remain at high strength, indicating a specific treatment effect [p. 83]'. Wolpe *et al.* (1964), on the other hand, argue that: 'The conditioning therapist differs from his colleagues in that he *seeks out* the precise stimuli to anxiety, and finds himself able to break down almost every neurosis into what are essentially *phobic systems* [p. 11].' The best controlled study (Lang and Lazovik, 1963) indicates that 'desensitization is very effective in reducing the intense fear of snakes held by normal subjects, though it can be questioned whether this is a phobia in the clinical sense'.

Thus, there seems to be some evidence that these *techniques* (as techniques and not as learning theory) are effective with certain conditions.[4] We feel that this bears stressing because psychotherapy has come to be narrowly defined in terms of dynamic, evocative, and nondirective methods, placing unnecessary limitations on the kind of patient suitable for psychotherapy. First, we must note that behavior techniques are not new (as Murray, 1964, points out in a recent article). Freud and Breuer used similar techniques prior to the development of psychoanalysis, Bagby described a number of these methods in 1928, and therapy based on techniques designed to eliminate undesirable responses was used for many years by Stevenson Smith at the University of Washington Clinic. While most of these techniques have been superceded by the various forms of dynamic psychotherapy, recent work (Frank, 1961) suggests that the time may be ripe for taking a fresh look at a variety of methods such as hypnosis, suggestion, relaxation, and other approaches of a more *structured nature* in which the therapist takes a *more active role*. Needless to say, this fresh look would best proceed unencumbered by an inadequate learning theory and with some minimal concern for control. As an example of a nondynamic approach to patient management, we refer to the work of Fairweather (1964) and his colleagues.

Reformulation

Up to this point our analysis has been primarily critical. We have tried to show that many of the so-called principles of learning employed by workers with a behaviorist orientation are inadequate and are not likely to provide useful explanations for clinical phenomena. In this section we will examine the potential

4. Just how many neurotics fit the phobia and/or specific symptom model is a complicated question, the answer to which depends in part on what one's own point of view leads one to look for. For example, an informal census of the first 81 admissions to the University of Oregon Psychology Clinic in 1964 revealed only 2 patients who could be so classified.

value of ideas from different learning conceptions. Before proceeding, however, we would like to discuss briefly the issue of the application of 'laws', principles, and findings from one area (such as animal experimentation) to another (such as neurosis and psychotherapy). The behaviorists have traditionally assumed that principles established under highly controlled conditions, usually with animal subjects, form a scientific foundation for a psychology of learning. Yet when they come to apply these principles to human learning situations, the transition is typically bridged by rather flimsy analogies which ignore crucial differences between the situations, the species, etc. Recently, Underwood (1964) has made the following comments concerning this problem:

Learning theories as developed in the animal-learning laboratory, have never seemed . . . to have relevance to the behavior of a subject in learning a list of paired associates. The emphasis upon the role of a pellet of food or a sip of water in the white rat's acquiring a response somehow never seemed to make contact with the human S learning to say VXK when the stimulus DOF was presented [p. 74].

We would add that the relevance is at least equally obscure in applications of traditional S-R reinforcement theory to clinical phenomena.

We do *not* wish, however, to damn any and all attempts to conceptualize clinical phenomena in terms of principles of learning developed outside the clinic. On the contrary, recent work in learning may suggest certain theoretical models which may prove useful in conceptualizing the learning processes involved in psychotherapy and the development of neuroses. Whether these notions can form the basis for a useful learning conceptualization of clinical phenomena will depend upon the ingenuity with which they are subsequently developed and upon their adequacy in encompassing the facts of neurosis and psychotherapy. Further, we would like to stress that their association with experimental work in the field of learning does not give them any *a priori* scientific status. Their status as explanatory principles in the clinical area must be empirically established within that area. In what follows, then, we will outline some ideas about learning and make some suggestions concerning their relevance to clinical problems.

Our view of learning centers around the concepts of information storage and retrieval. Learning is viewed as the process by which information about the environment is acquired, stored, and categorized. This cognitive view is, of course, quite contrary to the view that learning consists of the acquisition of specific responses; responses, according to our view, are mediated by the nature of the stored information, which may consist of facts or of strategies or programs analogous to the grammar that is acquired in the learning of a language. Thus, 'what is learned' may be a system for generating responses as a consequence of the specific information that is stored. This general point of view has been emphasized by Lashley (*see* Beach *et al.*, 1960), by Miller, Galanter, and Pribram (1960), in the form of the TOTE hypothesis, and by a number of workers in the cognitive learning tradition (Tolman, 1951; Woodworth, 1958). Recently it has even been suggested as a necessary formulation for dealing with that eminently S-R area, motor skills (Adams, 1964; Fitts, 1964).

This conception of learning may be useful in the clinical area in two ways: one, in formulating a theoretical explanation for the acquisition or development of neurosis, symptoms, behavior pathology, and the like, and, two, in conceptualizing psychotherapy as a learning process, and suggesting new methods stemming from this learning model.

A conceptualization of the problem of neurosis in terms of information storage and retrieval is based on the fundamental idea that what is learned in a neurosis is a set of central strategies (or a program) which guide the individual's adaptation to his environment. Neuroses are not symptoms (responses) but are strategies of a particular kind which lead to certain observable (tics, compulsive acts, etc.) and certain other less observable, phenomena (fears, feelings of depression, etc.). The whole problem of symptom substitution is thus seen as an instance of response substitution or response equipotentiality, concepts which are supported by abundant laboratory evidence.

Similarly, the problem of a learning conceptualization of unconscious phenomena may be reopened. Traditional S-R approaches have equated the unconscious with some kind of avoidance of a verbalization response. From our point of view, there is no reason to assume that people can give accurate descriptions of the central strategies mediating much of their behavior any more than a child can give a description of the grammatical rules which govern the understanding and production of his language. As a matter of fact, consciousness may very well be a special or extraordinary case – the rule being 'unawareness' of the mediating strategies – which is in need of special explanation, rather than the reverse. This view avoids the cumbersome necessity of having to postulate specific fear experiences or the persistence of anxiety-motivated behavior, as has typically been done by S-R theorists with regard to unconscious phenomena. It also avoids equating the unconscious with the neurotic, which is a virtue since there is so much that goes on within 'normal' individuals that they are unaware of. It further avoids the trap of attributing especially persistent and maladaptive consequences to painful experiences. As Solomon (1964) points out, the existing evidence does not support the view that punishment and pain lead unequivocally to anxiety and maladaptive consequences.

The view of learning we have outlined does not supply a set of ready-made answers to clinical problems that can be applied from the laboratory, but it indicates what sort of questions will have to be answered to achieve a meaningful learning conceptualization of neurosis and symptoms. Questions such as 'What are the conditions under which strategies are acquired or developed?' stress the fact that these conditions may be quite different from the final observed behavior. That is to say, a particular symptom is not necessarily acquired because of some learning experience in which its stimulus components were associated with pain or fear-producing stimuli. Rather, a symptom may function as an equipotential response, mediated by a central strategy acquired under different circumstances. As an example, consider Harlow's (1958, 1962) monkeys who developed a number of symptoms, the most striking being sexual impotence (a much better animal analogue of human neurosis than those typically cited as experimental neuroses [Liddell, 1944]). Their longitudinal record, or 'learning history', indicates that the development of this abnormal 'affectional system', as Harlow terms it, is dependent on a variety of non-isomorphic experiences, including the lack of a mother-infant relationship and the lack of a variety of peer-play experiences.

These brief examples are only meant to give a flavor of where a learning conception of neurosis which stresses the acquisition of strategies will lead. A chief advantage of this view is that it has *generality* built in at the core, rather than imported secondarily, as is the case with S-R concepts of stimulus and response generalization.

Let us now turn our attention to the very difficult problem of applying learning concepts to psychotherapy. Basically, we would argue that the development of methods and techniques is largely a function of the empirical skill and ingenuity of the individual-craftsman-therapist. Even a carefully worked-out and well-established set of learning principles (which we do not have at this time) would not necessarily tell us how to modify acquired strategies in the individual case – just as the generally agreed-upon idea that rewards affect performance does not tell us what will be an effective reward in any specific instance.

Bearing these cautions in mind, we might still address ourselves to the question of what applications are suggested by the learning approach we have presented. As a first suggestion, we might consider the analogy of learning a new language. Here we see a process that parallels psychotherapy insofar as it involves modifying or developing a new set of strategies of a pervasive nature. A careful study of the most effective techniques for the learning of a new language might yield some interesting suggestions for psychotherapy. Learning a new language involves the development of a new set of strategies for responding – new syntax as well as new vocabulary. Language learning *may or may not* be facilitated by an intensive attempt to make the individual *aware* of the strategies used, as is done in traditional language instruction which teaches old-fashioned grammar, and as is done, analogously, in those psychotherapies which stress insight. Alternatively, language learning sometimes seems most rapid when the individual is immersed in surroundings (such as a foreign country) where he hears nothing but the new language and where his old strategies and responses are totally ineffective.

Using this as a model for psychotherapy, we might suggest

something like the following process: First, a careful study should be done to delineate the 'neurotic language', both its vocabulary and its grammar, of the individual. Then a situation might be constructed (e.g., a group therapy situation) in which the individual's existing neurotic language is not understood and in which the individual must develop a new 'language', a new set of central strategies, in order to be understood. The detailed working out of such a procedure might very well utilize a number of the techniques that have been found effective in existing therapies, both group and individual, and in addition draw on some new techniques from the fields of psycholinguistics and language learning.

These are, of course, but initial fragmentary guesses, and they may be wrong ones. But we believe that the conceptions on which these guesses are based are sufficiently supported by recent learning research to warrant serious attention. Although this reconceptualization may not lead immediately to the development of effective psychotherapeutic techniques, it may at least provide a first step in that direction.

References

ADAMS, J. A. (1964), 'Motor skills', in P. R. Farnsworth (ed.), *Ann. Rev. Psychol.*, no. 15, pp. 181–202.

BAGBY, E. (1928), *The Psychology of Personality*, Holt, Rinehart & Winston.

BANDURA, A. (1961), 'Psychotherapy as a learning process', *Psychol. Bull.*, no. 58, pp. 143–59.

BEACH, F. A., HEBB, D. O., MORGAN, C. T. and NISSEN, H. W. (1960), *The Neuropsychology of Lashley*, McGraw-Hill.

BERLYNE, D. E. (1960), *Conflict, Arousal and Curiosity*, McGraw-Hill.

BLODGETT, H. C. (1929), 'The effect of introduction of reward upon the maze performance of rats', *University of California Publications in Psychology*, no. 4, pp. 113–34.

BRELAND, K. and BRELAND, M. (1961), 'The misbehavior of organisms', *Amer. Psychol.*, no. 16, pp. 681–4.

BROGDEN, W. J. (1939), 'Sensory preconditioning', *J. Exper. Psychol.*, no. 25, pp. 323–332.

BUGELSKI, B. R. (1956), *The Psychology of Learning*, Holt, Rinehart & Winston.

CHOMSKY, N. (1959), Review of B. F. Skinner, *Verbal Behavior*, *Language*, no. 35, pp. 26–58.

DEUTSCH, J. A. (1956), 'The inadequacy of human derivations of reasoning and latent learning', *Psychol. Rev.*, no. 63, pp. 389–99.

DOLLARD, J. and MILLER, N. E. (1950), *Personality and Psychotherapy*, McGraw-Hill.

ERIKSON, C. W. (ed.) (1962), *Behavior and Awareness*, Duke University Press.

EYSENCK, H. J. (ed.) (1960), *Behavior Therapy and the Neuroses*, Pergamon.

FAIRWEATHER, G. W. (1964), *Social Psychology in Treating Mental Illness: an Experimental Approach*, Wiley.

FORSTER, C. B., and SKINNER, B. F. (1957), *Schedules of Reinforcement*, Appleton-Century-Crofts.

FITTS, P. M. (1964), 'Perceptual-motor skill learning', M. A. W. Melton (ed.), *Categories of Human Learning*, Academic Press, pp. 244–85.

FRANK, J. D. (1959), 'Problems of controls in psychotherapy as exemplified by the psychotherapy research project of the Phipps Psychiatric Clinic', in E. A. Rubenstein and M. B. Parloff (eds.), *Res. Psychol.*, Am. psych. Ass.

FRANK, J. D. (1961), *Persuasion and Healing: a Comparative Study of Psychotherapy*, John Hopkins Press.

FROMM-REICHMANN, F. (1950), *Principles of Intensive Psychotherapy*, University of Chicago Press.

GIBSON, J. J. (1950), *The Perception of the Visual World*, Houghton Mifflin.

GONZALES, R. C. and DIAMOND, L. (1960), 'A test of Spence's theory of incentive motivation', *Amer. J. Psychol.*, No. 73, pp. 396–418.

GOODWIN, W. R. and LAWRENCE, D. H. (1955), 'The functional independence of two discrimination habits associated with a constant stimulus situation', *J. comp. phys. Psychol.*, no. 48, pp. 437–43.

GROSSBERG, J. M. (1964), 'Behaviour theory: a review', *Psychol. Bull.*, no. 62, pp. 73–88.

GUTHNE, E. R. (1935), *The Psychology of Learning*, Harper & Row.

GUTTMAN, N. (1963), 'Laws of behaviour and facts of perception', in S. Kodi (ed.), *Psychology: A Study of a Science*, McGraw-Hill, vol. 5, pp. 114–79.

HARLOW, H. F. (1958), 'The nature of love', *Amer. Psychol.*, No. 13, pp. 673–85.

HARLOW, H. F. (1962), 'The heterosexual affectional system in monkeys', *Amer. Psychol.*, no. 17, pp. 1–9.

HEBB, D. O. (1949), The *Organization of Behaviour: A Neurophysiological Theory*, Wiley.

HERBERT, M. J. and HORSH, C. M. (1944), 'Observational learning by cats', *J. Compar. Psychol.*, No. 37, pp. 81–95.

HILGARD, E. R. (1956), *Theories of Learning*, Appleton-Century-Crofts.

HULL, C. L. (1951), *Essentials of Behaviour*, Yale University Press.

KNIGHT, R. P. (1941), 'Evaluation of the results of psychoanalytic therapy', *Amer. J. Psychol.*, no. 98, p. 434.

KÖHLER, W. (1929), *Gestalt Psychology*, Liveright.

KRASNER, L. (1958), 'Studies of the conditioning of verbal behaviour', *Psychol. Bull.*, no. 55, pp. 148–70.

KRASNER, L. (1961), 'The therapist as a social reinforcement machine', in H. H. Strupp (ed.), *Second Research Conference on Psychotherapy*, Am. psychol. Ass.

KRECHEVSKY, I. (1932), 'The genesis of "hypotheses" in rats', *University of California Publications in Psychology*, No. 6, pp. 45–64.

LANG, P. J. and LAZOVIK, A. D. (1963), 'Experimental desensitization of a phobia', *J. ab. soc. Psychol.*, No. 66, pp. 519–25.

LAWRENCE, D. H. (1963), 'The nature of a stimulus: some relationships between learning and perception', in S. Koch (ed.), *Psychology: A Study of a Science*, McGraw-Hill, vol. 5, pp. 179–212.

LAWRENCE, D. H. and DeRIVIERA, J. (1954), 'Evidence for relational transposition', *J. comp. phys. Psychol.*, no. 47, pp. 465–71.

LAZARUS, A. A. (1963), 'The results of behaviour therapy in 126 cases of severe neurosis', *Behav. Res. and Ther.*, no. 1, pp. 69–80.

LEEPER, R. L. (1963), 'Learning and the fields of perception, motivation and personality', in S. Koch (ed.), *Psychology: A Study of a Science*, McGraw-Hill, vol. 5, pp. 365–487.

LEWIN, K. (1951), *Field Theory in Social Science*, Harper, ch. 4, pp. 60–86.

LIDDELL, H. S. (1944), 'Conditioned reflex method and experimental neurosis', in J. McV. Hunt (ed.), *Personality and the Behaviour Disorders*, Ronald Press.

LUNDIN, R. W. (1961), *Personality: An Experimental Approach*, Macmillan.

MACKINTOSH, N. J. (1963), 'Extinction of a discrimination habit as a function of overtraining', *J. comp. phys. Psychol.*, No. 56, pp. 842–7.

MILLER, G. A., GALANTER, E. H. and PRIBRAM, K. H. (1960), *Plans and the Structure of Behavior*, Holt, Rinehart & Winston.

MILLER, N. E. (1959), 'Liberalization of basic S–R concepts: extension to conflict behaviour, motivation and social learning', in S. Koch (ed.), *Psychology: A Study of a Science*, McGraw-Hill, vol. 2, pp. 196–292.

MOLTZ, H. (1960), 'Imprinting empirical basis and theoretical significance', *Psychol. Bull.*, no. 57, pp. 291–314.

MURRAY, E. J. (1964), 'Sociotropic learning approach to psychotherapy' in P. Worchel and D. Byrne (eds.), *Personality Change*, Wiley, pp. 249–88.

OLDS, J. and MILNER, P. (1954), 'Positive reinforcement produced by electrical stimulation of septal area and other regions of rat brain', *J. comp. phys. Psychol.*, no. 47, pp. 419–27.

OSGOOD, C. E. (1953), *Method and Theory in Experimental Psychology*, O.U.P.

POSTMAN, L. (1963), 'Perception and learning', in S. Koch (ed.), *Psychology: A Study of a Science*, McGraw-Hill, vol. 5, pp. 30–113.

RACHMAN, S. (1959), 'The treatment of anxiety and phobic reactions by systematic desensitization psychotherapy', *J. ab. soc. Psychol.*, no. 58, pp. 259–263.

RILEY, D. A. (1958), 'The nature of the effective stimulus in animal discrimination learning: transposition reconsidered', *Psychol. Rev.*, no. 65, pp. 1–7.

RITCHIE, B. F., AESCHLIMAN, B., and PEIRCE, P. (1950), 'Studies in spatial learning VIII. Place performance and the acquisition of place dispositions', *J. comp. phys. Psychol.*, no. 43, pp. 73–85.

ROTTER, J. B. (1954), *Social Learning and Clinical Psychology*, Prentice-Hall.

SCOTT, J. P. (1962), 'Critical periods in behavioural development', *Science*, No. 138, pp. 949–58.

SKINNER, B. F. (1938), *The Behavior of Organisms: an Experimental Analysis*, Appleton-Century-Crofts.

SKINNER, B. F. (1957), *Verbal Behavior*, Appleton-Century-Crofts.

SOLOMON, R. L. (1964), 'Punishment', *Am. Psychol.*, no. 19, pp. 239–53.

SPENCE, K. W. (1937), 'The differential response in animals to stimuli varying within a single dimension', *Psychol. Rev.*, no. 44, pp. 430–40.

STRICKLAND, B. R. and CROWNE, D. P. (1963), 'The need for approval and the premature termination of psychotherapy', *J. Cons. Psychol.*, no. 27, pp. 95–101.

THISTLETHWAITE, D. (1951), 'A critical review of latent learning and related experiments', *Psychol. Bull.*, no. 48, pp. 97–129.

TOLMAN, E. C. (1932), *Purposive Behavior in Animals and Men*, Appleton-Century-Crofts.

TOLMAN, E. C. (1933), 'Sign gestalt or conditioned reflex?', *Psychol. Rev.*, no. 40, pp. 391–411.

TOLMAN, E. C. (1951), *Collected Papers in Psychology*, University of California Press.

TOLMAN, E. C., and HONZIK, C. H. (1930), 'Introduction and removal of reward and maze performance in rats', *University of California Publications in Psychology*, no. 4, pp. 257–75.

UNDERWOOD, B. J. (1964), 'The representativeness of rote verbal learning', in A. W. Melton (ed.), *Categories of Human Learning*, Academic Press, pp. 47–78.

WATSON, A. J. (1961), 'The place of reinforcement in the explanation of behaviour', in W. H. Thorpe and O. L. Zangwill (eds.), *Current Problems in Animal Behavior*.

WOLPE, J. (1958), *Psychotherapy by Reciprocal Inhibition*, Stanford University Press.

WOLPE, J. (1960), 'Reciprocal inhibition as the main basis of psychotherapeutic effects', in H. J. Eysenck (ed.), *Behaviour Therapy and the Neuroses*, Pergamon, pp. 88–113.

WOLPE, J., SALTER, A. and REYNA, L. J. (eds.) (1964), *The Conditioning Therapies*, Holt, Rinehart & Winston.

WOODWORTH, R. S. (1958), *Dynamics of Behavior*, Holt Rinehart & Winston.

YATES, A. J. (1958), 'Symptoms and symptom substitution', *Psychol. Rev.*, no. 65, pp. 371–4.

ZENER, K. (1937), 'The significance of behavior accompanying conditioned salivary secretion for theories of the conditioned response', *Am. J. Psychol.*, no. 50, pp. 384–403.

Part Six
Contemporary Developments in Treatment

At the heart of most recent innovations in the treatment of those afflicted with psychological abnormality lies a shift from the exclusive dependence upon one therapist treating one patient at a time (as with the physician-patient relationship in physical medicine) to the use of all of the people in the patient's environment, whether 'professional' or not. Maxwell Jones, the British pioneer of the therapeutic milieu, began this movement and describes it in the first paper in this part of the present volume.

More recently, in the United States, the success of behavioural principles in restoring normal responses in hospital patients had led, by extension, to the large-scale use of these principles in ward management. Drs Atthowe and Krasner describe the operation of such a system.

Within the more traditional rubric of individual therapist-patient treatment, Dr Margaret Rioch and her colleagues at the National Institute of Mental Health have developed professional training programmes for university graduates and intelligent housewives. There is a notable economy of training time and, as the study reports, no evidence that the trainees are any less skilled than therapists who have gone through the more traditional and protracted curricula of the mental health professions.

16 A. A. Baker, M. Jones, J. Merry and B. A. Pomryn

A Community Method of Psychotherapy

A. A. Baker, M. Jones, J. Merry and B. A. Pomryn, 'A community method of psychotherapy', *British Journal of Medical Psychology*, vol. 26, 1953, pp. 222–44.

In this paper we shall attempt to describe some aspects of treatment which are in use in this therapeutic community. In particular we want to emphasize the technique in use at the daily meetings of the entire patient and staff population of the Unit, and to develop the concept of a therapeutic culture. This article is complementary to our recently published book (Jones, 1952).

Description of unit

The Social Rehabilitation Unit at Belmont Hospital has 100 beds and is part of the larger hospital. It was started in April 1947 for the specific purpose of studying the problem of adult character disorders. The patients are of both sexes, and come from all parts of the country being referred, in the main, from psychiatric out-patient departments or from the Courts. Patients are of all ages from eighteen to sixty, the majority being young adults. We have many cases of neurosis, but for the purposes of this article we are giving preference to those who give a history of a bad early environment, the early appearance of delinquency and various manifestations of antisocial behaviour in later life. Clinically they would be described as including criminal, aggressive and inadequate psychopaths, alcoholics and other forms of addiction, sexual perversions and such disorders as schizoid, paranoid, and hysterical personalities. Clearly character disorders of these kinds present a very difficult treatment problem. The vast majority are quite unsuited for the usual forms of treatment, including physical and psychoanalytic procedures. There has been a disturbance in their character development and their social adjustment. We have come to feel that the best approach to such problems is by the establishment of a therapeutic community. By this term we mean a community where each individual, whether patient or staff, has a definite role to play, and everything is done to help the individual to bring his emotional problems to the group. The patients not only expect the treatment for themselves but are afforded an opportunity to contribute to the treatment of other patients. The concept of a therapeutic culture will be discussed later.

The staff comprises four psychiatrists, two social workers, one clinical psychologist, two disablement rehabilitation officers seconded to us by the Ministry of Labour, five workshop instructors, three trained nurses and eleven social therapists. The latter are young women who have usually some form of social science training and are aiming at social work of one kind or another. They come to us from various countries in Scandinavia, Europe, or America and stay for six to twelve months. We have found these social therapists more useful to us than trained nurses as their social science background gives them a more objective approach to psychiatry, and they tend to have fewer prejudices than people with a medical training. Communication in the staff group is highly developed and there are few situations in which the staff does not think and act collectively. No important decision affecting the unit is ever taken without full discussion with the staff and, where relevant, the patient community too.

Activities
1 Therapeutic
We will now touch very briefly on the various therapeutic activities which occur during the day, reserving community techniques for more detailed study later.

(a) *Individual interviews*. The length of time spent in doctor/patient interviews varies greatly with different doctors and their individual patients; as far as possible each patient is seen alone by his doctor once a week, the length of interview being anything from a few minutes to an hour. Treatment is essentially supportive and aimed at strengthening or modifying the patient's defences and satisfying his need for assistance by actual guidance. Reference is frequently made to events outside the individual treatment situation which are known to the doctor because of the social structure and good communications of the therapeutic community. Details of the patient's ward, life, information from workshops and social situations generally can frequently be used to illustrate and explain aspects of the patient's emotional problems. Thus the emphasis is placed on the 'here and now'.

(b) *Therapeutic groups.* The technique used in therapeutic groups varies considerably with the personality and outlook of the different doctors. At least two-thirds of the patient population is in such a group treatment at any one time, and the groups meet from two to four times a week. No attempt will be made to give any detailed descriptions of group methods in use, as we are concerned here with community rather than group methods of treatment. It is important to mention, however, that tensions felt at community meetings frequently have a marked effect on the therapeutic group meeting later in the day.

(c) *The 8.30 a.m. meeting.* There is one meeting which requires particular attention because of its special function. This is called the '8.30 a.m. meeting', simply because it meets every morning at that hour; it lasts for thirty minutes. This meeting was initiated in July 1952 and has been running for four months. Prior to its inception doctors had raised any disciplinary problems involving their patients at an individual interview. There was an understandable resistance on the part of some doctors to undertake what was often an unpleasant role. The patients indicated in various ways that there was no consistent policy on the part of the different doctors toward the defaulters, although it was generally conceded that if anything was said it was intended to help the patient's treatment rather than punish him. The nurses and social therapists were not too happy about this rather vague policy, and felt that they were not always given adequate support by the doctors; their anxiety about anti-social behaviour amongst the patients tended to be raised at one of the 1 p.m. staff meetings. In order to try to improve an unsatisfactory situation a daily meeting of 'defaulters' was instituted. A record was kept of all patients who failed to conform to the simple rules of the Unit society. The social therapist went round with the Fault Book which contained the names of patients who had been absent from occupation, from the 9 a.m. meetings (see later), or who had come in late, drunk, etc., and invited them to attend the 8.30 a.m. meeting. At first the doctor sat at his desk and had the Fault Book in front of him, but after two or three days he sat in the circle and had no knowledge of the contents of the Fault Book. The social therapist who collected the patients usually stayed for the Group and might be joined by other social therapists. At first the patients were mainly resentful and regarded this meeting as the equivalent of any army defaulters' parade. They were on the defensive, demanded to know why they had been sent for, or had numerous excuses to explain their behaviour. Some refused to come to the meeting, while others left during the meeting apparently demonstrating their contempt for authority. Despite the fact that it had been stated clearly at a 9 a.m. meeting that this new group was intended to discuss the problems of patients who had difficulty in conforming to our simple community rules, it was clear that to begin with most people attending thought of it as being in some way punitive. The doctor was expected to play an authoritarian role and at first no one apparently contemplated any other possibility. After a few meetings, however, it began to dawn on some of the patients (several of whom had attended daily), that no punishment was being given. The doctor was behaving in much the same way as he did in any therapeutic group; moreover, he pointed out that although the patients seemed to be making certain assumptions regarding his role, he had no such preconceptions himself. The nature of the 8.30 a.m. meetings began to change. The social therapists noticed less resentment among the patients when they were asked to attend. The name 'defaulters' parade' became less popular and the noncommittal phrase '8.30 a.m. meeting' began to replace it.

To begin with, five or six aggressive psychopaths had appeared almost daily for various reasons, such as returning to hospital after the prescribed time, etc. This antisocial group had caused the administration considerable anxiety, and at the initial 8.30 a.m. meetings they were loud in their denunciation of the barrack-room methods which we were supposed to be using. At the fourth meeting of the 8.30 a.m. group one of these patients announced importantly that he had not been asked to attend by the social therapist, but had come as a visitor. The doctor made no comment and the remainder of the group did not seem to be displeased. The 'visitor' proceeded to show in the ensuing discussion that he had identified himself with the staff and was anxious to correct any misinterpretation of the function of the meeting which might be held by other members of the group. His example was followed by other patients and within a month the number of visitors attending was as great as the 'defaulters' who had been requested to attend. The visitors included all the aggressive psychopaths who had initially resented the meetings. The group structure was considerably altered by this change of events. The doctor was largely unaware of the different motivations for attending the group as the patients might be either 'defaulters' or 'visitors' and unless they chose to identify themselves he had no means of telling the difference. The 'visitors' did much of the talking and the meeting became something of a sociological seminar. The 'defaulters' frequently chose to speak of their difficulty in attending occupation, or their dislike of the 9 a.m. meetings, or their drunken behaviour, etc. They were under no obligation to do so but seemed to be driven by some inner compulsion. The group discussed the problem as though it had some inherent capacity to help the individual and was quite prepared to accept a supportive or even interpretative role.

One morning the social therapist asked six patients to come to the group meeting and all six arrived. Two men and one woman had been seen crossing the electrified railway the previous evening at 11 p.m. and when spoken to by one of the staff who had at first thought that they might be making a suicidal attempt, they had become abusive. They were clearly under the influence of drink and were taking a considerable risk crossing the railway where the live rail represented a serious hazard. One other couple had returned to the ward at 2 a.m. and the sixth patient returned to the ward at 1 a.m. Two social therapists and a doctor completed the group. Two of the male patients started talking at once and appeared to be under some pressure of anxiety. They both spoke about their desire to alter the current pattern of the unit and stay out late on Saturday night. They spoke enviously of other patients, who, because of the proximity of their homes, were able to go home on week-end pass. One of these men, severely crippled by an old poliomyelitis, said that he had always felt that rules were made to be broken, and he had already been discharged from three previous hospitals for anti-social behaviour. The other man, one of the two who had been drunk, and had crossed the railway line, talked of his mis-demeanour at some length and said that getting inebriated on a Saturday night was part of a pattern which he had developed while in hospital, but that he was now beginning to realize that his behaviour involved other people in situations which might have serious consequences. He said that he had not previously attended an 8.30 a.m. meeting, which he had felt was dominated by a group of 'intellectuals' and it was only now that he fully grasped the function of the meeting. He said that he felt considerable relief at having verbalized his guilt and had he not attended the meeting he would probably have felt miserable all day, and gone out drinking again that night. The polio case said that for the moment he had lost his desire to attack the hospital, and although he felt no loyalty to the community, he nevertheless felt concerned about the doctor's responsibility for the community and intended to mend his ways. One of the female patients said that she would find it easier to discuss her problem of late return with her doctor, but that she realized that her behaviour had significance not only for herself but also in relation to the community, and for this reason it was probably advantageous to discuss it in the group. This she did not do to any extent but the male patient with whom she had returned at 2 a.m. tended to blame himself for the situation on the grounds of his having been frustrated and fed up recently. He went on, however, to speak of the relief which the meeting afforded him, and that he approved of the method whereby the patient himself was made responsible for his behaviour. The meeting ended with a statement from the doctor regarding the function of the 8.30 a.m. meeting, and a restatement of the Unit's attitude to discipline. Two of the patients had not chosen to speak although they had clearly been on the verge of doing so on several occasions.

The individual was free to attend the group or not as he chose, and if he did he might or might not speak. The patient population came to understand slowly that within the unit, discipline rested with the individual. At the meeting it was often apparent that not only did the patient come to the group meeting expecting punishment but when this was not forthcoming, the patient had a feeling of disappointment. On the other hand, the patient frequently expressed relief at being allowed to verbalize his guilt without having to wait uneasily for something to happen. It would seem that the tendency was for the group to deal much more leniently with the patient's problem than did his own conscience. Even more important would appear to be the permissive attitude of the group and of the doctor in the group. The 8.30 a.m. meeting has come to be regarded as a useful barometer of social climate in the Unit. If patients choose to make use of it and understand it they indicate some awareness of our cultural aims.

(*d*) *The ward meeting*. The patients of each ward meet weekly for half an hour. Fifteen to thirty patients meet with the Sister of the Unit and the two social therapists allotted to the ward and a doctor. The meeting takes place in the ward; the members sitting informally in a group on beds and chairs. Free discussion is encouraged but emphasis is placed on topics relating to the ward community. Rivalry with the other wards is evident in discussions on ward cleanliness, participation in ward fatigues and in planning improvements on existing social activities. As far as possible patients are encouraged to seek their own solution to problems raised. Examples of these are untidiness in the ward or washroom and noisiness of patients after lights are extinguished. These problems are likely to be raised at successive ward meetings and defaulters named by patients so that the individual's difficulties in conforming may be discussed.

At these meetings the doctors can draw the attention of the active participants towards those who remain more passive. The problems of individual patients may also be raised. These will often have to be discussed against the wishes of the patient concerned. As an example, can be quoted the case of a young airman admitted because of repeated thefts since the age of seven. This had culminated in a sentence of two years' detention following entry into a Sergeants' Mess and robbery of cigarettes. The sentence had been altered so that he could enter hospital. He maintained that he could not resist the temptation to steal and feared that he might come into conflict with his fellow patients because of this. At the time of his admission there had been some petty pilfering in the ward. The patient, in individual interviews, indicated his reluctance to discuss his fears with other patients, but when at the ward meeting he was asked whether he would agree to the doctor doing so he acquiesced. His story was given in some detail, and related to the family circumstances in his early years of life. During this recital he became increasingly tense and restless and finally ran from the meeting and did not return. The other patients were clearly interested and indicated a belief that the stealing was symptomatic of his illness. The patient had feared ostracism in consequence of this meeting, but was much relieved to find that interest in his progress was maintained by other patients and there was no further evidence of pilfering in the ward.

(*e*) *Community discussions*. This term refers to the daily meetings of the total of patients and staff population at 9 a.m. At these meetings community projection techniques such as psychodrama are frequently employed and will be discussed later in this paper.

(*f*) *9.45 a.m. staff meeting*. The staff meets daily at 9.45 a.m. for half an hour to discuss the 9 a.m. community meeting and try to analyse if possible what the meeting has meant to the patients as a whole.

(*g*) *Lunch-time staff meetings*. The entire staff meets at lunchtime for three separate hours each week in an attempt to discuss individual and group problems and analyse some of the interpersonal and other difficulties which arise in the staff groups. Some of the time is spent by the doctor in charge giving information to the remainder of the group. In addition, many problems raised at community meetings with the patients have to be discussed and some attempt made to arrive at an attitude or concept with which the staff can identify itself. The structure of these staff meetings varies considerably, depending on how many important communications have to be made, but the major part of the three hours a week available is devoted to free discussion within the staff community, with any member being free to raise whatever topic he or she cares to initiate.

(*h*) *Tutorials for the social therapists*. These are held every day for periods varying from half to one hour. These tutorials are essentially for the interchange of information about the patients between doctor and social therapist. The form these meetings take is largely determined by the needs and anxieties of the social therapists, and they are concerned with clinical teaching, transference phenomena, and descriptions of social and work situations regarding the patients, etc.

(*i*) *Therapeutic group meetings for the social therapists*. These weekly therapeutic group meetings are held with the same doctor, and an attempt is made to make the social therapists conscious of some of their own tensions and unconscious motivations; in this way they have the opportunity to learn something of group dynamics at first hand.

2 Workshops

The working role has great significance to our patients, particularly to the male patients, most of whom were unemployed before coming to hospital. The workshops for the male patients comprise bricklaying, plastering, hairdressing, tailoring and gardening, each with its own instructor. No attempt is made to provide any training, and as far as possible the patients work as a group on a job which has value to the hospital community. Our aim is to make working conditions similar to those in outside workshops so that the patient is placed in a relatively unskilled work role and problems of adaptation, acceptance of authority, time-keeping, etc., will arise as they have done in the past under real working conditions; they can then be discussed in the community meetings. Hours of work are from 10 a.m. to 12 noon and 1 to 4 p.m., and everyone is expected to participate. If they do not attend no disciplinary action is taken but a certain amount of social pressure is brought to bear by the staff attitude and discussion groups generally. Non-attenders are invited to join the 8.30 meeting next morning. Problems arising from the work situations are frequently fed back to the community meetings, and there is much attention paid to the patients' attitude to work. Most of the men have a resistance to work and much can be done to help them to test out the possibility of a better work adjustment whilst still in hospital. They come to realize some of the support and understanding which they can obtain from other workmates and enjoy the opportunity for expression of hostility towards the instructor, etc. As far as possible the work produces obvious benefits to the community so that there is an opportunity for a feeling of mastery over the environment. In selected cases a certain amount of reality testing is possible. Patients can be tried out in jobs in the local community where they work for two to four hours a day on an unpaid basis. Over thirty employers in the Sutton district have helped us in this way, and this reality testing has been a very valuable additional aid to the psychologist and extends the field of vocational psychology. Finally some patients, who are still in hospital, are tried out in the local government training centre at Waddon, and if found suitable can go on to a full training in the appropriate trade after they leave hospital.

The women have a choice of dressmaking, cooking in the hospital kitchen, gardening or handicrafts, and once a week have a 'women's hour' spent on lecture-discussion on such topics as child-care, pregnancy, beauty-culture, i.e. the emphasis is upon the assumed 'normal' career of most women, to marry and have a home. In fact these meetings usually turn rapidly from the initial subject to discussion of such matters as social preference for men rather than women, the relation of this to homosexuality, sex-education, sexual relationships before marriage and similar problems which make a woman's role in our society difficult.

3 Social activities

A social role for the patients is given as much consideration as their occupational role. The more actively participant patients organize a very varied programme for the needs of the community, but there is always a small percentage of non-partici-pants. It is one aspect of the role of the social therapist to study the isolates' needs. She may make an individual approach to such a patient, as, for instance, by partnering him at dancing classes or by trying to evoke the help of other patients. The main goal in view is to study the individual patient and encour-age him to test out various possibilities of making social relation-ships. This process is greatly helped by the therapeutic activities such as the psychodrama. It is not infrequent for an inhibited shy patient to put on a psychodrama which clearly alters his relationship to the rest of the community, who now know some-thing of that patient's difficulties. This affords the other patients the opportunity to play a useful role in overcoming some of the inhibited patient's difficulties, and this in turn may lead to greater participation by them in social activities. The same pro-cess may operate in, say, the case of an alcoholic who discusses his social difficulties at an 8.30 a.m. meeting.

In the foregoing account we have attempted to show that the activities, whether specifically therapeutic, or in the workshops, or in the organized social programme, are all aimed at bringing the individual into closer harmony with the group and increas-ing the group sense of responsibility towards its individual mem-bers. The individual may come to find that the community deals with his problems in a more tolerant and understanding way than does his own conscience. An identification with the com-munity may give a patient a greater feeling of security.

Social structure of unit community

A role is a set of legitimate expectations of behaviour, and the cohesiveness of any social structure depends on the effective-ness of the performance of important roles.

The patients are given every opportunity to conceptualize their role in the daily discussion groups, and much of our time is spent in trying to get the patients to alter their attitude from that of passive dependence to active participation. Thus the aggressive and active patients tend to dominate the discussion groups and the 'silent members' tend to be overlooked. The patients tend to expect something to be done to treat them and frequently have little awareness of their own need to contribute if any change is to be effected. They have frequently come to blame the environment for all their difficulties and to disregard their own shortcomings. We want the patients to test out the beneficial results which may follow their own participation in even the simplest situations; for instance, in the ward meetings patients make complaints and expect the staff to deal with them. If this is not done they feel rejected and angry. If some patients cannot sleep because of a noisy door they will frequently continue to suffer the noise, feel angry with the staff and never contemplate correcting the problem for themselves. We want the patients to adopt a more constructive attitude to even the most simple situation. By discussion of problems, patients begin to adopt certain ways of meeting these problems in a more objective way. We expect the patients to resolve their own difficulties in so far as they are capable of doing so, and the contribution of the staff can only be complementary to their own contribution. In this sense the role of the patient has come to be increasingly therapeutic. Every effort is made to create situations in which the patient can play a useful part in the community life and even contribute to the betterment of the other patients. By having no overt discipline, the patient population is forced to face this problem and deal with its own defaulters. This helps the community to consider the meaning of antisocial behaviour and how these people can be helped to identify themselves more closely with the needs and aims of the group.

The social therapist has identified herself with both the patient and the staff community. Each social therapist is allotted to a ward of about thirty patients and knows each individual case fairly well. Moreover, the daily tutorials with the doctors afford an excellent opportunity for clarifying her concepts and lessening her anxiety in relation to the patients. As has already been mentioned, we have largely dispensed with the traditional nurse and, apart from the three senior nurses with medical training, the work is done by eleven social therapists who have a social science rather than medical background. So far it would seem that the social therapist is never completely accepted by the ward community and tends to be excluded from some of their more intimate social situations. This of course varies with the differing ward populations and with the personalities of the social therapists. The patient community still regards any member of the staff as being in a privileged position, and although they may turn to such a person for help they still tend to resent the discrepancy in their circumstances.

Perhaps a more difficult aspect of the social therapists' work is in relation to authority. There is no discipline in the conventional use of the term; all activities are voluntary but there are, nevertheless, clearly defined attitudes and expectations of behaviour. The social therapists are in a sense the carriers of the unit culture. They remind the patients that it is expected that they should go to the community discussion groups and to their occupations, etc. By playing such a role the social therapist feels the impact of the various antisocial trends which have brought the patient to hospital. She must try to remain objective and not become involved in an emotional situation for which, in many cases, the patient feels a need. She has to do much more than be pleasant or try to be liked by the patients, she has got to be realistic and remind the patient that he is going against the patterns of behaviour which have been agreed to by the patients themselves. As far as executive authority is concerned the social therapists indicate to a defaulter that he is expected to attend the 8.30 a.m. meeting the following day. The social therapists attend these meetings when possible and become thoroughly familiar with the aetiological approach to antisocial behaviour. They also become used to the concept of transference and their contact with the psychiatrists is on such an intimate day-to-day basis that the situations creating anxiety to the social therapists can largely be dealt with as they arise.

The social therapists participate in every aspect of the patients' activities and are expected to take as much interest in the patients in their work situations as in the social life of the wards, or in the organized social activities in the evening. They are in a position to feed back social problems to the community meetings if the patients concerned have been consulted and are agreeable to this procedure. For the doctors the social therapists perform many essential functions. As a result of the frequent discussion on patients' problems they will know how to handle any patient, which to encourage to join a committee, who needs to go to dancing classes, who needs, during a temporary crisis, more sympathy and attention. They also report back the daily occurrences on the ward to the doctor concerned who thus has much first-hand knowledge of recent patterns of behaviour.

The social therapists have a very difficult role to play. The patients are often suspicious of them, jealous of their ability to approach the doctors freely and afraid they will pass on 'bad' reports. However, the patients' need for human contacts, for affection and understanding or even for a willing listener to their tales of trouble, will usually overcome their doubts and fears. For patients who have hostility to women as a major problem the social therapists' persistent friendly and tolerant attitude is fundamental to a change of attitude – the patients' generalization that all women are bad or untrustworthy cannot last in the face of persistent evidence to the contrary.

As a group, the social therapists are doctor-centred and communicate directly with the psychiatrist concerned. The role of the Sister (charge nurse) has been considerably modified and, compared to the usual hospital role, she has come to have a largely integrative and interpretative function, trying to clarify the cultural concepts of the Unit to both social therapists and patients. She has avoided having an individual therapeutic relationship with the patients and has attempted to see the unit as a whole and relate particular events to the total structure.

The social workers, disablement resettlement officers, psychologist and instructors all attend the daily community meetings and the staff meetings. They have their own specific jobs to do, but in addition are conscious of their community role. They participate freely in the discussions and clarify their own roles when necessary or contribute to the discussion according to their own particular training or viewpoint. Such participation is not only beneficial to the community but is also educational. This applies particularly to the less trained personnel such as instructors who are afforded an opportunity to get some grounding in group dynamics and sociology. It also affords the patient population an excellent opportunity to express their feelings about the various individuals concerned and this in itself may bring about considerable modification of the various roles.

The doctors have a much closer contact with the patient population than is usual in a hospital. They meet their patients not only in individual interviews and therapeutic groups but also in the daily community meetings. They are continually called upon to express their views on different subjects and the personality of the individual doctor becomes relatively well known to the patient. They are the main recipients of the patients' aggression and set a pattern for the whole community in their handling of such situations. Their training and insight prepares them to meet such situations with a considerable degree of objectivity, and also allows them to make occasional interpretations when these are justified. There is no attempt to hide behind an aura of mystery or magic. On frequent occasions the doctors are forced to admit their ignorance, and it is part of a deliberate policy that the limitations of psychiatry should be freely admitted and the moderate therapeutic goal possible in the Unit's work constantly faced. The patients frequently indicate their desire for an authoritarian or even an omnipotent role; they want the doctor actively to resolve their problems while they wait passively for results. The discussion or re-enactment of current social problems in the community meetings afford excellent opportunities to demonstrate the unreality of such an attitude. We are still playing a largely intuitive role in the community meetings. The tendency is for all four doctors to participate if a discussion touches on some fundamental cultural concept so that the community has a clear demonstration of unity in outlook. In this sense they also tend to act as spokesmen for the entire staff and are more articulate in the main than are the other staff members.

The social structure of the Unit is being altered constantly with a view to achieving the best possible communication between various members. Clearly many individuals cannot make use of the opportunities afforded in a community meeting and, as far as possible, the opportunities for communication between any two individuals are made easily available, for instance, a patient may not only see his own doctor, but may ask to see one of the other doctors and such a request would be met; the doctor would however make it clear that any material would have to be made available to the patient's own doctor. The staff roles are constantly changing to meet changing needs and as a result of the new insights which result from the community meetings. It is hoped that the various roles are so well known by the staff members that in theory interchangeability of any of the existing roles could be conceived.

Community discussion

The entire Unit population meets each week-day at 9 a.m. for forty-five minutes. The meetings are attended by approximately sixty to eighty people who sit in a circle several rows deep. The meeting is not structured unless some particular projection technique is being employed, e.g. psychodrama is held every Friday and other techniques may be employed on other days as occasion arises. There is no formal leader in the meeting but the doctor acts as a sort of time-keeper, asking for any comments when the meeting starts and terminating the meeting at 9.45 a.m. It is unusual for the staff members to initiate any point for discussion, but it is clearly understood that they are there in their own particular roles and are just as free to communicate their views as are the patients. Our aim is to afford the patients the opportunity to verbalize their current problems and tensions. In such a meeting there is little opportunity for dealing with individual problems, although on occasion this may happen and a doctor may feel justified in making an interpretation in the light of material brought forward by one of his patients.

The meeting is more valuable in affording the opportunity for the appearance of disharmonious factions within the community. Most frequently the tension is between the staff and patient groups or in relation to a patient or group of patients who are assuming a leadership role in the patient community. The rivalries between two potential leaders may be acted out in front of everyone and the validity of their statements tested in a relatively objective way by the entire community. For example, a difference of opinion between two members of the patients' entertainments committee may come to be understood as essentially a problem of two individuals competing for a leadership role. In the same way complaints by the patients about neglect on the part of the staff can be tested against the known facts, and it may become clear that the problem is not one of neglect but is more related to the emotional problem of the patient.

The meeting can do much more than afford a setting for

reality testing. The patient population may be activated to tackle some of its own problems. The tendency is to feed back problems to the patient population if they do not raise them themselves. Take the problem of discipline. There is no executive authority on the Unit, and the current procedure is to invite those patients who fail to conform to the simple laws of our society to attend the 8.30 a.m. meeting. For instance, it may be that there is an increasing disregard of the rule that the patients are expected to be in pyjamas by 9 p.m. when the night staff come on duty. If this point is not raised by the patients themselves a staff member may bring it up at the community meeting. The patient population may show disinclination to act and imply that it is really the job of the staff to take action. The staff may remind the patients that partly to respond to their own wishes we have no formal disciplinary machinery. Various irrelevancies may be introduced to the discussion, and at this point it may be suggested that the patients are resisting assuming a responsible role which causes them some anxiety. If no positive step is taken by the community by the end of the meeting, it may be suggested that in view of the need for social order the topic should be raised at the next meeting.

On one such occasion no improvement had occurred in the patients' behaviour and no positive attitude had emerged after several days' discussion. An extraordinary meeting was called at 3.30 p.m. and the patients reminded of the need for a decision if the skeleton night staff were to fulfil their responsibilities to a sick population. This stimulated the more quiet and inarticulate section of the patients, who verbalized their annoyance with the small minority of defaulters for the first time. The defaulters themselves confessed to various feelings of guilt and promised improved behaviour. After several suggestions of a more strict disciplinary regime had been countered the meeting finally decided that in future the community meetings should be made compulsory instead of optional, so that those persons disregarding the ruling in question could be named and asked to account for their behaviour in front of the whole community. In addition, it was agreed that the social therapists when saying goodnight as they traditionally did at 9 p.m. should also make a note of any patients absent from the ward or not in pyjamas; those defaulters would then be expected to attend the 8.30 a.m. meeting where the group could discuss their difficulty in conforming to the social order. The meeting clearly felt, however, that treatment by discussion and a form of punishment in the direction of social censure should be complementary. The patients endorsed the need for a latent authority invested in the doctors which gave them the right to discharge patients if this was justified on clinical grounds, and was necessary to protect the community in the face of a serious threat to its existence or efficient function.

In the main, it might be said that the community meetings aim at resolving immediate tensions in the patient population and afford an opportunity for reality testing and free communication between patients and staff. To a lesser degree they would appear to achieve some clarification of social attitudes and ways of thinking with a view to helping the patient to a better social adjustment. As an extension to this largely educational process we have developed the group projection techniques which are described in the next section.

As an example of the way in which these community discussion meetings function the resolution of a rivalry situation will be described.

Two patients, Mr T. and Mr Q., were rivals for the leadership of a ward. This rivalry appeared in a number of situations. In a community discussion Mr T. had stated he had a problem to raise – the annoyance he felt at the intolerance of some patients towards Jews. Mr Q. stated that he assumed he was one of those referred to by Mr T. For five minutes these two patients argued with, and interrupted each other, the rest of the community watching. At the end of this time Mr Q. walked out, looking very angry. The rivalry situation was commented upon by both doctors present, who felt, however, that with one of the two concerned out of the meeting, little further progress would be made. In fact, the remainder of the meeting was inconclusive; there were two periods of silence, one patient was unusually aggressive in his comments about the staff and there was much more muttering than usual from the patients with few definite comments being made.

During the next week the community was disturbed by another problem and the rivalry seemed to be less obvious. On the day before the meeting just described, however, Mr T. had been elected chairman of the entertainments committee and Mr Q. was a ward representative on this committee. A week later, Mr Q. and one of the women's ward representatives resigned from the committee and this was reported to the community at 9 a.m. on the next day by Mr T. A doctor suggested that the reason for this should be discussed. Mr Q. then explained that he preferred to work on his own and not with the committee, though he still wanted to help them. Another patient suggested that the reason was that the committee could not work together, but Mr Q. denied this. At this point another doctor said he had some information to add. He knew that the women's ward representative had resigned because she felt that she had not received enough support from the other women. Mr Q. continued to deny that he had any animosity towards the other patients, or Mr T. on the committee, but a number of men from his own ward made comments showing that they did not agree with him. Mr T. made only one comment, that he too considered that there was no animosity between himself and Mr Q. 'The committee worked quite harmoniously', he said. At this point a doctor commented that the need to work by oneself was a common one among the patients, and that in fact several patients did entertainment work for the community but did not serve on the committee. For the next five minutes the doctor discussed this point with a number of those concerned and a patient then remarked that when outside (i.e. after leaving hospital) everyone had to work under somebody. The doctor agreed and then said that this was Mr Q.'s problem, that he was ambitious, wanted to succeed, but was intolerant of working with other people, or under authority because this seemed to hamper him. Mr Q. agreed with this, but another patient, who also was an individual worker, asked the doctor if this meant individual work was of no value. This point was elaborated by the doctor and several other patients, particularly one who had been on the entertainments committee previously and had identified himself, verbally at least, with the staff's attitude that all patients should work as a group rather than as individuals. The doctor then elaborated on the problem of rivalry situations, how they affected staff as well as patients and were in fact a universal problem which faced nations as well as individuals. He suggested that whereas in the past religion had tried to solve these problems now the social sciences were trying to make a contribution and our unit community life was an example of this. His statement lasted some six minutes. The patients listened attentively at first when the problem was clearly related to themselves but towards the end became restless and one murmured 'bosh'.

A woman patient now suddenly rose to her feet and asked what treatment she could have for her pain. This apparently irrelevant remark surprised the audience. A doctor commented, however, that this patient, like Mr Q., wanted to know how her individual needs could be fitted in with those of the community in general. Several patients now turned to Mr Q. and asked him in a most friendly manner to reconsider his decision and to serve again, on the committee. Mr T. joined this request and, after some hesitation, Mr Q. agreed. There was an obvious relaxing of tension and feeling of relief in the whole room at this. Mr T. now asked if the woman's representative would also continue. She, however, rejected his appeal. (She was a chronic depressive, who had spent several years in a mental hospital; her hostility to everyone was barely concealed beneath an apparent willingness to help.) The doctor who had first mentioned her problem earlier in the meeting pointed out that he felt her refusal was in part due to the unsettled state of the women's ward, and this could be profitably discussed at the women's ward meeting in the afternoon. The discussion then ended. Three members of the staff and fifteen patients had spoken.

As yet we have failed to achieve a satisfactory way of recording what goes on in the community. We have attempted to piece together what appears to be happening by reporting not only the community meetings but also the other meetings held throughout the day, along with any information the social therapists may report from the ward. This gives us some information, but we are fully aware of the limitations of this approach and feel the need for a social anthropologist who could devote his full time to the problem of studying the community reactions and to the assessment of cultural change.

We need a method of recording which will give us the maximum of objective information with the minimum of inaccuracy or unnecessary detail. Also since in our community everyone is expected to take an active part in discussion when necessary, the person doing the recording should find the method so simple that he can use it while taking part in discussion. In the present system squared paper is used, each square representing a minute. The following symbols are used:

S = statement.
I = came in.
$?$ = question.
M = muttering.
O = walk out.
A = answer.
$S/$ = statement interrupted.
S = person who interrupted.
S or $?$ = that one person spoke directly to
$/$ $/$
S A another rather than to the group as a whole.
$= = =$ means the statement lasted three minutes.

The influence of any individual on a group may be shown with clarity even by this crude method of recording. For example here is a record for part of the time in which one group discussed the same problem with and without individual X.

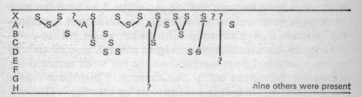

nine others were present

Without X the following pattern appears.

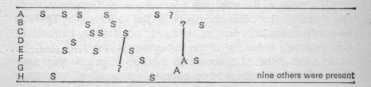

nine others were present

It can be seen that when X is present discussion is centred upon him, and takes place between him and other individuals. When he is absent the discussion is between individuals and the group as a whole. Also when X is present, because of his attitude fewer people can take part in the same discussion. Perhaps the group with X present can be described as a 'leader and followers' group, without him it becomes a free discussion group in which more can take part, there is greater freedom for reactions and one might suspect a more democratic, as opposed to authoritarian, attitude.

The recording technique was used for the morning community meeting already described in which the tension between Mr Q. (Patient 3) and Mr T. (Patient 2) was expressed. This meeting was recorded as follows:

Varieties in projection techniques
1 Psychodrama

During the five years that the unit has been in existence various projection techniques have been evolved. The oldest of these is the psychodrama which we had used for some years before the unit at Belmont was in existence. This technique has been employed by one of us (M.J.) for the last nine years. At that time we had no knowledge of Moreno's work (1946) and simply evolved a technique to meet a therapeutic need. The psychodrama has gone through various phases, and we shall describe its present structure. Each week a patient volunteers to present his problem in a dramatized form to the whole patient community. He chooses his own cast from patients or staff, and the group is excused from occupations for the week required for rehearsals before the actual performance. The patient relives certain incidents in his life and instructs the members of the cast and in so doing has to identify himself with the role of his father, mother, etc. This affords him the opportunity not only to reconstruct aspects of his own past life, but also to feel himself into the roles of the other members of the family, etc. There is usually some gain in perspective and in objectivity as a result of this process. Probably more important is the fact that the patient has gathered around him a group of people who have shown their willingness to co-operate.

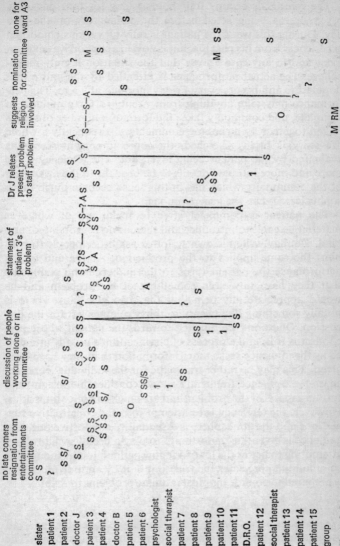

Figure 2 9 a.m. community meeting held on 14 October 1952

The rehearsals occupy four hours a day for four days, the psychodrama being acted before the community on the fifth day. During this week the patient is reliving various emotional experiences from his past life, but is now in a supportive environment and in any case knows that the situation is only make-believe. The actual performance is attended by the entire unit population and occurs every Friday morning at 9 a.m. The performance may take anything from twenty to forty minutes to complete, and commonly takes the form of a number of scenes linked together by a running commentary. Frequently a whole life story is briefly sketched, the more important scenes as evaluated by the patient being acted out. The tendency is for more and more intimate details to be brought to the awareness of the community which has in this sense become much more sophisticated than the general public.

The patient is completely free to make use of whatever material he cares to introduce and there is no censorship of any kind. He may write his own script or ask other people to help him: the same applies to the production. At the end of the performance the patient turns to the audience and comments that they have now seen something of his problem and he would appreciate any help that they can give him. There is usually something like twenty to thirty minutes left for the discussion. Questions are directed towards the patient whose psychodrama it is, and a process of clarification is usually attempted as the audience seeks more information than they have been given. This may be rather traumatic for the individual concerned as the audience frequently shows considerable insight into certain aspects of the problem and are quick to notice omissions. However, the tendency is to attempt to make constructive suggestions and the atmosphere is essentially a supportive one. The audience is given the opportunity to play a useful social role by attempting to better the lot of a fellow patient. It is as though the community appreciates the trust put in it by an individual who is prepared to confide his most intimate problems to them.

2 The out-patient clinic

We have at times employed a technique whereby the staff presents a problem set in a psychiatric out-patients' clinic. The problem is usually based on an actual case, preferably one in which the social factors are important, and where there is not an involved psychopathology. The audience witnesses an ordinary psychiatric interview, the psychiatrist playing his own role and bringing out the salient features of the case. He may then ask the out-patient nurse to bring in the relative who is in turn interviewed. It is possible to involve the other members of the psychiatric team, for example, the social worker or disablement resettlement officer, etc. At some point when the problem has been sufficiently developed the doctor turns to the audience and appeals to them as 'doctors' to continue treatment. Usually someone will volunteer to take over the doctor's role, and various patients may attempt to resolve or better the problem. This projection technique has certain advantages. It is very simple to prepare, as the doctor already knows the case and can guide the patient (usually played by a social therapist). The fact that the problem is based on a real case, the outcome of which is known to the doctor, gives it considerable interest to the patient population. They find it particularly easy to identify themselves with the patient and can readily be induced to identify themselves with the doctor's role, too; and so on with the social worker, psychologist and other members of the treatment team. In this way the patients are helped to understand better the meaning of treatment (limited to this simple type of counselling). By identifying themselves with the psychiatrist's role they come to see some of the problems which he has to face, and in particular the difficulties which result from an unco-operative or passive attitude adopted by the patient.

3 'Misfit' family

In this projection technique (*see* Baker, 1952) the staff present a brief family scene in order to 'warm up' the audience. In this scene a father, mother, brother and sister discuss some family problem, such as the son's late nights, the sister's boy friend, mother's illness or father's drunkenness, and show various family patterns, such as the inadequate or domineering parent, the sullen or rebellious child, sibling rivalry or other attitudes. The problem is discussed until tension is aroused, usually after a few minutes, when the scene will be broken off and the doctor turns to the audience for comments. After a few remarks from the audience which usually clarify the problem, four volunteers are asked to play the roles of the family. Usually volunteers are freely forthcoming and the scene is re-enacted either until some conclusion is reached or until an impasse occurs. The cast then return to their seats and the whole audience comments on the way the roles were played. It is important that the audience should discuss roles rather than persons since this minimizes the likelihood of offence being taken. In one community meeting from one to three families may take part, and at the end the doctor will summarize the problem and the efforts at finding a solution, usually taking a few minutes only. This technique emphasizes the family as the situation in which attitudes are developed and emotional habits formed. It provides the patient with an opportunity to try out his own behaviour pattern with a minimum of risk of personal humiliation. Patients can try to alter their patterns of behaviour and the effect of psychotherapy, or apparent 'insight' developed in other situations can be tested out. Even for those who are unable to play a role in the family, as one of the audience they can learn by observation and have a very real role to play by commenting upon the performance of others.

This technique is easily adapted to the presentation of any particular problem if it is known that one of the audience is able to make use of this method. For example the opportunity arose to use this technique as one aspect of the treatment in the case of a male patient, Mr X. We used the misfit family as a projection technique to bring out the difficulty of communication between patients and staff, and this meeting is reported verbatim; after this we will attempt to show how Mr X. was helped to apply certain aspects of the situation to his own problem.

This example is given verbatim and at some length because it indicates how the 'misfit family' or any other community techniques may be modified to suit a particular purpose and may be combined with other community methods if appropriate.

A 9 a.m. meeting using the 'misfit' family

Dr B: On Thursday we usually discuss some current problems in the Unit. We set a scene with mother, father, brother and sister.

Scene

BROTHER: When you told mother about that trouble last week how did she take it?

SISTER: Oh, she made a little scene, but it was not too bad. I'm very glad I told her. I didn't like it.

BROTHER: I don't want to tell if I can help it. Sh sh here they come.

    [*Enter mother and father.*]

The son asked the father if he had read the case in the paper about the man who had confessed to a crime, but had been tried and punished just the same.

FATHER: Serves him right.

BROTHER: Hum. (Silence.)

MOTHER: I wish you would be friendly and communicative like your father.

BROTHER: You can laugh, but you don't know what the trouble is.

MOTHER: Tell us, you are creating a bad atmosphere. Your father feels uneasy.

The scene ended by the son saying that he could not bring himself to confess.

    Some members of the audience wanted to know what he had actually done. Dr B. asked them what they thought he had done. A patient suggested that he had assaulted someone. Another patient said he might have been to see a psychiatrist! (laughter). She said he had something on his mind but could not discuss it. Another patient said that the most common trouble people get into a mess with is money.

DR B: This family seems to be uneasy. What is to be done?

PATIENT: Perhaps he was starting out in life full of ambition, and can't get there quick enough.

DR B: He might have been boasting of his success at home, whereas he might actually have got the sack.

A PATIENT: Perhaps he is afraid of being condemned by his parents. Parents should try to help bring it out by modifying their statements.

A PATIENT: His parents should make it clear that they will stand by their children when they are in trouble, and try to help them.

A PATIENT: It is rather difficult for the son to confess before a tribunal. It is difficult to confess in front of more than one person. If the father saw him alone he might confess more easily.

A PATIENT: What happens if you do make a confession in front of two or three people? They are likely to argue among themselves about it and so make a more chaotic atmosphere.

A PATIENT: It depends on what you have to confess and what punishment will be meted out.

A PATIENT: If you do have something to confess what does authority do except punish?

A PATIENT: You do not like to hurt people and do not like to see contempt on their faces.

MR X: You might hurt your wife by confessing, as in my own case.

DR B: It hurts some people much more to feel their parents are being hurt. You can be hurt very much if you see you have upset the family. Now we will try to make some different attitudes in the family.

A PATIENT: You are trying to single out one family.

DR B: Some families will handle this differently.

A PATIENT: The father should change his attitude.

A PATIENT: The sister said she didn't know what it was all about. She could help her brother more. She need not say she didn't know about it but could lead him on.

A PATIENT: The mother should have a stronger hand in leading him on.

They played the scene over again, but the son still couldn't confess although the mother had said they might be able to help him and the father said that it always helped to come out with things and that parents are left out of things far too much nowadays. When the son left saying that he could not confess a patient asked why someone didn't drag him back. It was made obvious that even when the family changed and was willing to help, the son still did not confide.

Another scene was played with two patients acting as the mother and father. At this point one of the female patients rushed out of the meeting. The scene started off as before.

MOTHER: You have to face up to things. If we talk about it and see what it is perhaps we can help you.

FATHER: Better get it off your chest.

MOTHER: We are your mother and father can't you tell us?

It was suggested that the son should go into another room and talk about it alone with the father.

A PATIENT: No, he wants to discuss it with the whole family. He may rather tell his mother or sister.

A PATIENT: Everybody knew about the chap in the paper, you were putting yourself on a level with this chap.

A PATIENT: I think the rest of the family should know. If the mother had said it was nothing to worry about, she could then explain it to the others.

A PATIENT: If it is stealing, and his first offence, he would probably get off with just a caution.

A PATIENT: He is not being very fair to the sister.

MR X: If it comes to a question you cannot discuss with your wife, mother or sister, what then?

A PATIENT: Tell one of the family and then come back and tell the rest.

A PATIENT: But the sister already knows.

A PATIENT: The mechanisms in most families show that the mother would take the son's part.

A PATIENT: He should go to the person with the most practical sense – usually the father.

Another scene by a fresh group of patients.

MOTHER: Can't you tell me? I am terribly worried and perhaps I can help you. Won't you try, you are worrying you father.

FATHER: You are my son, nothing you have done would make any difference.

A PATIENT: Suppose the father should say that he had done something and felt better when he had confessed.

DR B: Everybody has done something in their lives which

they regret. The parents are reasonable now and the real problem is the son himself.

DR B. then asked the audience for someone to play the part of the son and was met with silence, lasting several minutes.

A PATIENT: Someone has to know what the trouble is. I can't take the part because I do not know what he has done.

A PATIENT: Don't you think the sister would tell? In a family a woman can't keep things to herself, she would tell someone. If the son can't then she would have to do it.

A PATIENT: The sister should see the brother afterwards and ask if she could tell. He would say he would tell them himself, otherwise she would say he was a coward and not a man.

A PATIENT: If I were the father I wouldn't try to force it out. I think he would eventually tell him.

DR B: You are all thinking about things you have never been able to tell anyone. The family should stand by the son whatever he might have done.

A PATIENT: Brother and sister could arrange to tell their parents if they had any encouragement from their mother or father.

DR B: You may tell other patients things you wouldn't tell the staff. We should assure you that we should help you. When you face up to things they are not nearly so bad as you had thought.

Following this meeting it was agreed by the staff that the same misfit family should be repeated next day, as it was felt that Mr X might be encouraged to use this opportunity to bring his problem to the attention of the community. The plan for the misfit family was constructed with this possible end in view.

9 a.m. meeting next day

DR J: Yesterday we saw the difficulty which the 'children' had in telling the 'parents'. It was quite obvious that people wanted to say something but could not. They were only in need of help.

Scene as before

BROTHER: Ever since yesterday morning I have had a headache and I could not sleep last night.

SISTER: I think you should tell them about it. They have been wonderful every time we have done anything wrong. We ought to trust them. It would make you feel so much better.

BROTHER: Not this, though.

[Enter mother and father.]

MOTHER: You haven't slept very well.

FATHER: Come along and tell us what is on your mind.

BROTHER: It's not so easy as you think.

MOTHER: Everyone makes mistakes. We had all this yesterday. (To father) He is really worried.

BROTHER: How do you know? I have had this on my mind for weeks.

FATHER: Why not tell your mother?

MOTHER: You will be ill if you don't tell us.

BROTHER: I do not know where to start. Do you remember that chap I met at the holiday camp last year?

FATHER: Oh yes, he was a nice boy.

BROTHER: He is a bit of a funny chap. He lives in rooms in town. I got very friendly with him. Do you remember when I said I would be late home? I said I would spend the night with him. He is a homosexual. It seemed all right at the time but now I feel awful about it.

MOTHER: So this is the problem.

FATHER: If only you had told us about it long ago.

SISTER: He wanted to tell you days ago but he was afraid of being thought badly of.

FATHER: I have seen this happen over and over again. Why didn't you come and talk it over with me before?

BROTHER: Does it happen to other people?

FATHER: To everyone to a smaller or larger extent.

BROTHER: You never hear about it.

FATHER: No, of course there is convention about it.

BROTHER: It makes me feel very queer.

MOTHER: You have done right in telling us. It is a good thing to talk about it and get it out of your system. You have girl friends and you feel normal about that.

FATHER: Your mother is right. These things appear in the papers every night. It is something which every society has, you will pass through this. People are often faced with this problem, they can even marry and make a go of it.

BROTHER: You have helped a lot by talking about it.

A PATIENT [*interrupting*]: Society doesn't like it. You would be punished. If I told a policeman about it you would be punished.

A PATIENT: In fact, as long as you do not make a nuisance of yourselves in the district a policeman will not charge you, nothing will be done about it.

MR X: How would your wife take it?

DR J: Why don't we try it out? Have Sister as your wife.

At this point Mr X. who had had no warning that this situation would arise agreed to participate in an imaginary scene depicting his return home on weekend leave from the unit.

Scene on arrival at home for weekend leave

WIFE: Hello, how are things?

MR X: Not so bad. (*Sits on chair, head in hands.*)

WIFE: Have you got something on your mind?

MR X: No, I'm just tired. Where are the children?

WIFE: They are out playing down the road.

MR X: I wish I hadn't come home this weekend.

WIFE: Why don't you like coming home?

MR X: I do.

WIFE: Something is worrying you. What is the matter?

MR X: It is very hard to tell you what is on my mind.

WIFE: Well, try.

MR X: I am married and have three children.

WIFE: Surely being married so long we can trust each other.

MR X: Things haven't been the same since I have had this breakdown. Do I want things to go on as we are or get back to normal?

WIFE: What is so different?

MR X: I can't look at you or the children. I am ashamed to look at you.

WIFE: Why are you ashamed?

MR X: I am afraid you would not understand.

WIFE: Do you think I cannot understand?

MR X: If I told you you may want to get away. I would feel

like packing my bags. One side of me wants to stay at home and the other side wants to go away. Have you heard of homosexuals – when a man is keen on another man.

WIFE: Yes, you read about it in books, and newspapers.

MR X: Years ago I was interfered with by a man in a park. It brought on homosexual tendencies. I felt when I married you it would be plain sailing. I joined the army and found chaps with similar tendencies. It seems these things come on. It is something I am trying to fight. I tried to be a normal husband and father. Should I leave you, get away from all of you – how shall we carry on? I want to watch the children grow up. The other side wants to throw myself away. When I look at you it is all guilt because of this thing that is within me. Well, now you are told what are you going to do about it?

DR J: Here is a real difficulty. He has tried to work through his problem. It could go either way. It would be a struggle to start with. Mr X. has three children and he is at the stage where he is ashamed to meet his wife and children. What do you feel?

A PATIENT: I think his trouble is impotence. He has told me that the question of homosexuality exists only in his mind.

DR J: What do you suggest he does?

A PATIENT: I don't know.

MR X: I still feel strongly about my wife but we have had no intercourse since September. I really believe that the children sense this barrier. When I go home they cannot look at me. The point is – the question is that what I have been working for can crash and fall. This guilt feeling I have. I look at my elder girl and feel guilty. I want to get away, but I want to see the achievements of my family. Shall I ask to be put in a mental home?

A PATIENT: Go back to the family.

MR X: Am I condemned? ('No' from the audience.)

A PATIENT: Would your wife understand as sister did when she played the part?

MR X: She has been wonderful company. I do not know if she has some idea. I have had eleven years of breakdowns. I cannot tell her, somehow. I wonder what the outcome will be

SISTER: She will probably be very relieved. She has been speculating about this and will be glad to have things straightened out.

MR X: What does Dr J. think?

DR J: I think that your wife is aware that there is some big problem eating into the family structure. This is a problem that exists everywhere and is not a new thing. It is not a serious thing, but needs to be dealt with. Society has got an open attitude towards this and in the theatre, etc., it is commonplace. People we flock to see on the stage sometimes have difficulties of this kind, but may still be happily married. You have shown a change in attitude here. You have found it can be talked about. There are instincts that most people feel. Some people point a finger at homosexuals because they are so anxious to find someone else to be a scapegoat. I think your wife is a hard-working and fine woman and will try to understand you if you give her a chance.

A PATIENT: You read of cases in the paper – why are punishments so high?

DR J: Only for men, not for women for some unknown reason.

STAFF MEMBER: Do you think living in a male ward has highlighted it?

DR B: Men usually keep it from their wives because they don't want to worry them. The wife will usually respond to a frank discussion of the problem, and appreciate that her husband confides in her.

A PATIENT: She wouldn't mind hearing that as much as that he had had an affair with another woman.

STAFF MEMBER: From a woman's point of view – at least part of you wants to stay with your wife.

MR X: I wonder what the Unit thinks?

A PATIENT: We are not judges or juries.

MR X: Anyone can turn round and not speak to me.

A PATIENT: We think that people will think less of us in the Unit, but I don't think they do really. You are quite wrong in thinking people will think any less of you, it is an illness.

MR X: You see what I am up against. There are two sides of me, one wants to get away because I feel so guilty, more so since the children are grown up. My eldest girl knows about life – I can't face her. The other side wants to stay and see the children grow up. Where can I get away, into a mental home?

A PATIENT: We do not think it is an offence. You are convincing yourself more and more that you are guilty. I think you will tell your wife about it.

MR X: It's like something eating my mind away, my sanity.

A PATIENT: You are looking for sympathy now.

A PATIENT: How can being attracted to a man or a woman be an offence?

A PATIENT: You only feel guilty if you don't talk about it.

DR J: I think Mr X. has done the community a great service. It was a very difficult thing for him to have done. He deserves our confidence and respect.

Mr X attended Dr J.'s therapeutic group meeting at 11 a.m. and talked a great deal about his problem. One of the patients suggested that his wife should come and see the doctor and discuss her problem with both her husband and the doctor present. Mr X eagerly adopted this plan.

In view of the progress of Mr X it was decided to call an extraordinary meeting of the total community. This was held at 1 p.m. on the same day in order to avoid a weekend gap. In the meantime a female patient of Dr J.'s, Mrs B. had asked if she might help in some way because she herself was married to a homosexual. Mr X was given no warning that the following scene was contemplated.

Extraordinary community meeting a few hours after the previous meeting

DR J: I would like to ask for your help. This is a continuation of this morning's meeting at 9 o'clock. I want you to picture the Unit Club Room, with Mr X. sitting on his own, following this morning's meeting.

Scene

MRS B: Hello Mr X. May I sit down? I was very interested in what you said this morning, and I thought you were very brave. I wanted to say something to you, but there were too many people in the room. I thought I could help you. You see, I am married, and my husband is a homosexual. I do not think your wife would mind if you told her.

MR X: You're younger than my wife, age makes a difference. What is your attitude – how did you find out?

MRS B: I knew about it when I married him, actually before I married him. After we were married we lived a normal sex life. He has a boy friend whom I know and am also fond of.

MR X: Surely you have a feeling of repulsion. If your husband sleeps with another man, there must be a feeling of repulsion against your husband.

MRS B: No, I cannot say there is. Why should I feel that way about it?

MR X: What gave you the feeling in the first place?

MRS B: I don't understand.

MR X: You found out in some way. Perhaps by some of his mannerisms. These things are very difficult to talk about in a normal community as a whole. You say you heard me talking about it and you felt you could help me. I find it interesting to have a member of the opposite sex taking the point of view I would like my wife to take.

MRS B: It is going to be very difficult for her as she did not know before, but once she gets used to the idea I do not think she will feel repulsed.

MR X: You have no feeling of repulsion against me?

MRS B: No, in fact I am very pleased in a lot of ways that my husband has this boy friend. It is not like having to be jealous of another woman taking him away.

MR X: I feel it is impossible to regard other women with interest. They do not appeal to me at all and having affairs would be out of the question. It is a question of loyalty to my wife. If by chance another man came along, I would go with him. But I have this feeling of guilt whenever I look at my wife. She is twice as old as you. Will she have the same feeling if I confess to her. I have carried the burden for years. She has stayed by me while I was in and out of work.

DR J: Thank you very much Mrs B. for carrying this problem further. Mr X. did not know what Mrs B. was going to raise. She volunteered, and Mr X. was as much in the dark as the rest of us. Mr X. has decided that he will raise this question on Sunday with his wife. I think we should have a rehearsal of the scene that we expect to take place with his wife on Sunday.

There followed a scene with Dr J. and Mr X. and Sister taking the part of Mrs X. One patient stood up and wished Mr X. the best of luck for the future. Mr X. said that Sister was only playing a part and that he still did not know what his wife's actual reaction would be, but that he would have to face it sooner or later. It would have to go one way or the other. Either his wife would stand by him, or she would not. He said 'How am I going to face her when she knows what I am like?'

A PATIENT: She may be more upset than Sister has been, at first, but in the end she will understand. You have not done anything wrong.

MR X: To some people it is a great wrong.

STAFF MEMBER: You may have a clue to how she reacted to things in the past. Has she criticized you because you do not go home at the weekend? Or does she want you to go back home?

MR X: She wants me to go home.

DR J: I have seen her three times. There is no question about her integrity or consistency. She accepted the fact that he has been ill and she would only be too glad to see him as a husband and a wage earner once again.

STAFF MEMBER: You do have something to go on. It is not just guesswork, you know what her attitude has been in the past.

MR X: But I don't know how she is going to take this sort of thing.

STAFF MEMBER: You are not quite right there. She has a certain amount of feminine intuition. She may have some idea. She would rather know exactly what it is.

A PATIENT: A lot depends on the way you tell her.

DR J: What about the way we have approached it? Does it meet with general agreement? Is there some other way we can put it?

A PATIENT: It will be a shock, but if one thinks enough of a person one can make a fresh start. It is not like the competition of another woman.

A. A. Baker *et al*. 385

MR X: You are not the guilty person. I shall still feel guilty.
A PATIENT: You emphasize the word 'guilt', you must face your guilt.
A PATIENT: Because you have kept it to yourself for so long it has grown out of proportion.
MR X: I have been trying to lead a normal married life but my guilt forces me back.
A PATIENT: Do you think she might leave you?
MR X: I should have to leave her because I could not face her afterwards.
A PATIENT: This question should be brought out with your wife.
MR X: I have been evading the issue. I have brought it up in the group, but I feel that unless this comes out of me, I shall lose my reason. This is how I felt last night. I tried to bring it out to the group yesterday. The opportunity was given to me this morning to bring it out to the community. Now the most serious problem is on Sunday. This is something which affects her sex life. I make excuses for not indulging, the point is that when I get back I have no excuse. I have got to face the facts, I have got to resume my normal married life. I cannot go home unless my wife knows what is causing the trouble. I am prepared to take the risk, she must know about me, so that I can live with her again.
A PATIENT: You expect her to condemn you because you condemn yourself. If you cannot come to terms with yourself you cannot solve the problem.
A PATIENT: May I suggest to you that what you really feel guilty about is the fact that you did not want to have intercourse with her, not about your homosexuality.

Mr X left hospital a week after this meeting. During this period he discussed his problem with his wife in the presence of Dr J. The meeting followed very closely on the lines of the interview acted out previously when Sister took the part of Mrs X. The Social Worker paid a follow-up visit three months after Mr X. had left hospital at the request of the doctor to ascertain patient's adjustment to the resumption of work and home life since his discharge from hospital.

Mr and Mrs X live in a four-roomed council house which is

adequately though not comfortably furnished. Mr X. was at home with two of his daughters when I called, and his wife, who works till eight each evening, came in during my visit.

Mr X looks a different man since his discharge from hospital. His face has filled out, he no longer averts his eyes when speaking to one, and his carriage is more erect. He states that he feels better than he has for years and that, as the doctor suggested he would, he is improving each week. Although he still gets tired sometimes, he feels quite capable of carrying out his present job and hopes soon to be able to resume a heavier one. Mrs X agreed that her husband had changed a great deal since his treatment in hospital, and mentioned that she couldn't give him enough to eat now, where before he had often left a meal untouched. She felt the children were responding to having their father at home again, and though Mr X was occasionally irritable it was nothing like the old days.

Mrs X seemed rather tired; she works mornings and evenings and is really worn out by the time she returns home about half past eight. It is apparently essential for Mrs X. to work in the meantime; the financial difficulty of keeping the two older children at Grammar School (where they must wear school uniform and so on) is also Mr X's main reason for wanting to resume a heavier and better-paid job. He hopes to come down to Belmont to get his doctor's advice on this.

Mr and Mrs X are planning to come to Belmont during their fortnight's holiday in September to take part in a group discussion and to see a psychodrama. Mr X. would like to tell the patients how very beneficial he found the treatment and thinks it might be helpful for them to see how very greatly improved he is. He could not sufficiently nor frequently enough express his gratitude for what has been done for him, and said that he still missed the morning meetings, and in particular the groups which he often thought about at eleven o'clock.

His colleagues at work are amazed at the change in Mr X in both appearance and manner, and their frequent remarks about this are a great encouragement to him, as they reinforce his own impression as to his increasing return to health. He is unhesitatingly recommending the treatment in the Unit to those whom he thinks require it!

The concept of a therapeutic culture

In the foregoing sections we have attempted to describe the various activities of the Unit with particular reference to its social structure and community methods of treatment. We have attempted to structure the community in such a way as to achieve the maximum degree of communication between all its members and to establish certain cultural concepts. By the culture of the unit we mean its customary and traditional ways of thinking and of doing things which are shared to a greater or lesser degree by all members. New members must learn and at least partially accept these ways of thinking and acting in order to belong to the community. Psychiatric treatment of an individual kind will frequently bring about changes in the individual's attitude to society, but it is felt that society as represented by the Unit community can itself act as a therapeutic agent. As far as possible we want the individual to verbalize his problems in the community with a view to obtaining a more objective awareness of his difficulty, but also to test out public opinion. This is particularly important in a community such as ours where the majority of patients feel that they are social outcasts. Under these circumstances the patient's attitude is usually a mixture of resentment towards the social order and a feeling of guilt. If he can only be brought to the point where he can test out the community's reaction to his problem, he may find that they are much more helpful and understanding than he would have anticipated, and much less punitive than his own conscience. This point was illustrated by the case of Mr X already referred to when discussing the 'misfit' family.

The unit community has attempted to define its attitudes to most of the common social problems with which it is confronted. The difficulty is that such attitudes may be clarified at a time when the topic is of particular interest, but its perpetuation within the culture will rest with the staff rather than with the patients. This is because such concepts are on the whole better understood by the staff and because there is a rapid turnover of the patient population. The staff cultural concepts are constantly changing or being modified. Take for instance the question of discipline which has already been discussed when describing the

8.30 a.m. meetings. At one time the discipline of the unit was largely the concern of the doctor in charge. More recently there has been no overt discipline and the goal has been to make each individual patient responsible for his own behaviour in relation to the needs of the unit.

The assumption is that the Unit Culture will help the patients in preparing them to lead relatively normal lives outside hospital. The culture is found most positively in the staff community, and the patients assimilate it in varying degrees. In order to aid this process of assimilation and education there are daily meetings of the total patients and staff. Various acting techniques are utilized which all aim to raise the patients own individual and group problems for discussion.

The discussion may be made more vivid by impromptu acting to test out the validity of a proposed solution. The patients have come to accept that free participation in discussion and acting a role are part of the ordinary means of communication approved by the Unit society. Social difficulties such as the resistance to employment in the workshops, dislike of the doctors' authority, or the nurses' favouritism, are typical of the problems raised. The aim is to see each problem as objectively as possible and to try to get some understanding of the various motivations and mental mechanisms involved, be they projection, displacement, or rationalism, etc. Real understanding or insight may be rare but the very process of acting out or verbalizing feelings and attitudes gives definition to them and in so doing modifies them. There is also the degree to which the group appears to accept a particular attitude which may then become an integral part of the group culture.

These various community methods afford the patients the opportunity to consider their group problems, and at the same time they are made aware of the staff attitude to these problems. In this way the staff culture may be considerably modified by the patients' attitudes, but much more frequently the patients come to accept in part at least, the more formulated cultural attitudes of the staff.

The general process would appear to be discussion, conceptualization and adoption of various social attitudes on the part of the staff and a repetition of this process within the total community, the whole process having a circular form because the problems are frequently raised in the first instance by the patients themselves.

The structure of the community is designed to enable the best possible human relationship to develop. The basis of any good relationship is that there should be mutual understanding and tolerance and free expression and discussions of difference to enable the needs of all concerned to find as much satisfaction as possible. Our patients' needs for affection, self-respect and status in any community have all been thwarted by their past life, and we hope that by living in the unit they may be able to discover afresh that it is possible to find a way of living with people that brings satisfaction instead of discouragement.

References

BAKER, A. A. (1952), 'The misfit family', *Brit. J. med. Psychol.*, vol. 25, pp. 235–43.

JONES, M. (1952), *Social Psychiatry*, Tavistock Publications.

MORENO, J. L. (1946), *Psychodrama*, Beacon House.

17 J. M. Atthowe, Jr and L. Krasner

Preliminary Report on the Application of
Contingent Reinforcement Procedures (Token Economy)
on a 'Chronic' Psychiatric Ward

J. M. Atthowe, Jr and L. Krasner, 'Preliminary Report on the
Application of Contingent Reinforcement Procedures (Token Economy)
on a "Chronic" Psychiatric Ward', *Journal of Abnormal Psychology*, vol.
73, 1968, pp. 37–43.

Although investigators may disagree as to what specific strategies or tactics to pursue, they would agree that current treatment
programs in mental hospitals are in need of vast improvement.
Release rates for patients hospitalized five or more years have
not materially changed in this century (Kramer, Goldstein,
Israel and Johnson, 1956). After five years of hospitalization,
the likelihood of release is approximately 6 per cent (Kramer *et
al.*, 1956; Morgan and Johnson, 1957; Odegard, 1961), and, as
patients grow older and their length of hospitalization increases,
the possibility of discharge approaches zero. Even for those
chronic patients who do leave the hospital, more than two out
of every three return within six months (Fairweather, Simon,
Gebhard, Weingarten, Holland, Sanders, Stone and Reahl,
1960). There is certainly need for new programs of demonstrated
efficiency in modifying the behavior of long-term hospitalized
patients.

In September 1963 a research program in behavior modification was begun which was intimately woven into the hospital's
ongoing service and training programs. The objective was to
create and maintain a systematic ward program within the on-
going social system of the hospital. The program reported here
involves the life of the entire ward, patients, and staff, plus
others who come in contact with the patients. The purpose of
the program was to change the chronic patients' aberrant
behavior, especially that behavior judged to be apathetic, overly
dependent, detrimental, or annoying to others. The goal was to
foster more responsible, active, and interested individuals who
would be able to perform the routine activities associated with

self-care, to make responsible decisions, and to delay immediate reinforcement in order to plan for the future.

The ward population

An eighty-six bed closed ward in the custodial section of the Veterans Administration Hospital in Palo Alto was selected. The median age of the patients was fifty-seven years and more than one-third were over sixty-five. Their overall length of hospitalization varied from three to forty-eight years with a median length of hospitalization of twenty-two years. Most of the patients had previously been labeled as chronic schizophrenics; the remainder were classified as having some organic involvement.

The patients fell into three general performance classes. The largest group, approximately 60 per cent of the ward, required constant supervision. Whenever they left the ward, an aide had to accompany them. The second group, about 25 per cent, had ground privileges and were able to leave the ward unescorted. The third group, 15 per cent of the patients, required only minimal supervision and could probably function in a boarding home under proper conditions if the fear of leaving the hospital could be overcome.

In order to insure a stable research sample for the two years of the project, sixty patients were selected to remain on the ward for the duration of the study. The patients selected were older and had, for the most part, obvious and annoying behavioral deficits. This 'core' sample served as the experimental population in studying the long-term effectiveness of the research program, the token economy.

The token economy

Based on the work of Ayllon and his associates (Ayllon, 1963; Ayllon and Azrin, 1965; Ayllon and Houghton, 1962; Ayllon and Michael, 1959) and the principle of reinforcement as espoused by Skinner (1938, 1953), we have tried to incorporate every important phase of ward and hospital life within a systematic contingency program. The attainment of the 'good things in life' was made contingent upon the patient's performance.

If a patient adequately cared for his personal needs, attended his scheduled activities, helped on the ward, interacted with other patients, or showed increased responsibility in any way, he was rewarded. The problem was to find rewards that were valued by everyone. Tokens, which could in turn be exchanged for the things a patient regards as important or necessary, were introduced. As stated in the manual distributed to patients (Atthowe, 1964):

The token program is an incentive program in which each person can do as much or as little as he wants as long as he abides by the general rules of the hospital, *but*, in order to gain certain ends or do certain things, he must have tokens. . . . The more you do the more tokens you get [p. 2].

Cigarettes, money, passes, watching television, etc., were some of the more obvious reinforcers, but some of the most effective reinforcers were idiosyncratic, such as sitting on the ward or feeding kittens. For some patients, hoarding tokens became highly valued. This latter practice necessitated changing the tokens every thirty days. In addition, the tokens a patient still had left at the end of each month were devaluated 25 per cent, hence the greater incentive for the patient to spend them quickly. The more tokens a patient earned or spent, the less likely he would be to remain apathetic.

In general, each patient was reinforced immediately after the completion of some 'therapeutic' activity, but those patients who attended scheduled activities by themselves were paid their tokens only once a week on a regularly scheduled pay day. Consequently, the more independent and responsible patient had to learn 'to punch a time card' and to receive his 'pay' at a specified future date. He then had to 'budget' his tokens so they covered his wants for the next seven days.

In addition, a small group of twelve patients was in a position of receiving what might be considered as the ultimate in reinforcement. They were allowed to become independent of the token system. These patients carried a 'carte blanche' which entitled them to all the privileges within the token economy plus a few added privileges and a greater status. For this special status, the patient had to work twenty-five hours per week in special vocational assignments. In order to become a member of the 'elite group', patients had to accumulate 120 tokens which entailed a considerable delay in gratification.

The token economy was developed to cover all phases of a patient's life. This extension of contingencies to all of the patient's routine activities should bring about a greater generality and permanence of the behavior modified. One criticism of conditioning therapies has been that the behavior changed is specific with little evidence of carry-over to other situations. In this project plans were incorporated to program transfer of training as well as behavior change, per se. As a major step in this direction, token reinforcements were associated with social approval.

The attainment of goals which bring about greater independence should also result in strong sustaining reinforcement in and of itself. The aim of this study was to support more effective behavior and to weaken ineffective behavior by withdrawal of approval and attention and, if necessary, by penalties. Penalties comprised 'fines' of specified numbers of tokens levied for especially undesirable behavior or for *not* paying the tokens required by the system. The fines can be seen as actually representing a high token payment to do something socially undesirable, for example, three tokens for cursing someone.

Method

The research program was initiated in September of 1963 when the senior author joined the ward as the ward psychologist and program administrator. The remainder of 1963 was a period of observation, pilot studies, and planning. Steps were taken to establish a research clinic and to modify the traditional service orientation of the nursing staff. In January 1964, the base-line measures were begun. The base-line or operant period lasted approximately six months and was followed by three months in which the patients were gradually prepared to participate in the token economy. In October 1964, the token economy was established and, at the time of writing, is still in operation. This report represents results based on the completion of the first year of the program.

The general design of the study was as follows: A six-month base-line period, a three-month shaping period, and an eleven-month experimental period. During the baseline period, the frequency of particular behaviors was recorded daily, and ratings were carried out periodically. The shaping period was largely devoted to those patients requiring continual supervision. At first, the availability of canteen booklets, which served as money in the hospital canteen, was made contingent upon the amount of scheduled activities a patient attended. It soon became clear that almost one-half of the patients were not interested in money or canteen books. They did not know how to use the booklets, and they never bought things for themselves. Consequently, for six weeks patients were taken to the canteen and urged or 'cajoled' into buying items which seemed to interest them (e.g., coffee, ice cream, pencils, handkerchiefs, etc.). Then all contingencies were temporarily abandoned, and patients were further encouraged to utilize the canteen books. Next, tokens were introduced but on a noncontingent basis. No one was allowed to purchase items in the ward canteen without first presenting tokens. Patients were instructed to pick up tokens from an office directly across the hall from the ward canteen and exchange them for the items they desired. After two weeks the tokens were made contingent upon performance and the experimental phase of the study began.

Within a reinforcement approach, the principles of successive approximation in gradually shaping the desired patient behavior were utilized. Once the tokens were introduced, shaping procedures were reduced. It would be impossible to hold reinforcement and shaping procedures constant throughout the experimental period or to match our ward or our patients with another ward or comparable group of patients. Consequently, a classical statistical design does not suit our paradigm. It is much more feasible, in addition to reducing sampling errors, to use the patients as their own controls. Therefore, we first established a base line over an extended period of time. Any changes in behavior from that defined by the base line must be taken into account. The effects of any type of experimental intervention become immediately obvious. We do not have to rely solely on the inferences teased out of statistical analyses.

Other than an automatic timer for the television set, the only major piece of equipment was the tokens. After a considerable search, a durable and physically safe token was constructed. This token was a $1\frac{3}{4} \times 3\frac{1}{2}$ inch plastic, nonlaminated, file card which came in seven colors varying from a bright red to a light tan. Different exchange values were assigned to the different colors. The token had the appearance of the usual credit card so prevalent in our society.

Whenever possible, the giving of the tokens was accompanied by some expression of social approval such as smiling, 'good', 'fine job', and a verbal description of the contingencies involved for example, 'Here's a token because of the good job of shaving you did this morning.'

Results

There has been a significant increase in those behaviors indicating responsibility and activity. Figure 1 shows the improvement in the frequency of attendance at group activities. During the base-line period, the average hourly rate of attendance per week was 5·85 hours per patient. With the introduction of tokens, this rate increased to 8·4 the first month and averaged 8·5 during the experimental period, except for a period of three months when the reinforcing value of the tokens was increased from one to two tokens per hour of attendance. Increasing the reinforcing value of the tokens increased the contingent behavior accordingly. With an increase in the amount of reinforcement, activity increased from 8·4 hours per week in the month before to 9·2 the first month under the new schedule. This gain was maintained throughout the period of greater reinforcement and for one month thereafter.

Thirty-two patients of the core sample comprised the group-activity sample. Nine patients were discharged or transferred during the project, and the remaining patients were on individual assignments and did not enter into these computations. Of the thirty-two patients, eighteen increased their weekly attendance by at least two hours, while only four decreased their attendance by this amount. The probability that this is a significant difference is ·004, using a sign test and a two-tailed estimate. Of those patients going to group activities, 18 per cent changed to the more token-producing and more responsible

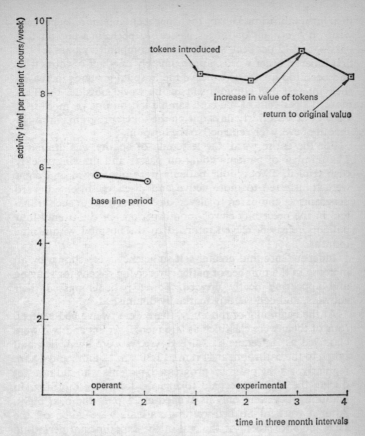

Figure 1 Attendance at group activities

individual assignments within four months of the onset of the token economy.

A widening of interest and a lessening of apathy were shown by a marked increase in the number of patients going on passes, drawing weekly cash, and utilizing the ward canteen. Of the core sample of sixty patients, 80 per cent had never been off the hospital grounds on their own for a period of eight hours since their hospitalization. During the experimental period, 19 per cent went on overnight or longer passes, 17 per cent went on day passes, and 12 per cent went out on accompanied passes for the first time. In other words, approximately one-half of those who had been too apathetic to leave the hospital grounds increased their interest and commitment in the world outside. Furthermore, 13 per cent of the core sample left on one or more trial visits of at least thirty days during the token program, although six out of every ten returned to the hospital.

For the entire ward, the lessening of apathy was dramatic. The number of patients going on passes and drawing weekly cash tripled. Twenty-four patients were discharged and eight were transferred to more active and discharge-oriented ward programs as compared to eleven discharges and no such transfers in the preceding eleven-month period. Of the twenty-four patients released, eleven returned to the hospital within nine months.

Independence and greater self-sufficiency were shown by an increase in the number of patients receiving tokens for shaving and appearing neatly dressed. Fewer patients missed their showers, and bed-wetting markedly diminished.

At the beginning of the study, there were twelve bed-wetters, four of them were classified as 'frequent' wetters and two were classified as 'infrequent'. All bed-wetters were awakened and taken to the bathroom at 11 p.m., 12:30 a.m., 2 a.m., and 4 a.m. regularly. As the program progressed, patients who did not wet during the night were paid tokens the following morning. In addition, they were only awakened at 11 p.m. the next night. After a week of no bed-wetting, patients were taken off the schedule altogether. At the end of the experimental period no one was wetting regularly and, for all practical purposes, there were no bed-wetters on the ward. The aversive schedule of being awakened during the night together with the receiving of tokens for a successful non-bed-wetting night seemed to instigate getting up on one's own and going to the bathroom, even in markedly deteriorated patients.

Another ward problem which had required extra aide coverage in the mornings was the lack of 'cooperativeness' in getting out of bed, making one's bed, and leaving the bed area by a specified time. Just before the system of specific contingency tokens was introduced, the number of infractions in each of these areas was recorded for three weeks. This three-week base-line period yielded an average of seventy-five 'infractions' per week for the entire ward, varying from seventy-one to seventy-seven. A token given daily was then made contingent upon not having a recorded infraction in any of the three areas above. This token was given as the patients lined up to go to breakfast each morning. In the week following the establishment of the contingency, the frequency of infractions dropped to thirty and then to eighteen. The next week the number of infractions rose to thirty-nine but then declined steadily to five per week by the end of nine weeks (see Figure 2). During the last six months, the frequency of infractions varied between six and thirteen, averaging nine per week.

A significant increase was shown in measures of social inter-action and communication. A brief version of the Palo Alto Group Psychotherapy scale (Finney, 1954) was used to measure social responsiveness in weekly group meetings. The change in ratings by one group of raters one month before the introduc-tion of tokens compared with those of a second group of raters four months later was significant at the ·001 level. A simple sign test based upon a two-tailed probability estimate was used. Neither set of raters knew which of their patients was included within the core sample. The later reliability of the scale is ·90 (Finney, 1954). Evidence of enhanced social interaction was dramatically shown by the appearance of card games using tokens as money among some of the more 'disturbed' patients and an increased frequency in playing pool together.

Discussion and conclusion

A detailed description of the entire procedures and results is in preparation. However, we wish to point out in this paper the usefulness of a systematic contingency program with chronic patients. The program has been quite successful in combating institutional behavior. Prior to the introduction of tokens most patients rarely left the ward. The ward and its surrounding grounds were dominated by sleeping patients. Little interest was shown in ward activities or parties. Before the tokens were introduced, the ward was cleaned and the clothing room operated by patients from 'better' wards. During the experimental period the ward was cleaned and the clothing room operated by the patients of this ward themselves. Now, no one stays on the ward without first earning tokens, and, in comparison to prior standards, the ward could be considered 'jumping'.

Over 90 per cent of the patients have meaningfully participated in the program. All patients do take tokens, a few only infrequently. However, for about 10 per cent, the tokens seem to be of little utility in effecting marked behavior change. With most patients, the changes in behavior have been quite dramatic; the changes in a few have been gradual and hardly noticeable. These instances of lack of responsiveness to the program seem to be evident in those patients who had previously been 'catatonically' withdrawn and isolated. Although most of the patients in this category were favorably responsive to the program, what 'failures' there were, did come from this type of patient. Our program has been directed toward all patients; consequently, individual shaping has been limited. We feel that the results would be more dramatic if we could have dealt individually with the specific behavior of every patient. On the other hand, a total ward token program is needed both to maintain any behavioral gains and to bring about greater generality and permanence. Although it was not our initial objective to discharge patients, we are pleased that the general lessening of apathy has brought about a greater discharge rate. But, even more important, the greater discharge rate would point to the generalized effects of a total token economy.

The greater demands on the patient necessitated by dealing with future events and delaying immediate gratifications which were built into the program have been of value in lessening patients' isolation and withdrawal. The program's most notable contribution to patient life is the lessening of staff control and putting the burden of responsibility, and thus more self-respect, on the patient himself. In the administration of a ward, the program provides behavioral steps by which the staff can judge the patient's readiness to assume more responsibility and thus to leave on pass or be discharged.

The program thus far has demonstrated that a systematic

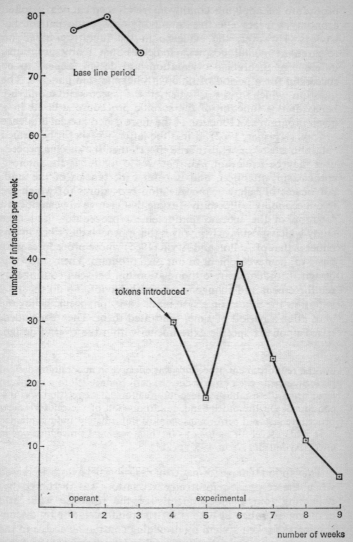

Figure 2 Number of infractions in carrying out morning routines

procedure of applying contingent reinforcement via a token economy appears effective in modifying specific patient behaviors. However, the evidence in the literature based on research in mental hospitals indicates that many programs, different in theoretical orientation and design, appear to be successful for a period of time with hospitalized patients. The question which arises is whether the success in modifying behavior is a function of the specific procedure utilized in a given program or a function of the more general social influence process (Krasner, 1962). If it is the latter, whether it be termed 'placebo effect' or 'Hawthorne effect', then the specific procedures may be irrelevant. All that would matter is the interest, enthusiasm, attention, and hopeful expectancies of the staff. Advocates of behavior-modification procedures (of which the token economy is illustrative) argue that change in behavior is a function of the specific reinforcement procedures used. The study which most nearly involves the approach described in this paper is that of Ayllon and Azrin (1965) whose procedures were basic to the development of our own program. Their study was designed to demonstrate the relationship between contingency reinforcement and change in patient behavior. To do this they withdrew the tokens on a systematic basis for specific behaviors and, after a period of time, reinstated them. They concluded, based upon six specific experiments within the overall design, that

. . . the reinforcement procedure was effective in maintaining desired performance. In each experiment, the performance fell to a near-zero level when the established response-reinforcement relation was discontinued. On the other hand, reintroduction of the reinforcement procedure restored performance almost immediately and maintained it at a high level for as long as the reinforcement procedure was in effect [Ayllon and Azrin, 1965, p. 381].

They found that performance of desirable behaviors decreased when the response-reinforcement relation was disrupted by: delivering tokens independently of the response while still allowing exchange of tokens for the reinforcers; or by discontinuing the token system by providing continuing access to the reinforcers; or by discontinuing the delivery of tokens for a previously reinforced response while simultaneously providing tokens for a different, alternative response.

In the first year of our program we did not test the specific effects of the tokens by withdrawing them. Rather, we approached this problem in two ways. First, we incorporated within the base-line period of nine months a three-month period in which tokens were received on a noncontingent basis. During this period patients received tokens with concomitant attention, interest, and general social reinforcement. This resulted in slight but nonsignificant change in general ward behavior. The results of the experimental period were then compared with the base line which included the nonspecific reinforcement. The results indicate that the more drastic changes in behavior were a function of the specific procedures involved. The other technique we used was to change the token value of certain specific activities. An increase in value (more tokens) was related to an increase in performance; return to the old value meant a decrement to the previous level of performance (see Figure 1).

We should also point out that the situation in the hospital is such that the token economy did not mean that there were more of the 'good things in life' available to these patients because they were in a special program. The patients in the program had had access to these items, for example, extra food, beds, cigarettes, chairs, television, recreational activities, passes, before the program began, as had all patients in other wards, free of charge. Thus we cannot attribute change to the fact of more 'good things' being available to these patients and not available to other patients.

Thus far, a contingent reinforcement program represented by a token economy has been successful in combating institutionalism, increasing initiative, responsibility, and social interaction, and in putting the control of patient behavior in the hands of the patient. The behavioral changes have generalized to other areas of performance. A token economy can be an important adjunct to any rehabilitation program for chronic or apathetic patients.

References

ATTHOWE, J. M. Jr. (1964), *Ward 113 Program: Incentives and Costs – a Manual for Patients*, Veterans Administration Hospital.

AYLLON, T. (1963), 'Intensive treatment of psychotic behaviour by stimulus satiation and food reinforcement', *Behav. Res. and Therapy*, vol. 1, pp. 53–61.

AYLLON, T. and AZRIN, N. H. (1965), 'The measurement and reinforcement of behaviour of psychotics', *J. exp. anal. Behav.*, vol. 8, pp. 357–84.

AYLLON, T. and HOUGHTON, E. (1962), 'Control of the behavior of schizophrenic patients by food', *J. exp. anal. Behav.*, vol. 5, pp. 343–52.

AYLLON, T. and MICHAEL, J. (1959), 'The psychiatric nurse as a behavioral engineer', *J. exp. anal. Behav.*, vol. 2, pp. 323–34.

FAIRWEATHER, G. W., SIMON, R., GEBHARD, M. E., WEINGARTEN, E., HOLLAND, J. L., SANDERS, R., STONE, G. B. and REAHL, J. E. (1960), 'Relative effectiveness of psychotherapeutic programs: a multi-criteria comparison of four programs for three different patient groups', *Psychol. Monog.*, vol. 74 (5, Whole No. 492).

FINNEY, B. C. (1954), 'A scale to measure interpersonal relationships in group psychotherapy', *Group Psychotherapy*, vol. 7, pp. 52–66.

KRAMER, M., GOLDSTEIN, H., ISRAEL, R. H. and JOHNSON, N. A. (1956), 'Application of life table methodology to the study of mental hospital populations', *Psychol. Res. Rep.*, vol. 5, pp. 49–76.

KRASNER, L. (1962), 'The therapist as a social reinforcement machine', in H. H. Strupp and L. Luborsky (eds.), *Res. in Psychol.*, Am. Psych. Ass., pp. 61–94.

MORGAN, N. C. and JOHNSON, N. A. (1957), 'The chronic hospital patient', *Am. J. Psychol.*, vol. 113, pp. 824–30.

ODEGARD, O. (1961), 'Current studies of incidence and prevalence of hospitalized mental patients in Scandinavia', in P. H. Hoch and J. Zubin (eds.), *Comparative Epidemiology of the Mental Disorders*, Grune & Stratton, pp. 45–55.

SKINNER, B. F. (1938), *The Behavior of Organisms*, Appleton-Century-Crofts.

SKINNER, B. F. (1953), *Science and Human Behavior*, Macmillan.

18 M. J. Rioch, C. Elkes, A. A. Flint, B. S. Usdansky, R. G. Newman and E. Silber

National Institute of Mental Health Pilot Study in Training Mental Health Counselors

M. J. Rioch, C. Elkes, A. A. Flint. B. S. Usdansky, R. G. Newman and E. Silber, 'National Institute of Mental Health Pilot Study in Training Mental Health Counselors', *American Journal of Orthopsychiatry*, vol. 33, 1963, pp. 678–89.

In the spring of 1960 a pilot study was begun in the Adult Psychiatry Branch of the National Institute of Mental Health to explore one means of alleviating the shortage of trained workers in the mental health field and of filling some of the community's needs for low-cost psychotherapy. The idea behind the experiment is that, even as the Public Health nurse can perform many duties with and for patients, thereby freeing the medical officer for tasks requiring greater training, so also a corps of workers could be trained in the mental health field, thereby freeing a significant amount of the psychiatrist's time.

One of the best reservoirs of people gifted for this kind of work consists of married women of about forty who are looking for a constructive activity outside the home to take the place of the job of child rearing. To exploit this gold mine of psychological talent would be to kill two birds with one stone: The need for low-cost therapy could be alleviated and the mature woman's need to be useful could in some cases be filled. This latter would not be a salvage operation for neurotic middle-aged ladies, but rather the appropriate deployment of people who have performed successfully in one phase of life and who are now passing to another. These women have an inestimable advantage over the usual beginning psychotherapist; they have resided for a considerably longer time on this planet and have been engaged in the highly complex interpersonal training ground of child rearing and family living. By virtue of this they are less self-absorbed than their more youthful counterparts and have a larger pool of experience from which to draw.

The objective of this study is in line with the recommendation of the Report of the Joint Commission on Mental Health and Illness:

... that nonmedical mental health workers with aptitude, sound training, practical experience and demonstrable competence should be permitted to do general, short-term psychotherapy – namely, the treating of persons by objective, permissive, nondirective techniques of listening to their troubles and helping them resolve these troubles in an individually insightful and socially useful way.

The experiment can be divided into four phases. The first two, Recruitment and Selection, have been completed. The third, Training, is in process. The fourth, Evaluation, has been accomplished for the first year's work, and will be repeated with variations for the second year, in June 1962. A follow-up study is being planned for the years following the experiment itself.

The hypothesis, which was tested in the recruitment stage, was that there is a large unexploited reservoir of talent among middle-aged women, waiting and eager to be used. This was amply demonstrated, at least for the Washington area.

The recruitment lasted approximately six weeks. During this short period by means of sixty telephone calls and six short public speeches, eighty women became sufficiently interested to request application blanks. Forty-nine applications were returned filled out. No blank was sent out before a ten-minute telephone conversation had taken place with the applicant, explaining the program and emphasizing its experimental character. Applicants were told that there would be no financial recompense during the two-year training period, and that there was no guarantee of success, or of future employment. The insecurity that we were obliged to emphasize with regard to our experimental program limited its appeal to people who could and would take a risk. They were all from the middle class and most of them had been to college. We thought the program might well appeal to many from the lunatic fringe, but, of the forty-two women who came to the NIH for the selection procedures, at most three might be thought to fall into this category: Even including these, all were capable people whose services could and should be used in some form in the community.

We began the selection phase by asking for an autobiography of about 1,500 words from each applicant. The forty-two women who complied with this request were invited to come to the National Institutes of Health in groups of approximately eight for a day of group procedures, including tests and discussions. On the basis of these, the Committee of Selection chose twenty who were given individual interviews and tests and from whom eight were finally chosen as the successful candidates. Their median age was forty to forty-four. One was widowed; all the others were living with their husbands. All had children, the average number being 2·4. Their husbands were all either professionals or executives. They were all college graduates; three had advanced degrees. Of their undergraduate majors, four were in the behavioral sciences, three in the humanities, one in biology. Six had held paying jobs at a professional level. Four had been psychoanalysed.

The hypothesis to be tested by this phase was that, by the various group and individual procedures used, a number of candidates could be selected who would have good general intelligence, perceptiveness, integrity and sufficient emotional maturity to be able to operate effectively together and to cope with the stresses of psychotherapeutic work. To be complete, this hypothesis should include the statement that the selectors were for the most part the teachers in the Training Program.

This hypothesis has proved correct at least to the extent that all eight of the selected candidates have remained in the program and intend to continue in this field.[1] Further, the staff has not wished to recommend dismissal of any one of them. It cannot, of course, be claimed that the procedures used selected the best of the applicants. We have no way of knowing how much better some of the rejectees may have been than the selected candidates.

The training began in September, 1960, and is to run officially for four semesters. Actually, from what we know of the eight women in this experiment, they will continue their training indefinitely in one form or another. The two years we are offering them constitute only a beginning of their awareness of them-

1. One was absent from the city during the second semester, which she had told us might occur. She returned for the second year.

selves as therapeutic instruments. This report will deal with the two semesters completed in June, 1961.

In planning our program, we had to decide at the start whether we were training professionals or technicians. In other words, should we expose our students to a variety of theories and practices with the intention of helping them gradually to find their own way, or should we teach them to follow directions according to a set method? We agreed on the former course. The statement was made explicitly to the students that there is no one 'right way' to do therapy but that each person develops his own style, which is right for him because it is an integral function of his own personality. The instructors, including the consultants, are people with a variety of backgrounds: Some are psychoanalysts, some psychiatrists, some psychologists. All of them hold a broad, more or less eclectic point of view with regard to theory and practice. We are unable to make a sharp distinction between counseling and therapy. Our students are called Mental Health Counsellors for lack of a better term. What they do in their interviews varies a great deal from one to another, from one phase of their development to another, and from one patient to another. Sometimes they listen sympathetically and supportively; sometimes they 'represent reality' or give common-sense advice; sometimes they engage in a process of exploration of the patient's feeling and attitudes with a view to a better understanding of them; and occasionally they are able to draw out into the open some aspect of a patient to which he had previously been blind, and to help him become more aware and accepting of this aspect. In our teaching we have emphasized that the patient's problem has something to do with distorted perceptions of himself and others and that he would be able to see more clearly if the anxiety in these areas were reduced. We have also emphasized the need to listen to the patient on more than one level, to hear the unspoken messages and to respond to them as well as to the spoken ones. And we have stressed above all the importance of self-awareness.

Our training is narrow but intensive; it is sharply focused on psychotherapy, and only on psychotherapy. This differentiates it from training for social work, psychology and psychiatry. Members of all three of these professions engage in psychotherapy, but their education includes many other things. Our hypothesis is that the intensive training offered to carefully selected applicants can produce in a relatively short time people qualified to do this particular task for which the need is so great.

In setting up our program we tried to allow ourselves maximum flexibility, but we did have certain notions about how it would be structured. One was that the students should be thoroughly and frequently supervised and supported in their work; a second was that they should be given a broad, undogmatic point of view with as little jargon as possible. A third was that the work would be primarily practical, on-the-job training, and only secondarily theoretical. These have all been carried out.

We had some other intentions, however, which have been modified. First, we planned that the training would be twenty hours a week, or half time for two years. But the students have worked so hard that they have turned it into what is now practically a full-time program. Second, we thought that we would limit the type of patient to be seen, so that the training would be more intensive in one area. We chose college students partly because of the already existing interest in the Adult Psychiatry Branch; partly because we thought they would be easy to treat and by and large not so very sick, and thus appropriate for a first experiment; and partly because, from the general mental health point of view, this seemed like a good age for preventive psychiatry. For practical reasons having to do chiefly with geography and transportation, we were unable to carry out this intention. Not enough college students were available to the out-patient service at the NIH, so we included high school students and their parents. Then other adults came seeking help, bringing the age range of our patients to between fifteen and fifty-five. There has been a preponderance of adolescents and their parents, however, and we have emphasized in our course work the problems of this developmental phase.

Third, we intended to have our students see patients with relatively minor disturbances. This intention has gone the way of unrealistic expectations, since practically none of the patients who have sought out our services has been really easy to treat. We think that in general it is best to screen out those patients who are schizophrenic, those who act out a great deal and those who would probably develop a very demanding and possessive sort of transference relationship. In some cases we have taken a calculated risk because there was no other possibility for treatment. In some cases in which our screening was faulty, the trainee performed the useful service of helping the patient and his family, through a series of introductory interviews, to accept more intensive and experienced therapy than we could offer.

Fourth, we intended to screen all patients for the trainees. While this still occurs consistently at NIH, initial interviewing is now being done by some of the trainees in their community placements.

The training covered the following five areas:

1. The first was practical work at NIH. This consisted of interviewing normal subjects and patients, group therapy for adolescents and their parents, individual and group supervision including listening to the playback of the trainees' own tape-recorded interviews. This was the most important part of the work.

The trainees began by interviewing the normal control subjects who live at the Clinical Center of the NIH and are studied by the various institutes. Most of them were college students. It was a great advantage to have this resource in the initial period, especially in an untried pilot program. Since a number of these 'normal' people had very serious problems, we became aware that our trainees were able to cope with a greater degree of emotional disturbance than we had originally intended to have them handle. Before the end of the first semester each trainee had been assigned at least one real patient.

From the very beginning all the interviews were tape-recorded. Each trainee listened to her own interviews, not only by herself and with a supervisor, but with the whole group. One of the remarkable aspects of the first year's work was the way in which an atmosphere of mutual support developed among the students, making it possible for them to expose their floundering and blundering to each other without essential loss of self-esteem.

The supervision took place at scheduled times both individually and in groups of four or eight. In addition, it was made clear that the supervisors were always available to their students in case of need. The need might be a matter of supporting the trainee in dealing with a demanding patient, answering a practical question of how to refer a patient's relative to a psychiatrist or sitting down for an extra session with the tape recording and working through the anxiety about a given situation. It is fair to say that the trainees felt confident that they could rely upon their supervisors for prompt assistance in a crisis and for a generally benign attitude in dealing with their difficulties. This does not imply that the supervisors were uncritical or that the process of supervision was anxiety-free. It does imply that we had a fair measure of success in establishing what might reasonably be called a therapeutic environment, although no formal therapy (group or individual) of the trainees was ever undertaken in the program. It should be mentioned here, however, that during this first year one trainee continued until late winter her previously begun analysis. Two returned to therapists with whom they had earlier terminated. One began therapy for the first time. This indicates that the program stirred up considerable anxiety. It is our opinion that this was by and large constructive in that it led the trainees to work through problems that would otherwise have limited their effectiveness as therapists. Those who were or had been in therapy learned at first hand what it is like to be a patient. If the students had been unable, for financial or other reasons, to arrange treatment for themselves when needed, it would have been advisable to proceed differently. Group therapy could be made part of the regular schedule, or the program could be maintained at a lower level of anxiety. In the latter case there might be some loss in effectiveness.

2. The second area of training was observation of group, family and individual therapy.

3. The third consisted of lectures and seminar discussions.

4. The fourth was outside reading and report writing.

5. And the fifth was community placements. These were arranged partly to broaden the experience of the trainees and partly to open doors that might lead to future employment. This was the beginning of a feeling-out process to see how the

community would react to the trainees and how the trainees would fit and function in the community. We met with a remarkably open-hearted and open-minded welcome on the part of most, though not all, of the agencies with which we had contact. Only two of the ten agencies we approached declined to accept any trainees. The placements for the first year were in one federal probation office, two juvenile courts, three clinics, one university counseling center and one social service agency. The trainees were especially warmly welcomed and well thought of in the probation office, the juvenile courts, and two of the clinics. In one clinic the attitudes of the staff were mixed and shifting. The university was very warmly hospitable but not enthusiastic about future employment. The social service agency turned out to be an unsuitable placement. For the second year we have trainees placed in seven clinics, two public high schools, one public junior college, two universities and one college.

The evaluation phase of the work will not, of course, be complete until the second year of training is over. The follow-up study will, we hope, present additional material. The results of the first year's evaluation are being presented now as part of a progress report.

We are aware that there is no recognized standard method of measuring the amount learned in this field or the degree of competence of a psychotherapist or the success of anyone's therapeutic endeavors. We have tried to approach the problem in five different ways.

1. In an effort to obtain an objective judgment of the trainees' work, uncolored by the personal investment of the teachers in the project, we obtained the services of four raters from outside the Washington area who, without knowing anything about the program or the background of the trainees, agreed to do blind ratings of tape-recorded therapeutic interviews. After listening to and rating each tape, the rater was to open a sealed envelope containing an autocriticism of the interview by the trainee. This also was to be rated on several criteria, as well as on global impression. The results of this procedure are summarized in Tables 1, 2 and 3. Two ratings on each of two interviews are not enough to represent a valid judgment of any one interviewer,

but the average of twenty-eight judgments is a reasonable assessment of the group of trainees as a whole.[2]

The average rating on the global impression of all the interviews was 3·0, that is, in the middle range of the scale. The aver-

Table 1 Rating of interview

Name of rater: Code number of interview:	excellent 5	good 4	satisfactory 3	passable 2	poor 1
1. Global impression of interview	3	5	12	4	4
2. Respect for the patient	2	15	8	1	2
3. Interest in the patient	4	14	7	3	0
4. Understanding of the patient	4	4	9	8	3
5. Success in drawing out affect	2	5	6	11	3
6. Beginning of interview	1	3	7	10	4
7. End of interview	1	7	2	10	4
8. Professional attitude	3	18	4	3	0
9. Skill in using patient's cues	1	7	4	10	6

	Very easy	Easy	Medium	Difficult	Very difficult
Patient's accessibility to therapy (i.e., an easy or difficult patient)	2	3	7	14	1
Remarks:					

Tables 1 and 2 are reproductions of the rating blanks sent to the raters. The numbers in each box represent the number of times a rating was assigned to that box. Totals are not always the same because occasionally a rater did not rate, if the recording was not clear enough to allow him to form a judgment.

Table 2 Rating of autocriticism

Name of rater: Code number of interview:	excellent 5	good 4	satisfactory 3	passable 2	poor 1
1. Global impression	5	10	10	2	1
2. Shows awareness of major weakness or weaknesses	5	6	9	5	2
3. Shows awareness of the main points at which communication broke down	7	4	8	6	2
4. Shows awareness of how and where communication was facilitated	3	10	6	5	3
5. Shows awareness of her own 'inner workings'	4	12	5	5	2
Remarks:					

2 We owe the clear formulation of this idea to a personal communication from Dr Roy Grinker.

Table 3

Rating of interviews	average score
1. Global impression of interview	3·4
2. Respect for the patient	4·0
3. Interest in the patient	4·0
4. Understanding of the patient	3·4
5. Success in drawing out affect	3·2
6. Beginning of interview	2·7
7. End of interview	2·9
8. Professional attitude	4·2
9. Skill in using patient's cues	3·0

Rating of patient's accessibility to therapy
(i.e., an easy or difficult patient)   3·2
5. very easy
4. easy
3. medium
2. difficult
1. very difficult

Rating of autocriticism

1. Global impression	4·0
2. Shows awareness of major weakness or weakness	3·7
3. Shows awareness of main points at which communication broke down	3·7
4. Shows awareness of how and where communication was facilitated	3·6
5. Shows awareness of her own 'inner workings'	3·8

Table 3 shows the average scores on the blind ratings, first year: 5 – excellent; 4 – good; 3 – satisfactory; 2 – passable; and 1 – poor.

It is important to remember that the 'reference interview' done by a professional therapist was given an average rating of 3 by six judges.

age rating on the global impression of the autocriticisms was 3·6. Since no one's average rating was below 2, or passable, and since 3, or the middle range of the scale, represents satisfactory performance, this part of our evaluation procedure has shown positive results.

2. We have tried to assess the changes that took place in the patients seen by the trainees at NIH, considering at the same

time the kind of patient and the degree of difficulty of the treatment. Table 4 summarizes the work. As in all such assessments of change under therapy, there is no way of knowing how much of this might have occurred without any intervention whatsoever.

There were in all forty-nine patients – eighteen males, thirty-one females, twenty-one adolescents, twenty-eight adults. Each trainee saw an average of seven patients once a week. The diagnoses were distributed as follows: twenty personality trait disorder, twelve neurotic reaction, six schizoid or borderline schizophrenic, five immature or unstable personality, four adjustment reaction of adolescence, two diagnosis doubtful. None of these patients changed for the worse. In nineteen there was no change. Thirty, or 61 per cent, showed some change. Seventeen showed a slight improvement; ten showed a moderate improvement; three, marked improvement. In evaluating the results it is important to remember that 69 per cent of the patients were 'difficult or very difficult to treat', and that the length of treatment at the time of our evaluation was in no case more than six months and, on the average, ten weeks. That the patients themselves were favorably impressed is demonstrated by the fact that of those who came asking for help, only one dropped out of therapy.

3. We asked the supervisors in ten community placements to rate the trainees who worked with them. The ratings are shown in Table 5. The general results here are highly favorable. The average rating is 'good', and none is lower than 'satisfactory'.

4. We asked the trainees themselves to evaluate the program. There was general agreement on their part that it had been important to have one systematic, very well-given background course in personality development. There was general appreciation of a 'human' attitude on the part of instructors who were willing to expose their own fears and failings, especially in their therapeutic work. They liked it particularly when theory and practice were brought close together, as in a course on family interaction patterns that was integrated with the group therapy for adolescents and their parents. The practical work was considered the 'guts' of the program and wishes were expressed for

Table 4 Overall summary of work with NIH patients by all seven trainees

	N	%
Number of patients		
Males	18	
Females	31	
Young adolescents, ages 15–16	7	
Older adolescents, ages 17–19	14	
Young adults, ages 20–25	5	
Mature adults, ages 30–55	23	
Average number of patients per trainee	7	
Total number of patients	49	
Number of interviews		
Average number of interviews by each trainee	77	
Range of number of interviews with a single patient	1 to 26	
Average number of interviews with a single patient	10	
Total no. of interviews	539	
Diagnosis of patients		
Personality trait disorders	20	
(14 of these were patients who came for help ostensibly because of their children)		
Neurotic reaction	12	
Schizoid or borderline schizophrenic	6	
Immature or unstable personalities	5	
Adjustment reaction of adolescence	4	
Diagnosis doubtful	2	
Rating of patients' improvement or in the course of therapy		%
Marked improvement	3	6
Moderate improvement	10	20
Slight improvement	17	35
No change	19	39
Rating of patients according to difficulty of treatment		
Very difficult	13	
Difficult	21	
Medium	10	
Easy	5	
Very easy	0	

more opportunities to listen with the supervisors to selected tapes of their own interviews and to observe more interviews by experienced therapists. Some of the placements were considered useful; some, more or less time wasting.

For all of the trainees the program has been an important step in their lives. Although they were warned *ad nauseam* that it is an experiment with no guarantee of success or future employment, they are, without exception, looking forward to using this training in serious work. They have raised the question whether a degree or certificate of some kind might be obtained that would enable them to identify themselves in any community in which they might live as being equipped to do the kind of work for which they have been trained. For all of them, the program supplied something they needed in that it filled satisfyingly a vacuum left by their children's growing up.

Table 5

Name of agency: Name of trainee:	excel- lent 5	good 4	satis- factory 3	pass- able 2	poor 1	insuffi- cient infor- mation	average score
The trainee did the work assigned to her in a way which was: (Please use other students in training as a yardstick)	4	4	1				4·3
The trainee fitted into this agency in a way which was:	4	4	1				4·3
The trainee made progress during the time she was with this agency in a way which was:	4	1	4				3·9
Comments:							

Signature:

This table reproduces the blank sent to the supervisors in the various agencies, except that the last column on the right has been added to represent an average rating. The numbers in each box represent the number of times it was checked by a supervisor with regard to one trainee. One supervisor placed no check marks giving as the reason: 'Assignments for direct service were so limited (due to limitations in time she was available and suitable assignments for a beginning trainee) that I feel it impossible to make an appraisal of patterns of her relating to families, staff and supervisor.'

The table is incomplete since one supervisor has not yet returned his rating. Some trainees had more than one placement during the year.

5. The teachers in the program have reported their impressions. Not all of the instructors are in a position to pass judgment on the clinical competence of all the trainees, but there has been a consensus on the part of those who have worked with them that they are a responsive, intelligent, conscientious group of people. During the first semester, comments were made several times to the effect that their 'receptors' were good although the 'broadcasting' was often awkward. From the beginning they impressed observers with their perceptiveness. One of the consultants observed with pleased surprise that when he asked for a description of a patient he really got it, in full detail.

As therapists they have all performed some useful services to patients during this past year, and none of them has done anyone any harm. They have improved considerably since the beginning of the course in their ability to draw out troublesome material and to respond appropriately to patients' cues.

Their greatest fault has been a tendency to follow the dictates of polite society. In other words, they pleasantly reassure, protect and sympathize when it would be better to question more deeply and seriously. A second fault is a tendency to try to deal on a surface, common-sense level with problems that are soluble only by eliciting unconscious conflicts.

We do not contend that the work of the trainees with their patients was highly skillful. Some of it was skillful; some was adequate; some was awkward. The fact of the matter is that favorable change sometimes occurred in spite of awkward, blundering work.

It is, of course, not yet possible to form a judgment about the degree of usefulness these women will demonstrate when they have finished the two-year course and are away from the protection of the group and their familiar teachers. Their future employment is uncertain and the quality of their performance will no doubt depend upon the kind of settings in which they find themselves, as well as upon what they will take with them at the end of the course. We hope to arrange a weekly seminar for them for the years following the training, not only for the purpose of continuing education, but also because it will be important from the point of view of morale so long as their identity in the field is an uncertain one.

What, now, are the implications of this pilot study for the general field of mental health?

First, there is a potential reservoir of workers in the age group we have tapped that is not presently being exploited. There may well be others, such as retired persons, who could also be used in various ways.

Second, we have anecdotal evidence to the effect that the forty-year-old married woman with children is reluctant to embark upon the regular training programs set up for young graduate students, and in some cases she is not welcomed in them. She does respond eagerly to a program tailored flexibly to her situation.

Third, there is the large and complex question of whether there is need and space for a new profession in the field of mental health. Many people have been concerned that the training for psychotherapy as a major professional activity is not optimally served in psychiatry, psychology or social work. The present study is not by any means an attempt to prepare doctors of psychotherapy who would be licensed to practice independently. Our goal is a far more modest one. If such people as our trainees can perform useful services to patients – and in their first year of training they have done just that – then it should be possible for departments of psychiatry, psychology or social work to offer a subcurriculum something like this one, with emphasis upon practical work, which would train people in psychotherapy. The students in such curricula would no doubt arrive at varying levels of competence, ranging from listening sympathetically and giving common-sense advice, to skillful therapeutic interviewing with optimal use of unverbalized messages, and so on. They could be employed in settings in which they need not work above or beyond the limits of their competence. There will, of course, be no rigorous proof that this NIH pilot project can be replicated unless and until it is tried elsewhere. But there is no essential element in our program that could not be reproduced in other centers with good universities and clinics. A double purpose would be served if this could occur: More patients could be seen and more people could find a constructive use for their talents.

Acknowledgements

Permission to reproduce the Readings in this volume is acknowledged to the following sources:

1 American Psychological Association
2 *British Journal of Psychiatry*
3 *Canadian Journal of Psychology*
4 American Psychological Association
5 *Journal of Mental Science*
6 British Psychological Society
7 *British Journal of Psychiatry*
8 American Psychological Association
9 *American Journal of Orthopsychiatry*
10 C. V. Mosby Co.
11 Society for Psychophysiological Research
12 *Psychosomatic Medicine*
13 *Psychosomatic Medicine*
14 Stanford University Press
15 American Psychological Association
16 British Psychological Society
17 American Psychological Association
18 *American Journal of Orthopsychiatry*

Author Index

Subject Index

duodenal ulcer study, 255–71
emotion/attitude study of,
  273–86
see also Asthma; duodenal ulcer;
  migraine
Psychotherapy,
  see Behaviour therapy;
  desensitization; hospital
  practice; psychodynamics
Punishment unnecessary in
  community therapy, 352

Raynard's disease, 277, 283
Reinforcement,
  centres in brain function, 88–90
  in behaviour learning, 308, 313
  by reward,
    in learning, 320–25, 342
    in psychotherapy, 339, 391–403
Reliability/validity of
  classification, 27–30
Response,
  as behaviour symptom, 32
  in learning, 314–16
  in psychopath study, 232–49
Reticular over-activity, 111–18
Retrospective reconstruction
  criticized, 150–52, 179–81
Rhinitis, 273, 278, 280
Risk of schizophrenia, 173–91

Schizophrenia,
  causal factors,
    environment, 77–9, 129–31,
      186, 188
    family interaction, 147,
      152–68
    genetic study in fostered
      children, 134–46
    see also Schizotaxia; schizotype
  in classification, 24–5, 127–9
  and creative ability, 174–5

diagnosed in comparative study,
  48, 49
drug induced, 68–9, 116–17
as illness,
  aversiveness, 84–8, 92, 97, 100
  compared with psychopathy,
    199, 201
  compensation in, 85–8
  phases of, 103–9
  thought disorder, 82–4
  violence, 181–2
and mental deficiency, 142–3
need for research, 11–12
personality, 87, 95, 107
prevention, 182–3, 190–92
risk, 173–8, 180
theory,
  cognitive slippage, 82–4, 87, 88,
    91–4
  Gestalt, 103, 109
  overinclusion, 120–25
  reticular over-activity, 110–17
Schizophrenic mother, 84, 85–7,
  143, 163–4
Schizotaxia, 84–5, 87–100
Schizotype, 85, 87, 94, 100
Self-sufficiency encouraged,
  in community therapy, 354–60
  in token reward system, 391–8,
    403
Serial invalidation theory, 121
Skin conductance, see
  electrodermal measurements
Skinnerian learning, see operant
  learning
Social
  activities in community
    therapy, 358–9
  environment stress, 257
  interaction encouraged by
    reward, 399, 403
  status as schizophrenic risk, 186,
    188

Social – *continued*
  therapists in community units,
    357, 360–62
Sociopath, *see* psychopathy
Specific dynamic configuration
    theory, 275
Staff, in community therapy, 350,
    356–7, 360–64
Stimulus
  in learning, 312, 314–16
  in psychopath study,
    autonomic activity, 232–9
    conditioning, 239–49
Stress
  in psychosomatic disorder, 12,
    255
  in schizophrenia, 129–31
Symptoms in classification, 32–3,
    35–7

Taxonomy, 21–2
Tension,
  nervous, 256–7, 283
  resolution in community
    therapy, 364–71
Terminal phase of schizophrenia,
    108–9
Tests, *see* assessment tests
Therapist,
  social, in community units, 357,
    360–62
  unsatisfactory recording
    instrument, 149–50
  women trained as, 405–19
Therapy, *see* psychotherapy

Thought disorder in
  schizophrenia, *see* Cognitive
  slippage; Gestalt theory;
  Overinclusion; Reticular
  over-activity
Tonic activity, 230–34
Token reinforcement procedure,
    391–403
Tone as shock
  in autonomic responsivity study,
    233, 235–9
  in conditioning learning, 242–3
Total quality property, 105–6
Transposition in learning, 314
Trema phase of schizophrenia,
    104, 108, 109, 113, 118
Twin studies, 79–80, 269

Urticaria, 277, 280, 283

Validity
  of classification, 28–30
  of experimental variables, 65,
    66–7
Variables in experimental
    psychopathology, 64–5
Violence, 181–2
Vomiting, 278–9, 280, 285–6, 294

World Health Organization, 17,
    43, 225
Women trained as psychotherapy
    counsellors, 405–19
Work in community therapy
    units, 357–8

Human Ageing
Sheila M. Chown

We all age and we all alter as we age. Even if it were possible to keep ourselves in perfect physiological order, could we avoid psychological ageing?

Dr Chown, an international authority, looks at the question through two pivotal ideas – cognition and personality. Cognition is examined in four sections: first, 'pure ageing', second, 'intelligence', third, 'factors affecting intellectual activity', which identifies particular sources of difficulty for the old; and fourth, 'learning and memory', which includes papers both identifying deficits and describing remedial measures.

The field of personality has been separated into three. First, age differences found on personality tests; secondly, the theory that the old withdraw into themselves is examined; and the third section looks at the reactions to stresses imposed by the environment.

Dr Chown writes, 'The book is intended to whet the reader's appetite.' She has therefore picked the research papers that have done that for her and concentrated on features of normal rather than pathological ageing.

Sheila M. Chown is Lecturer in Psychology at Bedford College, University of London.

'Penguin Modern Psychology Readings should be of inestimable value to psychology students, to students in other social sciences, and for that matter to the educated general reader.' *The Times Educational Supplement*

Introducing Psychology

D. S. Wright, Ann Taylor, D. Roy Davies, W. Sluckin,
S. G. M. Lee and J. T. Reason

Introducing Psychology was specially commissioned by Penguin
Education from some of the staff of the Department of Psychology
at the University of Leicester; their collaboration provides a wide
range of specialist views within the coherence of a common
framework and a consistent style.

After an introductory Part One on the scope of the book and on
observational and experimental method in psychology ('the strongest
unifying bond of the present book'), Part Two relates heredity,
maturation and physiology to behaviour. A discussion of perceptual
processes is followed by chapters on the effects of early experience,
learning processes, the development of skills, and remembering.
This last chapter leads on to the discussion of symbolic processes,
which is the concern of the chapters on language and thinking
in Part Four. In Part Five the authors explore methods of measuring
individual differences, and discuss the motions of intelligence,
personality and normality. In Part Six a chapter on some
mechanisms of social influence describes recent work, in which
basic principles of learning have been extended to the two person
situation. This is followed by a review of certain aspects of
socialization and the book ends with a chapter on persuasive
communications and the determining influence of group
membership upon and individual's behaviour.

'*Introducing Psychology* deserves a special welcome. It is well
organized, sensibly illustrated, clearly written and properly
documented.' *New Scientist*

'It is a pleasure to note the clarity of exposition in the Leicester
book, which amply demonstrates that serious writing does not have
to be jargon-ridden in order to be scientific, nor colloquial
in order to be readable . . . the Leicester book is heading for
nomination as "Best Buy" in the *Which?* sense. Quite apart from its
positive merits, its price even for a paperback is amazingly low.'
British Journal of Psychology

Maternal Deprivation Reassessed
Michael Rutter

Twenty years have passed since 'maternal deprivation' was
first greeted with a storm of controversy. Some early views have
been modified, but the basic proposition – that lack, loss or
distortion of child care have a very important effect on
psychological development – has received substantial support.

Why and how are children adversely affected? Dr Rutter reviews
the qualities of mothering needed for normal development and
both the short term and long-term effects of 'maternal
deprivation' are considered. Dr Rutter concludes that the term
covers a wide range of *different* experiences with quite *different*
effects on development.

What is now needed, Dr Rutter argues, is a more precise
description of the different aspects of 'bad' care and 'bad'
effects. In starting on these tasks and in reappraising briefly
and clearly the whole concept of 'maternal deprivation',
Dr Rutter has written a book which will be necessary reading for all
those concerned with the upbringing, care, teaching or
treatment of children.

Michael Rutter is a Reader in Child Psychiatry at the Institute of
Psychiatry, University of London. He is also Honorary
Consultant Child Psychiatrist at the Maudsley Hospital, London.

'Psychology is now a part of innumerable courses, throughout
all levels of higher education. . . . Up to now, reading lists have
tended to consist . . . of weighty, expensive and rapidly
obsolescent volumes. . . . The Penguin Science of Behaviour is
going to blow this whole unsatisfactory situation sky-high
within a fairly short time.' *Higher Education Review*

Psychometric Assessment of the Individual Child

R. D. Savage

Psychometric Assessment of the Individual Child covers the assessment of intellectual, educational, personality and motor-perceptual characteristics, and is completed by examples of the comprehensive assessment undertaken on some typical clinical educational problem children. 'The aim,' the author writes, 'has been to be up to date, yet not too technical, accurate, but not too precise, and comprehensive without being too lengthy.'

'Psychology is now a part of innumerable courses, throughout all levels of higher education. . . . Up to now, reading lists have tended to consisit . . . of weighty, expensive and rapidly obsolescent volumes . . . The *Penguin science of behaviour* is going to blow this whole unsatisfactory situation sky-high within a fairly short time.' *Higher Education Review*

'Dr Savage emphasizes the dangers of misinterpretation of psychometric results. His book, as valuable for the teacher or social worker as for the psychologist, should help to reduce this very real danger.' *The Times Educational Supplement*

'The need of teachers and other non-psychologists is for a clear and concise text that will enable them to read psychological reports and interpret results with knowledge and understanding. . . . Dr Savage's book goes a long way towards answering this need.' *Special Education*

R. D. Savage is Lecturer in Applied Psychology in the Department of Psychological Medicine, Royal Victoria Infirmary and the University of Newcastle upon Tyne.